A Clinician's Guide to Otolaryngology

A Clinician's Guide to Otolaryngology

Edited by **Donald Murphy**

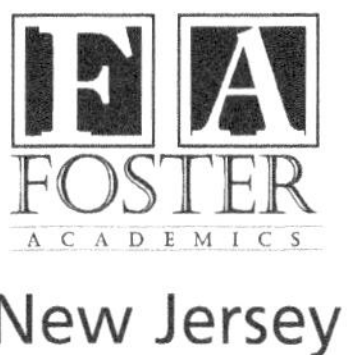

New Jersey

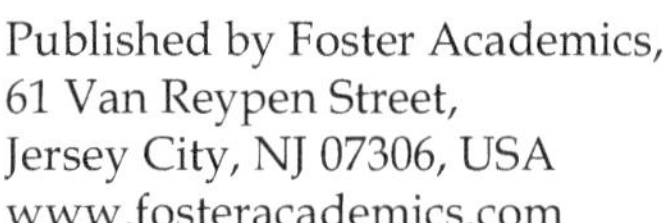
Published by Foster Academics,
61 Van Reypen Street,
Jersey City, NJ 07306, USA
www.fosteracademics.com

A Clinician's Guide to Otolaryngology
Edited by Donald Murphy

International Standard Book Number: 978-1-63242-441-9 (Hardback)

Printed in the United States of America.

Contents

Preface

Otolaryngology is a field of medical science that deals with the diagnosis and treatment of disorders related to ear, neck, throat (ENT) and base of skull. This field examines the problems in the ENT region and treats them with the help of surgery and various medicines. This book discusses the various techniques and new advancements in this field. It will include contributions from experts and scientists which will provide in-depth knowledge of this subject. A number of researches and case studies from all over the globe have been included in this book which makes it a complete source of knowledge. Coherent flow of topics, reader friendly language and extensive examples make this is an invaluable reference source for those interested in this subject.

This book unites the global concepts and researches in an organized manner for a comprehensive understanding of the subject. It is a ripe text for all researchers, students, scientists or anyone else who is interested in acquiring a better knowledge of this dynamic field.

I extend my sincere thanks to the contributors for such eloquent research chapters. Finally, I thank my family for being a source of support and help.

Editor

1

Role of Videonystagmography (VNG) in Epley's Maneuver

Saloni Shah[1*], Rajesh Vishwakarma[2]

[1]Civil Hospital, B.J. Medical College, Ahmedabad, India
[2]ENT Department, Civil Hospital, B.J. Medical College, Ahmedabad, India
Email: [*]drsaloni155@gmail.com

Abstract

Aims and Objectives: To study benefit of videonystagmography in confirmation of canalolith repositioning in patients with Benign Paroxysmal Positional Vertigo after Epley's manouver. Study Design: Prospective study of 35 cases of BPPV. Materials and Method: 35 patients of BPPV presenting at vertigo clinic of ENT department at Civil Hospital Ahmedabad were treated with canalolith repositioning procedure and improvement in nystagmus was studied and confirmed by VNG. Observation: 31 patients out of 35 patients were improved with 1st CRP, 2 out of 3 patients improved with 2nd CRP and 1 patient improved with 3rd CRP. This improvement is confirmed using VNG. Conclusion: Videonystagmography is a very useful tool for ensuring the otolith repositioning by the canalith repositioning manouver. It is a confirmatory adjunct to visual analysis.

Keywords

BPPV, Epley's Manouver, Videonystagmography

1. Introduction

BPPV (Benign Paroxysmal Positional Vertigo) is the most common cause of vertigo. It is typically described as a brief, intense sensation of spinning that occurs when there are changes in the position of the head with respect to gravity. An individual may experience BPPV when rolling over to the left or right, upon getting out of bed in the morning. It is due to the presence of normal but misplaced calcium crystals called otoconia, which are normally found in the utricle and saccule (the otolith organs) and are used to sense movement. If they fall from the utricle and become loose in the semicircular canals, they can distort the sense of movement and cause a mismatch between actual head movement and the information sent to the brain by the inner ear, causing a spinning

[*]Corresponding author.

sensation. It affects vestibulo-ocular reflex and produce nystagmus [1]-[4].

Head movement -> SCC moves -> signal via 8th nerve to vestibular nuclei -> send impulse to 6th nerve to medial rectus -> cause eye movements [4].

Videonystagmography (VNG) is useful to test balance system and record nystagmus by a camera. There are neural connections that stretch balance mechanisms in inner ear to muscles of eye. Any disorder of balance mechanism produces small eye jerks that can only be detected by computer and frenzel's goggles [5] [6]. It can be monitored by putting body in different positions by Dix Hallpike's test and Roll Over test. VNG is a test used to determine whether or not dizziness may be due to inner ear disease. It also assesses the function of the vestibular end organs, central vestibulo-occular pathway and oculomotor processes.

Most commonly involved SCC is horizontal due to its anatomical location. During Dix Hallpike's test the rotatory nystagmus, in the form of twitching movements directed towards the affected ear, is seen after 5 to 10 seconds and it disappears in 45 seconds [7] [8].

Epley's maneuver (canalith repositioning procedure—CRP) [1]-[3] [9]-[11] is to reposit otoconia from abnormal position of SCC to normal in utricle. This maneuver was developed by Dr. John Epley and first described in 1980.

Several articles have been published on efficacy and utility of CRP for treatment of BPPV [12]. It is widely accepted that CRP can result in substantial benefit with very low recurrence rate on short- and long-term outcomes basis. The common factors responsible for recurrence are hormones, calcium metabolism and trauma.

2. Aims and Objectives

To study the benefit of use of videonystagmography for confirmation of repositioning of otolith by Epley's manouvere by noting the improvement in nystagmus and vertigo in patients with BPPV [13]-[16].

3. Materials and Method

- In this prospective study 35 patients suffering from BPPV presented in vertigo clinic at our institute between July 2012 to April 2014 were enrolled.
- Inclusion criteria: positive history of positional vertigo, confirmed with Dix hallpike's test and nystagmus is recorded with VNG.
- Exclusion criteria: patients with spinal disease, hypertension/hypotension, heart disease, neurological diseases, central lesions confirmed on history, physical examination in the form of neurological tests-reflexes, cranial nerve examinations, X-ray, CT or MRI.

4. Procedure

- Patients were first allowed to sit for 5 mins to get relaxed from anxiety.
- Patients were left in position during Dix Hallpike's test for 45 seconds and provoked nystagmus is recorded on VNG.

  Then CRP was done and VNG recording was continued to see improvement in nystagmus.

  Patient was advised to take bed rest, not to bend over and no head shaking movements.
- Follow up done on 7th, 14th, 21st day to see improvement of nystagmus and if provocative maneuver was positive on follow-up evaluation, the CRP was repeated and follow up VNG done.
- Patients which improved were followed up every three monthly.
- Some patients came for follow up for 6 months to 1 year and then were lost for follow up.

5. Results

- At the time of presentation, duration of symptoms varied from 3 months to 1 year.
- VNG showed improvement in nystagmus immediately in 31 patients after 1st CRP.
- 3 patients showed improvement on VNG with 2nd CRP and 1 with 3rd CRP (see **Figure 1**).

Table 1 and **Graph 1** show that 88.5% patients improved with 1st CRP which was recorded on VNG, 8.5% patients improved with 2nd CRP and 2.8% patients improved with 3rd CRP.

Table 2 and **Graph 2** show that out of 35 patients 31 patients shows improvement both clinically and in videonystagmography after 1st CRP.

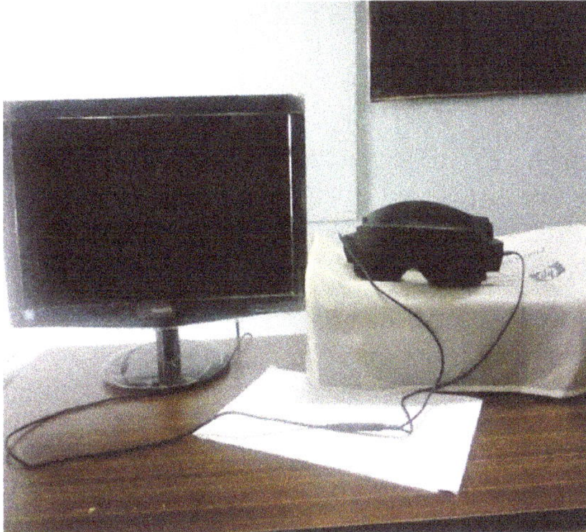

Figure 1. VNG machine.

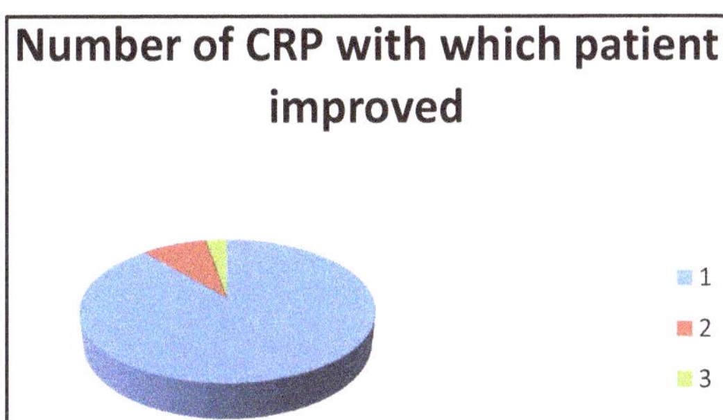

Graph 1. Graphical presentation of above table.

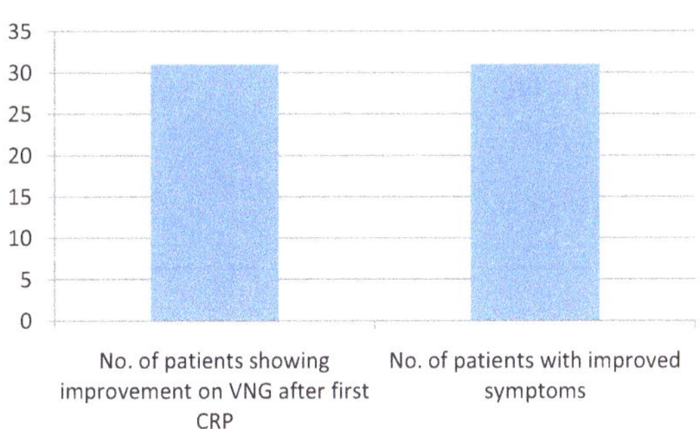

Graph 2. Graphical presentation of above table.

Table 1. Improvement with number of canalith repositioning procedure—CRPs observed in videonystagmography.

Number of patients (n = 35)	Number of CRP with which patient improved
31 (88.5%)	1
3 (8.5%)	2
1 (2.8%)	3

Table 2. Patients showing improvement both clinically and in videonystagmography after first canalith repositioning procedure—CRP.

No. of patients showing improvement on VNG after first CRP	No. of patients with improved symptoms
31	31

Table 3 and **Graph 3** show that out of remaining 3 patients 2 patients shows improvement both clinically and in videonystagmography after 2nd CRP.

Immediate adverse effects after 1st CRP were light headedness and nausea for few hours (1 - 2) seen in 15 patients.

2 patients out of 3 improved with 2nd CRP were older than 65 yrs. 1 patient improved with 3rd CRP had history of head trauma [9]-[11].

6. Interpretation of VNG

Electrical signals from the data obtained from the infrared camera (VNG) are fed into the computer to create a digital readout. On the horizontal channel, movement up indicates an eye movement to the right and movement down indicates an eye movement to the left. On the vertical channel, movement up indicates an eye movement up and movement down indicates an eye movement down (shown in **Figures 2-4**) [5] [6].

Table 3. Patients showing improvement both clinically and in videonystagmography after second canalith repositioning procedure—CRP.

No. of patients showing improvement on VNG after second CRP	No. of patients with improved symptoms
3	2

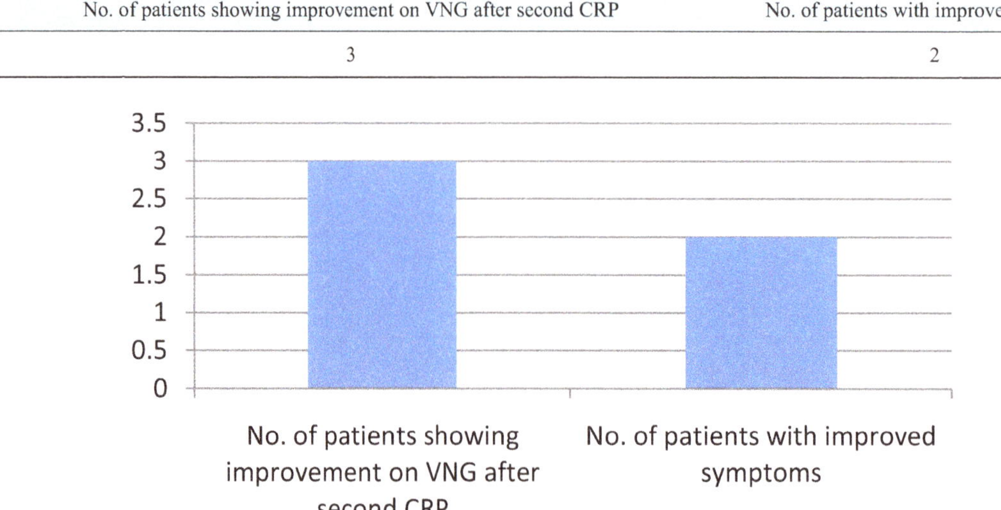

Graph 3. Graphical presentation of above table.

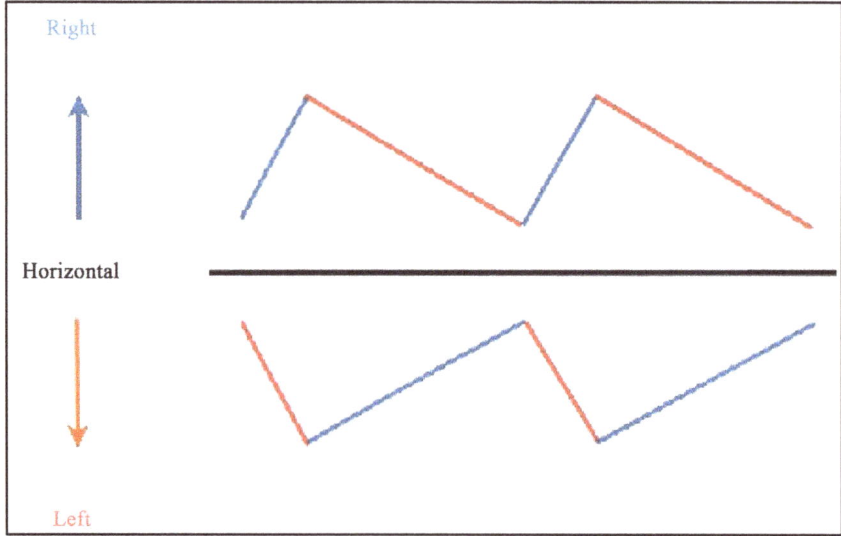

Figure 2. Interpretation of horizontal channel nystagmus.

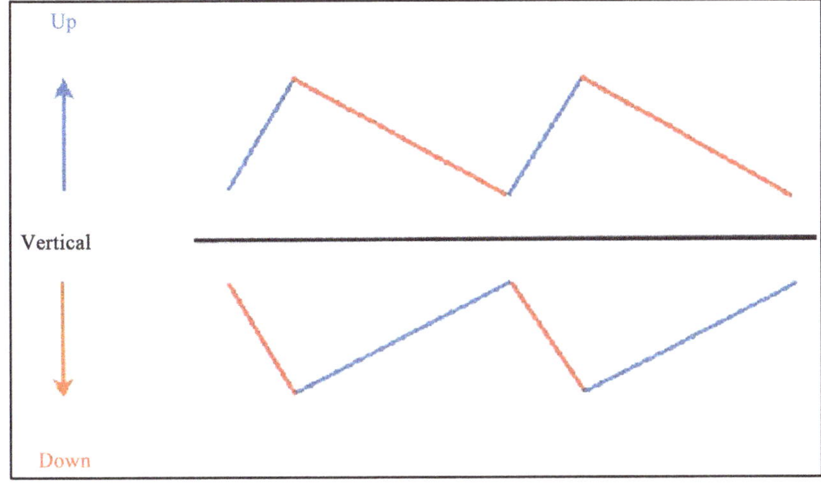

Figure 3. Interpretation of vertical channel nystagmus.

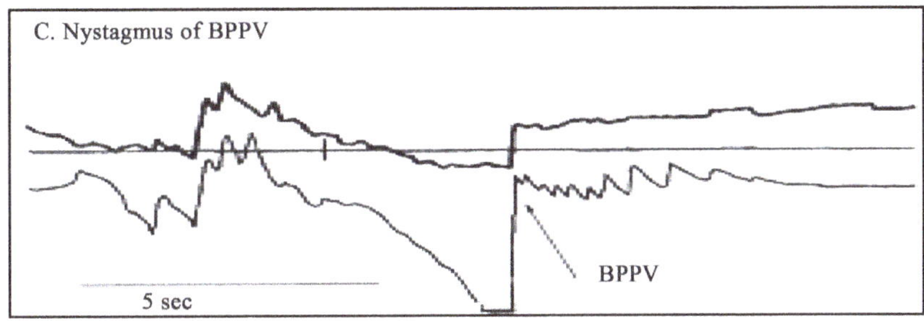

Figure 4. Nystagmus of BPPV [8].

Graph 4 shows nystagmus (arrow) after 7 seconds in a patient with BPPV which lasted for around 45 seconds.

Then CRP was done, followed by repeat VNG.

Graph 5 is post CRP VNG showing improvement in nystagmus (arrow).

7. Discussion

The canalith theory suggests that the gravity dependent movement of heavier otoconial debris from utricle to lateral semicircular canal is responsible for vertigo. The crystals themselves can adhere to a semicircular canal cupula making it heavier than the surrounding endolymph. The semicircular canal is weighted down by the dense particles thereby inducing an immediate and maintained excitation of semicircular canal afferent nerves. This condition is termed as cupulolithiasis. Recent concept has suggested that major pathologic change in BPPV is degeneration of vestibular neurons. This results in loss of inhibition of otolith organs on canal activation. The recurrence rate of BPPV is 27%, and relapse largely occurs in the first 6 months [1]-[4].

VNG can record spontaneous, positional, gaze and optokinetic nystagmus as well as saccadic movements [5] [6]. Dix hallpike's test can check posterior canal of lower ear, anterior canal of opposite ear and lateral canals of both the ears at 45 degree. While the patient is in supine position and head moves to one side, a direction changing nystagmus is observed and it is indicative of,

- Horizontal canal BPPV-nystagmus intense with long duration.
- Central BPPV-verticle component of nystagmus with less duration.

Minimum duration of observation for nystagmus is 20 seconds. It is observed that lateral semicircular canal stimulation gives horizontal nystagmus and anterior or posterior semicircular canal stimulation gives torsional nystagmus.

Positional test performed with patient in sitting and supine position with Dix hallpike's test. The following results are seen.

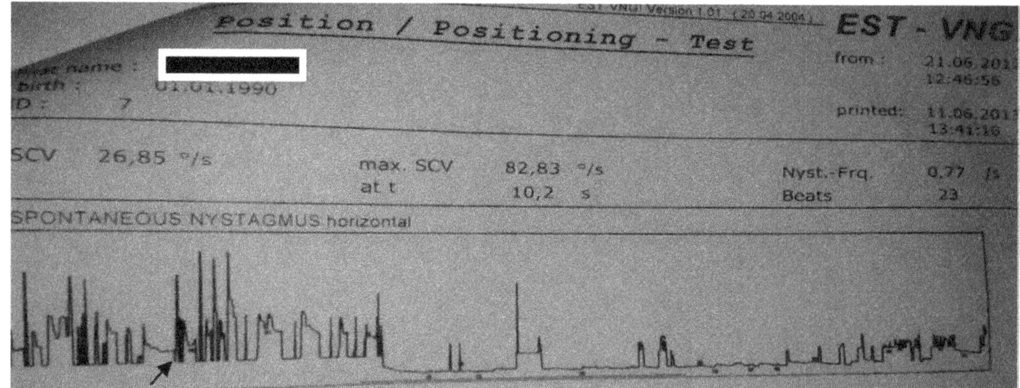

Graph 4. Nystagmus (arrow) after 7 seconds in a patient with BPPV (benign paroxysmal positional vertigo).

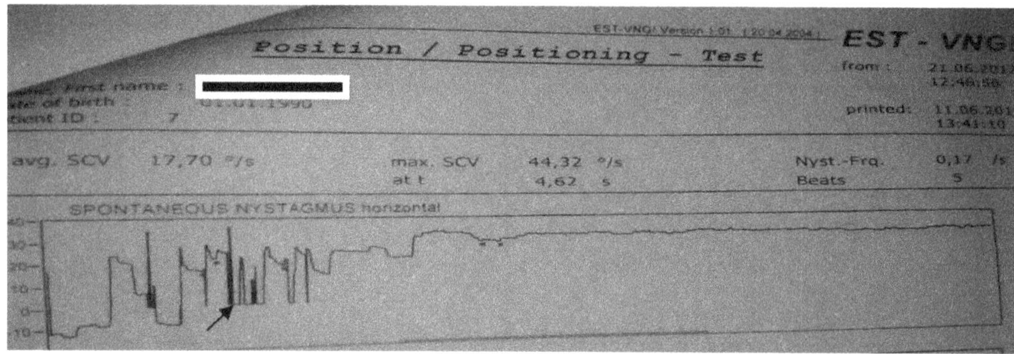

Graph 5. Post canalith repositioning procedure—CRP, videonystagmography.

- Direction changing-Horizontal canal BPPV.
- Direction fixed-uncompesated unilateral vestibular pathology.

Central positional nystagmus does not have a central component and it is not inhibited by fixation [8] [11] [12].

In our patients out of 35 patients 31 improved and 4 patients didn't improve. This may be due to increased age of patients, multiple canaloliths, non-repositioning of otoliths, inefficient CRP or other co-morbidities.

The ENG test relies on the corneoretinal potential to detect the changes in eye position, where as the VNG uses infrared cameras to detect the same. Thus the ENG is an indirect evaluation of the ocular motility, where as the VNG is a direct one [17]-[20].

References

[1] Brandt, T., Steddin, S. and Daroff, R.B. (1994) Therapy for Benign Paroxysmal Positioning Vertigo, Revisited. *Neurology*, **44**, 796-800.
http://vestibular.org/understanding-vestibular-disorders/types-vestibular-disorders/benign-paroxysmal-positional-vertigo#sthash.WngZxHF9.dpuf
http://dx.doi.org/10.1212/WNL.44.5.796

[2] Fife, T.D., Iverson, D.J., Lempert, T., Furman, J.M., Baloh, R.W., Tusa, R.J., Hain, T.C., Herdman, S., Morrow, M.J. and Gronseth, G.S. (2008) Practice Parameter: Therapies for Benign Paroxysmal Positional Vertigo (an Evidence-Based Review): Report of the Quality Standards Subcommittee of the American Academy of Neurology. *Neurology*, **70**, 2067-2074.
http://vestibular.org/understanding-vestibular-disorders/types-vestibular-disorders/benign-paroxysmal-positional-vertigo#sthash.WngZxHF9.dpuf
http://dx.doi.org/10.1212/01.wnl.0000313378.77444.ac

[3] Epley, J.M. (1992) The Canalith Repositioning Procedure: For Treatment of Benign Paroxysmal Positional Vertigo. *Otolaryngology—Head and Neck Surgery*, **107**, 399-404.

[4] Gacek, R.R. (2003) Pathology of Benign Paroxysmal Positional Vertigo Revisited. *Annals of Otology, Rhinology Laryngology*, **112**, 574-582.
http://www.mm3admin.co.za/documents/docmanager/6e64f7e1-715e-4fd6-8315-424683839664/00021518.pdf

[5] Vitte, E. and Sémont, A. (1995) Assessment of Vestibular Function by Videonystagmoscopy. *Journal of Vestibular Research*, **5**, 377-383. http://dx.doi.org/10.1016/0957-4271(95)00008-4

[6] Mekki, S. (2014) The Role of Videonystagmography (VNG) in Assessment of Dizzy Patient. *Egyptian Journal of Otolaryngology*, **30**, 69-72. http://dx.doi.org/10.4103/1012-5574.133167

[7] Fife, T.D. (2009) Benign Paroxysmal Positional Vertigo. *Seminars in Neurology*, **29**, 500-508.
http://www.medscape.com/viewarticle/714335_3
http://dx.doi.org/10.1055/s-0029-1241041

[8] Hain, T.C. (2009) The Dix-Hallpike Test, Definitive Diagnostic Test for Benign Paroxysmal Positional Vertigo (BPPV). http://www.dizziness-and-balance.com/disorders/bppv/dix%20hallpike.htm

[9] Prokopakis, E., Vlastos, I.M., Tsagournisakis, M., Christodoulou, P., Kawauchi, H. and Velegrakis, G. (2013) Canalith Repositioning Procedures among 965 Patients with Benign Paroxysmal Positional Vertigo. *Audiology and Neurotology*, **18**, 83-88. http://dx.doi.org/10.1159/000343579

[10] Prokopakis, E.P., Chimona, T., Tsagournisakis, M., Christodoulou, P., Hirsch, B.E., Lachanas, V.A., Helidonis, E.S., Plaitakis, A. and Velegrakis, G.A. (2005) Benign Paroxysmal Positional Vertigo: 10-Year Experience in Treating 592 Patients with Canalith Repositioning Procedure. *Laryngoscope*, **115**, 1667-1671.
http://dx.doi.org/10.1097/01.mlg.0000175062.36144.b9

[11] Tevzadze, N. and Shakarishvili, R. (2007) Effectiveness of Canalith Repositioning Manoeuvers (CRM) in Patients with Benign Paroxysmal Positional Vertigo (BPPV). *Georgian Medical News*, **148-149**, 40-44.

[12] Bhattacharyya, N., Baugh, R.F., Orvidas, L., Barrs, D., Bronston, L.J., Cass, S. and Haidari, J. (2008) Clinical Practice Guideline: Benign Paroxysmal Positional Vertigo. *Otolaryngology—Head & Neck Surgery*, **139**, S47-S81.
http://dx.doi.org/10.1016/j.otohns.2008.08.022

[13] Furman, J.M. and Cass, S.P. (1999) Benign Paroxysmal Positional Vertigo. *The New England Journal of Medicine*, **341**, 1590-1596. http://dx.doi.org/10.1056/NEJM199911183412107

[14] Campbell, K. (1997) Essential Audiology for Physicians. Singular Publishing Group, San Diego.

[15] Jacobson, G.P., Newman, C.W. and Kartush, J.M. (1993) Handbook of Balance Function Testing. Singular Publishing Group, San Diego.

[16] Barber, H.O. and Stockwell, C.W. (1976) Manual of Electronystagmography. Mosby, St. Louis.

[17] The Role of Videonystagmography (VNG), American Academy of Audiology. A Comparison between ENG and VNG.

[18] Ganança, M.M., Caovilla, H.H. and Ganança, F.F. (2010) Electronystagmography versus Videonystagmography. *Brazilian Journal of Otorhinolaryngology*, **76**. http://dx.doi.org/10.1590/S1808-86942010000300021

[19] McCaslin, D.L. and Jacobson, G.P. (2009) Current Role of the Videonystagmography Examination in the Context of the Multidimensional Balance Function Test Battery. *Seminars in Hearing*, **30**, 242-253.

[20] McCaslin, D.L. PhD. Electronystagmography/Videonystagmography (ENG/VNG).

2

ENT Pathologies Screening in Woodworkers in Parakou, Benin

Spero H. Raoul Hounkpatin[1], Fabien A. C. Gounongbe[1], Sonia Lawson Afouda[2], Marius C. Flatin[1], Karl A. F. B. Dossou-Kpanou[1], François Avakoudjo[2], Elvire Dossoumou[1], Wassi Adjibabi[2]

[1]Faculté de Médecine, Université de Parakou, Parakou, Benin
[2]Faculte des Sciences de la Santé de Cotonou, Université d'Abomey-Calavi, Cotonou, Bénin
Email: speraoul@yahoo.fr

Abstract

Wood dust may induce health risks on exposed timber or wood workers, one of which is ENT disorders. This article aimed to detect ENT pathologies found among woodworkers in Parakou. It was a cross-sectional descriptive study carried out from 1st March to 31st May, 2012 in Parakou, North-Benin. It involved 703 carpenters and sawyers operating in timber workshops in Parakou, regardless of age and sex. The mean age of the wood-workers was 26.14 ± 7.77 years. Their seniority in the timber profession was on average 4.9 ± 2.64 years. All of them were males. It had been noticed that 81.6% of them did not comply with any safety measure for their protection. ENT pathology had been diagnosed in 60.3% of the timber workers. Rhinitises came first and affected 43.1% of the workers, followed by pharyngitises (14.1%). The histological nature of the only case of tumor observed in Parakou could not have been specified, as the patient refused to undergo anatomo-pathological examination. Measures should be taken to get Parakou timber workers to protect themselves.

Keywords

Timber/Wood-Workers, Occupational Rhinitis, ENT Pathologies

1. Introduction

Timber dust may induce pathologies like respiratory disorders in particular, including ENT-related ones on exposed timber workers [1]. The carcinogenic effects of wood dusts are well-known for many years and their responsibility in nose and sinus cancers is well established [1]-[3]. Wood dust is also responsible for non-carcinogenic diseases like rhinitises. Several studies had been globally dedicated to non-carcinogenic respiratory pathologies induced by occupational exposure to wood dust [4] [5].

In Africa where the working conditions are different from those of developed countries in which most of the studies are conducted, few articles have been devoted to the diseases induced by occupational exposure to wood dust. In Benin, up to this day, any study of screening of ENT disease among woodworkers has been realized. This one was carried out in order to screen the ENT pathologies found among Parakou timber workers in the north of Benin.

2. Methods

The study was a cross-sectional study with descriptive purpose based on a collection of prospective data. It was conducted from 1st March to 31st May, 2012 in the District of Parakou. The target population consisted of carpenters and sawyers working in workshops in Parakou, regardless of age and sex. In Parakou, carpenters and sawyers work in open-air workshops spread out over the town, by the streets or in empty compounds.

Using membership register, all the 749 wood-workers who were members of the three trade unions of the town were selected for the study. However only 703 wood-workers were included in the study; 46 wood-workers refused to participate because according to them, the study would disturb their work and was not profitable for them.

Data were collected, on the one hand, through an individual questionnaire submitted to timber workers, and on the other hand, through the ENT clinical examination of the latter. The clinical examination had particularly explored the ear canal and the eardrum with an otoscope, then the nasal cavity by means of anterior rhinoscopy as well as the oropharynx.

The studied variables were socio-demographic data (age, sex, type of timber work, seniority in the profession), ENT history, presence of ENT pathologies and the suggested diagnosis. Epi-info 3.5.1 software was used for the processing of collected data.

3. Results

3.1. Socio-Demographic Profile of Participants

The 703 timber workers selected for the study based on inclusion criteria were all males. There were 607 carpenters (86.3%) and 96 sawyers (13.7%). The mean age of the timber workers was 26.14 ± 7.77 years with extremes from 9 years and 60 years and a median of 26 years. **Table 1** reports workers' distribution according to age.

Most of the timber workers (79.2%) were aged from 15 to 34 years. Only 9.8% were 34 year old and above.

3.2. Respondents' Seniority in the Profession

The respondents' seniority in wood work was on average 4.9 ± 2.64 years with extremes of 1 month and 25 years. The median was 5 years. **Table 2** represents the distribution of the investigated workers according to their seniority.

3.3. Knowledge of the Risks Related to Timber Professional Activity and Protection Measures

Among the 703 respondents, 549 (78.1%) were aware of the risks related to their professional activity and 154

Table 1. Distribution of wood-workers according to age.

	Number	Percentage (%)
Under 15 years	77	11
15 - 24 years	244	34.7
25 - 34 years	313	44.5
35 - 44 years	59	8.4
45 years and above	10	1.4
Total	703	100.0

Table 2. Distribution of wood-workers according to seniority.

	Number	Percentage (%)
Under 1 year	18	2.6
1 - 5 years	259	36.8
6 - 10 years	237	33.7
Above 10 years	189	26.9
Total	703	100.0

(21.9%) ignored about them. However 582 timber workers *i.e.* 81.6% did not observe any safety measure for their protection. A bib was used as a protection measure by 117 timber workers (16.6%). The other protection measures used (1.8%) were glasses and a headset, each by one timber worker. Two timber workers used a combination of the three protection measures.

3.4. History of Morbidity among the Respondents

Out of the 703 respondents, 315 (44.8%) reported having suffered at least once from an ENT pathology. **Table 3** summarizes the distribution of wood/timber workers according to ENT pathological history.

Almost nine wood workers out of ten had a previous history of rhinitis.

3.5. Pathologies Diagnosed in the Respondents

Among the 703 respondents, 60.3% were diagnosed as carriers of an ENT disorder. **Table 4** summarizes the distribution of respondent workers according to the diagnosed ENT pathology.

The main ENT pathologies diagnosed were rhinitis and pharyngitis.

4. Discussion

The wood-workers of our cohort were young with a mean age of 26.14 years. They were younger than their counterparts from Lille in France (mean age: 35.4 years), from Italy (mean age: 37.8 years) [6] [7]. The Parakou timber workers' young age could be explained by many factors: youthfulness of the Benin population in general, early school dropout and the fact that in Benin, many craftsmen or skilled workers leave their profession to perform other more profitable activities at the earliest opportunity. The great physical effort required by timber work in the developing countries due to lack of adequate tools for this work may justify the absence of female workers. In Lille, Frimat *et al.* reported 2% of female timber workers [6]. In a Lithuanian cohort, Smailyte *et al.* had found a higher female presence (29%) [8]. In the south-east of Nigeria, neighboring and developing country like Benin, Aguwa *et al.* reported 491 men and 50 women but the latter were busy with collecting and selling sawdust generated by men's work [9].

Nearly half of the workers indicated having ENT case history and among the reported pathologies, rhinitis came well ahead followed by anginas. The rate of ENT pathologies (associated or not with sawdust) detected in Parakou's timber workers based on the questionnaire and ENT clinical examination, was relatively significant (60.3%). An Italian study carried out in 2007 by Belvilacqua *et al.* in a population of timber workers, reported a 32.7% rate of ENT affections in timber workers [7]. This difference could a priori be associated with the absence of individual and collective protection among Parakou timber workers as is the case in the developed countries but also with the fact that all the ENT pathologies had been taken into account, whether related or not to timber work.

Rhinitises came first among ENT pathologies as well as ENT case history in Parakou timber workers. Rhinitis is a pathology which is often reported in timber workers [5]-[7] [9]. According to Garnier [10], rhinitis is one of the most common occupational diseases. As it causes little disability, it is often neglected by the concerned persons. It is generally misunderstood by physicians, whose knowledge of occupational pathologies and their causes is frequently insufficient. It is due not only to sawdust but also to timber-related allergens. In Parakou, rhinitis rate is close to the one of the developed countries [7] [11] [12]. It is significantly lower than the one found by Aguwa in Nigeria where timber workers are gathered in timber work markets consisting of poorly ventilated workshops and without any method for sawdust removal [9]. In Parakou, almost all the workshops are

Table 3. Distribution of wood-workers according to ENT history.

	Number (N = 315)	Percentage
Rhinitises	277	87.9
Anginas	22	7.0
Otitises	13	4.1
Sinusitises	3	1.0

Table 4. Distribution of wood-workers according to the diagnosed ENT pathology.

	Number (N = 703)	Percentage
Rhinitis	303	43.1
Pharyngitis	99	14.1
Ear wax	43	6.1
Deafness suspicion*	24	3.4
Average chronic otitis	10	1.4
Otitis externa	6	0.9
Acute otitis media	3	0.4
Nasal tumor**	1	0.1
No pathology screened	279	39.7%

*Only with sawyers. **Histological examination not done, as the patient refused to do it.

installed in the open air, on street corners and isolated. This helps reduce substantially sawdust concentration in the air (which we did not measure), but at the expense of the environment.

A pharyngitis case had been found in 14% of timber workers in Parakou. In Italy, Veneri *et al.* reported 17.1% of pharyngitis cases and found a statistically significant relationship with sawdust [11].

The histological nature of the only tumor case observed in Parakou could not have been specified, since the patient refused to undergo the anatomo-pathological examination. However, we assume it was a non-malignant tumor considering its clinical characteristics, and not an adenocarcinoma. Moreover, in the studies where naso-sinusal cancers in timber workers had been reported, workers have always been exposed for a long period. Thus, in their studies, Mayr *et al.* as well as Bimbi *et al.* reported average exposure duration of 32.3 years in patients suffering from cancer associated with timber [13] [14]. The duration of average exposure of timber workers to sawdust in our study was 4.9 years, which does not give enough ground to associate the tumor observed to timber work.

We suspected 6% of deafness in timber workers, especially sawyers only. This deafness could be associated with a long and frequent exposure to noise insofar as only two patients among the workers protected themselves from noise.

In general, the other ENT pathologies screened in this study (ear wax and otitises) are not considered as an outcome of the exposure to sawdust.

5. Conclusion

ENT pathologies are relatively frequent among timber workers in Parakou. Among those pathologies, the most frequent ones are cases of rhinitis and sinusitis the relationship of which with wood work is well known. Everything still remains to be done as regards protection and prevention in this profession, both at individual and collective levels. At least wood workers should be encouraged to use dust masks; they should wet regularly the floor of their workshops to prevent the dust to be airborne. For this purpose, information and awareness/sensitization programmes should be implemented and protection standards imposed by public authorities.

References

[1] Mirza, S. (2010) Risks to the Health of Wood Workers: What Can Be Done? *Zigazag Journal of Occupational Health and Safety*, **3**, 1-8. http://www.zjohs.eg.net/pdf/vol3no1/1.pdf

[2] Hemelt, M., Granström, C. and Hemmenki, K. (2004) Occupational Risks for Nasal Cancer in Sweden. *Journal of Occupational and Environmental Medicine*, **46**, 1033-1040. http://dx.doi.org/10.1097/01.jom.0000141653.30337.82

[3] Imbernon, E. (2003) Estimation of the Number of Some Cancer Cases Attributable to Occupational Factors. http://fulltext.bdsp.ehesp.fr/Invs/Rapports/2003/rapport_cancer_pro.pdf

[4] Jacobsen, G., Schaumburg, I., Sigsgaard, T. and Schhüssen, V. (2010) Non-Malignant Respiratory Disease and Occupational Exposure to Wood Dust. Part I. Fresh Wood and Mixed Wood Industry. *Annals of Agricultural and Environmental Medicine*, **17**, 15-28.

[5] Jacobsen, G., Schaumburg, I., Sigsgaard, T. and Schhüssen, V. (2010) Non-Malignant Respiratory Disease and Occupational Exposure to Wood Dust. Part II. Dry Wood Industry. *Annals of Agricultural and Environmental Medicine*, **17**, 29-44,

[6] Frimat, P., Leroyer, A., Beuneu, A., Dubrulle, F., Larroque, G., Fontaine, B., *et al.* (2002) Screening of Nasosinusal Pathologies in Employees Exposed to Sawdusts. National Days for Occupational Health in the Construction and Public Works Sector, Lille, 79-64.

[7] Bevilacqua, I., Magnavita, N., Becchetti, G., De Matteis, B., Giunta, G., Lancia, F., *et al.* (2007) Vigilance on Health Surveillance in Wood Sector. *Giornale Italiano di Medicina del Lavoro ed Ergonomia*, **29**, 794-795.

[8] Smailyte, G. (2012) The Incidence of Cancer among Workers Exposed to Timber Dust in Lithuania. *Journal of Occupational and Environmental Medicine*, **69**, 449-451. http://dx.doi.org/10.1136/oemed-2011-100253

[9] Aguwa, F., Okeke, T. and Asuzu, M. (2007) The Prevalence of Occupational Asthma and Rhinitis in Woodworkers in South-Eastern Nigeria. *Tanzania Health Research Bulletin*, **9**, 52-55. http://dx.doi.org/10.4314/thrb.v9i1.14293

[10] Garnier, R., Villa, A. and Chataigner, D. (2007) Occupational Rhinitises. Respiratory Disease Review. *Revue des Maladies Respiratoires*, **24**, 205-220. http://dx.doi.org/10.1016/S0761-8425(07)91043-8

[11] Veneri, I., Caso, M.A., Ravaioli, M., Albonetti, A., Ghini, P., Mazzavillani, M., *et al.* (2007) Study on the Prevalence of Respiratory Upper and Lower Tract with Carpenters, Data Monitoring Reports and Medical Records of Exposure. *Giornale Italiano di Medicina del Lavoro ed Ergonomia*, **29**, 833-835.

[12] Milanowiski, J., Góra, A., Skorska, C., Krysińska-Traczyk, E., Mackiewicz, B., Sitkowska, J., *et al.* (2002) Work-Related Symptoms among Workers in Furniture Factory in Lublin Region (Eastern Poland). *Annals of Agricultural and Environmental Medicine*, **9**, 99-103.

[13] Mayr, S.I., Hafizovic, K., Waldfahrer, F., Iro, H. and Kutting, B. (2010) Characterization of Clinical Symptoms and Risk Factors for Sino-Nasal Adenocarcinoma: Results of a Case-Control Study. *Archives of Environmental and Occupational Health*, **83**, 631-616. http://dx.doi.org/10.1007/s00420-009-0479-5

[14] Bimbi, G., Saraceno, M.S., Riccio, S., Gatta, G., Licitra, I. and Cantù, G. (2004) Adenocarcinoma of Ethmoid Sinus: An Occupational Disease. *Acta Otorhinolaryngologica Italica*, **24**, 199-203.

3

Assessment of Fine Structure Processing Strategies in Unilaterally Deafened Cochlear Implant Users

Dayse Távora-Vieira[1,2], Gunesh P. Rajan[1,2]

[1]Otolaryngology, Head & Neck Surgery, School of Surgery, University of Western Australia, Perth, Australia
[2]Fremantle Hospital, Fremantle, Australia
Email: dayse.tavora@health.wa.gov.au

Abstract

This study aimed to investigate the speech perception and subjective preference of unilaterally deafened cochlear implant users for two different speech coding strategies. Thirteen subjects who received a cochlear implant were provided with 2 maps that differed in the speech coding strategy, FS4 or FS4-p (MED-EL). Subjects were requested to alternate between the two maps daily for two weeks and to complete a questionnaire daily. Speech perception testing was performed using the adaptive Bamford-Kowal-Bench speech-in-noise test (BKB-SIN) after two weeks of alternating FS4/FS4-p use. The subjective benefit of FS4-p was significantly greater than the subjective benefit of FS4 on all five questions of the questionnaire. There was a significant improvement in speech perception scores over time under the S_0/N_0, S_0/N_{HE}, S_{CI}/N_{HE} test conditions. There was no significant difference between the speech perception scores obtained with FS4 and FS4-p coding strategies. For this group of cochlear implant recipients, assessment of the subjective preference for the speech coding strategy is likely to enhance motivation, compliance and consequently, outcomes.

Keywords

CI, Unilateral Deafness, FS4, FS4-p

1. Introduction

The technology and surgical techniques for auditory implants have advanced rapidly in recent years enabling us to treat various types and degrees of hearing loss. In addition, there is a continuous interest in improving signal processing and speech coding strategies. The improvements are designed not only to improve cochlear implant (CI) users' speech understanding in quiet and in noise, but also to enhance appreciation of music, and speech understanding in tonal languages.

Various speech coding strategies have been developed, all of which aim to provide CI users with the clearest and most natural sound possible given the constraints of the limited stimulation representation of the implant electrodes. Envelope representation of an incoming sound signal is a common theme in many speech-encoding strategies, examples of which include Continuous Interleaved Sampling (CIS) [1], HiResolution (HiRes) [2], and Advanced Combination Encoder (ACE) [3]. One of MED-EL's (Innsbruck, Austria) coding strategies, called Fine Structure Processing (FSP) [4], uses envelope representation (High Definition-CIS) and low frequency temporal information to improve subtle pitch discrimination and temporal cues in the low frequencies [5] (reviewed by Moore *et al.* [6]). There are reports of a general subjective preference for FSP over CIS+ coding strategies as well as a better appreciation of music using FSP [7]. The presentation of the fine structure is thought to enhance CI users' music appreciation, and speech understanding in noise [8]. Arnoldner *et al.* [9] reported that speech and music perception was improved with FSP when compared to CIS in the early stage of the study, but this improvement was not statistically significant at the 12-month follow up [10]. FS4 and FS4-p, developments of the FSP coding strategy, both have fine structure information delivered to designated low-frequency apical channels which can span 70 Hz - 950 Hz. While FS4 can stimulate just one low-frequency fine structure channel at any point in time, FS4-p can simultaneously stimulate two of the four fine structure channels at any given time and can thus provide the temporal code specific to each of the two channels with higher accuracy. Recently, Riss *et al.* [11] compared FS4 and FS4-p with FSP in terms of speech perception, sound quality and subjective preference. It was found that there was no significant difference among the three strategies for speech performance in noise. At the end of the study, 20 out 33 participants chose FS4 or FS4-p over FSP.

In the last few years, several studies have investigated the benefits of cochlear implantation in individuals with unilateral deafness (UD). There is a growing literature demonstrating that cochlear implantation decreases tinnitus disturbance associated with UD, improves speech understanding in noise, enhances localization ability and improves patients' self-perception of hearing performance [12]-[19].

Unilaterally deafened subjects commonly expect to match the hearing from the CI to their normal hearing in the contralateral ear. However, to best of our knowledge, there are no studies that address whether unilaterally deafened CI users demand different mapping techniques or modification of map parameters.

Unilaterally deafened CI users are in the unique position of being able to assess and compare the quality of speech coding strategies directly with the correlating sound percepts of their normal hearing ear. In this study, it was proposed that subjective evaluation of sound quality, and ease/effort of listening should also be explored, as the speech perception tests in isolation are insufficient to address these dimensions of hearing. Therefore, the present study sets out to evaluate how unilaterally deafened CI users subjectively perceive and rate sound when using two different speech coding strategies. It aimed to investigate if the differences between FS4 and FS4-p had a subjective benefit for unilaterally deaf cochlear implant users. We expected subtle differences between FS4 and FS4-p, and therefore formulated an open questionnaire that aimed to obtain information regarding the subjective perception.

2. Material and Methods

Thirteen adult subjects (7 males, 6 females) with post-lingual UD who received a MED-EL implant were recruited for this study. The mean age at implantation was 56 years (range 39 - 74). Further demographic data is presented in **Table 1**. The better hearing ear had a pure tone average ($PTA_{0.5-4\,kHz}$) of ≤32 dB and the ear to be implanted had a ($PTA_{0.5-4\,kHz}$) of ≥72 dB. A hearing aid was fitted to the poorer ear if any functional hearing was present, and if this was unsuccessful, a patient was considered for a CI. Prior to implantation, all patients were offered a two week trial of both a conventional contra-lateral routing of signal amplification (CROS) hearing aid and a bone anchored hearing aid (Baha) mounted on a headband. Standardized pre-operative evaluation of the subjects included high-resolution computed tomography (CT) and magnetic resonance imaging (MRI) of the temporal bones and brain to rule out the presence of any inner ear anomalies or cochlear nerve pathologies that might constrain electrical stimulation by a CI. The audiological evaluation consisted of immitance measures, audiometry and speech discrimination in quiet using Arthur Boothroyd (AB) words [20].

Speech perception testing was performed using the adaptive Bamford-Kowal-Bench speech-in-noise test

Table 1. Subject demographic data.

Subject	Duration of deafness (years)	Age at implantation (years)	Ear	Pure tone average (0.5, 1, 2 and 4 kHz)—non implanted ear in dB*	Pure tone average (0.5, 1, 2 and 4 kHz)—implanted ear in dB*
1	1.5	73	L	21	>110
2	1	57	L	25	76
3	5	71	R	30	74
4	4	39	R	19	>110
5	2.5	74	L	21	>110
6	7	53	R	24	95
7	1	57	L	32	80
8	0.5	42	L	10	92
9	1.5	47	R	21	87
10	1.0	53	L	18	90
11	3.0	76	R	27	77
12	1.5	39	R	13	>110
13	4.5	44	L	18	86

PTA = pure tone average at 0.5, 1, 2 and 4 kHz. R = right; L = left. *Before cochlear implantation.

(BKB-SIN) [21] which investigates the signal to noise ratio needed to achieve 50% speech perception. Tests were performed in a free-field with the subject seated 1 meter away from loudspeakers located at angles of 0, −90 and +90 degrees. The following spatial configurations were used: S_0/N_0-speech and noise presented from the front; S_0/N_{HE}-speech presented from the front and noise to the normal hearing ear; and S_{CI}/N_{HE}-speech presented to the implanted ear and noise to the side of the normal hearing ear.

All subjects were implanted with a FLEX^{SOFT} electrode (MED-EL, Austria) and received an OPUS 2 speech processor. Subjects were fitted with their speech processors 2 weeks after cochlear implantation. Mapping sessions took place weekly for the first four weeks. All patients had 3 months of CI experience prior to the experiment, and were using the FSP speech coding strategy since CI activation.

Three months post-CI activation, after giving written consent to participate in this study, subjects were provided with 2 maps called program 1 (P1) and program 2 (P2) that differed only in the coding strategy, FS4 or FS4-p, respectively. The subjects were blind to the different settings P1 and P2, and were not provided with any information regarding the differences between the two programs. The subjects were requested to alternate between the two maps daily for two consecutive weeks and to complete a non-standardized 10 point scale questionnaire at the end of each day, and return it to the audiologist. The patients' scores were averaged for each question for each program (P1 and P2). The questionnaire comprised of 5 questions:

1) How similar is the sound from the cochlear implant to the other ear? In this question the scale varied from 1 = "very different" to 10 = "very similar".

2) How is the clarity of sounds? The scale varied from 1 = "very unclear" to 10 = "very clear".

3) How easy is it to hear in quiet? The scale varied from 1 = "very difficult" to 10 = "very easy".

4) How easy is it to hear in noise? The scale varied from 1 = "very difficult" to 10 = "very easy".

5) How do you like the sound? The scale varied from 1 = "not at all" to 10 = "very much".

Speech perception in noise test was performed at the end of the two weeks. The sequence of the test (P1/P2) was randomized. The audiologist performing the test was blind to the settings of the speech processor.

This study was designed and conducted in accordance with the Declaration of Helsinki, and ethical approval was obtained from the relevant ethics and institutional review committees.

Wilcoxon signed-rank test was used to determine the difference between the coding strategies for all 5 questions and for the speech perception in noise scores. A repeated measure ANOVA was performed to see if there was a significant improvement from preoperative to postoperative speech perception scores on the 3 spatial conditions.

A p-value of <0.05 was considered statistically significant. IBM SPSS Statistics 19 (IBM, Armonik, New

York) software was used for the data analyses. Graphs were created using Microsoft Office Excel 2010 (http://www.microsoft.com).

3. Results

Figure 1 illustrates the difference between FS4 and FS4-p for each question presented to the unilaterally deafened CI users. The speech coding strategy FS4-p scored significantly higher than FS4 for all 5 questions. The results are shown in **Table 2**.

There was a significant improvement across all test intervals in the BKB-SIN under the S_0/N_0 test condition ($p < 0.001$) (**Figure 2**). The improvement in the BKB-SIN under the S_0/N_0 test condition was significant between pre-operative testing and the P1 program test ($p = 0.001$); and significant between pre-operative testing and the P2 program test ($p = 0.001$). There was no significant difference between P1 and P2 in the BKB-SIN under the S_0/N_0 test condition ($p = 1.000$).

There was a significant improvement across all test intervals in the BKB-SIN in the S_0/N_{HE} test condition ($p = 0.002$) (**Figure 2**). The improvement in the BKB-SIN under the S_0/N_{HE} test condition was significant between pre-operative testing and the P1 program test ($p = 0.005$); and significant between pre-operative testing and the P2 program test ($p = 0.007$). There was no significant difference between the P1 and P2 in the BKB-SIN under the S_0/N_{HE} test condition ($p = 0.763$).

There was a significant improvement across all test intervals in the BKB-SIN in the S_{CI}/N_{HE} test condition ($p < 0.001$) (**Figure 2**). The improvement in the BKB-SIN under the S_{CI}/N_{HE} test condition was significant between pre-operative testing and the P1 program test ($p = 0.002$); and significant between pre-operative testing and the P2 program test ($p = 0.002$). There was no significant difference between the P1 and P2 in the BKB-SIN under the S_{CI}/N_{HE} test condition ($p = 0.157$). The majority of the patients (10 out of 13) kept either FS4 or FS4-p at the end of the study.

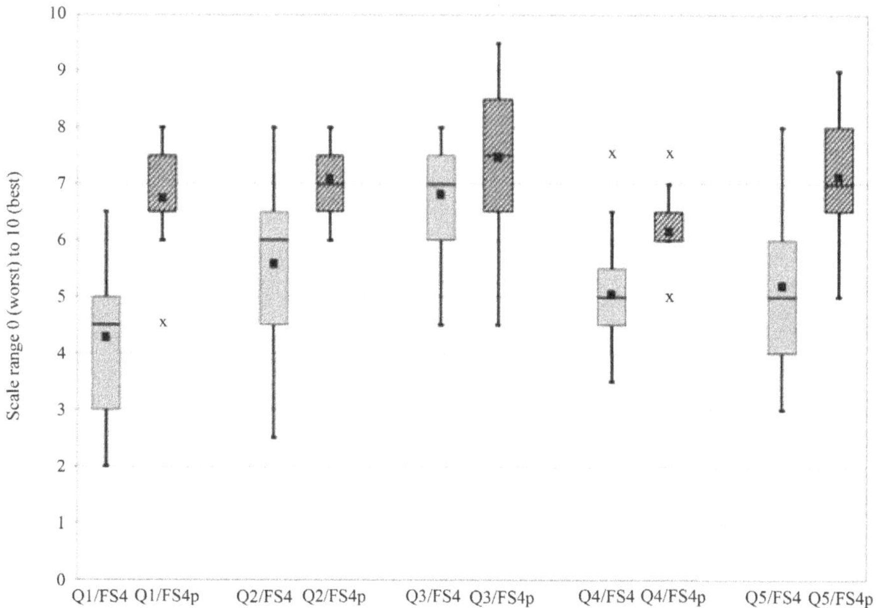

Figure 1. The group results for each of the five questions. FS4 is shown in grey boxes. FS4-p is shown in diagonally lined boxes. Mean values are depicted as black squares, median as horizontal lines, and asterisks are the outliers (calculated as 1.5 to 3 times box height above the 75th percentile).

Table 2. Wilcoxon signed-rank test results for questions 1-5.

	Q1	Q2	Q3	Q4	Q5
Z	−3.195	−2.632	−1.906	−2.562	−2.874
p-value (2-sided)	0.001	0.008	0.057	0.010	0.004

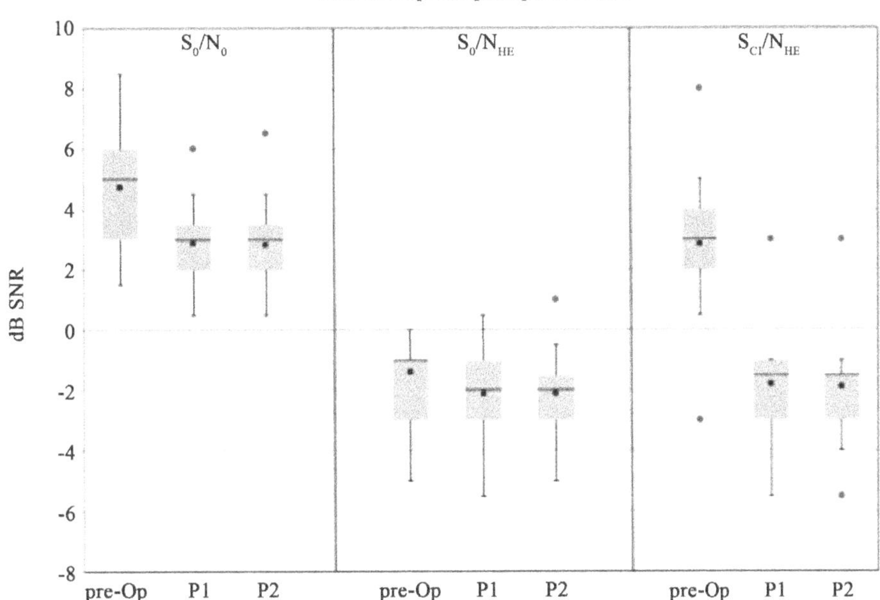

Figure 2. Results of the Bamford-Kowal-Bench speech-in-noise (n = 13) with speech presented from the front and noise presented from the front (S_0/N_0); speech presented from the front and noise presented from the side of the normal hearing ear (S_0/N_{HE}), and; speech presented from the side of the cochlear implant and noise presented from the side of the normal hearing ear (S_{CI}/N_{HE}). Mean values are depicted as black squares, median values as horizontal lines, and dots signify outliers (1.5 to 3 × box height above the 75th percentile).

4. Discussion

Several studies have demonstrated that cochlear implantation is a suitable hearing rehabilitation option for adults with unilateral profound deafness. Among the hearing devices used in the rehabilitation of UD subjects, CI is the only option that provides ear specific information and thus potentially the benefits of binaural hearing. The studies have investigated the effects of cochlear implantation on tinnitus, subjective perception of improvement, speech understanding in noise and localization ability [12]-[19]. A review of the literature by Vlastarakos *et al.* [22] has emphasized that self-assessment questionnaires were commonly used to assess the patients' perception of improvement in daily listening conditions. In fact, Stelzig *et al.* [16] reported that the subjective rating of outcomes tended to be more positive than the objective measures which could be related to an inadequacy of speech perception test for the unilaterally deafened CI users.

To date, there is no literature that addresses whether the patients with unilateral deafness demand any different mapping strategies or mapping parameters. This study addressed this issue by comparing the speech coding strategies FS4 and FS4-p in terms of patients' performance in the adaptive speech in noise test and the patients' responses to a non-standardized questionnaire. The questionnaire was developed by the authors and aimed to determine the subjective perception of sound from the CI.

The results showed a significant improvement in speech perception in noise scores when speech and noise are presented from the front (S_0/N_0), and when speech is presented from the front (S_0/N_{HE}), or from the CI side (S_{CI}/N_{HE}) with the noise presented to the normal hearing ear. This was true for both speech coding strategies. Riss *et al.* [11] found that there was no significant difference among the three strategies FSP, FS4 and FS4-p using an adaptive sentence test in noise. Similarly, in this study, there was no significant difference between FS4 and FS4-p in the speech understanding measures. These finding were expected as the difference between FS4 and FS4-p is subtle.

Outcome performance studies (which investigated the superiority of one speech coding strategy over another) have predominantly focused on speech perception, for which objective speech perception testing is appropriate. Unilaterally deafened CI users are in the unique position of being able to assess and compare the quality of speech coding strategies directly with the correlating sound percepts of their normal hearing ear. Therefore, it was proposed that subjective evaluation of sound quality and ease/effort of listening should be added to the evaluation protocol with the final objective to facilitate patients' acclimatization to electrical stimulation.

The results indicated that FS4-p was rated significantly superior to FS4 in all five questions answered by the unilaterally deafened CI users. As per question 1, it appears that unilaterally deafened CI users perceived that FS4-p mimicked the sound quality of the normal hearing contralateral ear significantly better than FS4. This was reinforced by the rating in question 5, since the patients reported to like the sound provided by the CI more when using FS4-p. The explanation for these results is not clear. As the patients alternated between the two strategies daily, they had the same experience with both settings and thus it unlikely that the patients have acclimatized to one setting in particular. To avoid any bias, the audiologist performing the speech in noise test was blind to which speech coding strategy was being used.

The FSP strategy with its fine structure coding [23] aims to improve pitch perception, which is thought to improve speech discrimination, sound localization, and music appreciation [7]. The original FSP strategy provides fine structure processing in 1 - 3 apical channels up to 470 Hz. The newer developed FS4 and FS4-p provide it to the 4 most apical low-frequency channels. FS4 stimulates the apical channels sequentially, while FS4-p simultaneously stimulates 2 of the 4 designated low frequency apical channels from 70 - 950 Hz, and this is thought to further enhance temporal information. This may explain why CI users preferred FS4-p to FS4.

The subjective results in this study differ from those reported by Riss *et al.* [11] since our group of unilaterally deafened subjects rated FS4-p superior to FS4. This difference might be linked to the variability of the subjects between the studies. The subjects with UD might have rated the sound in comparison to normal acoustic hearing, while patients with bilateral hearing loss may rate the sound quality based solely on their auditory memory and/or an input from acoustic amplification on the contra-lateral ear.

The results of this study need to be interpreted with caution, as it used a non-validated questionnaire and a small number of subjects. However, it is the first to provide some insights about the mapping strategies to be considered for patients with unilateral deafness. Combined with speech perception testing, assessment of the patients' subjective preference for a specific speech coding strategy may assist in the rehabilitation program for unilateral deafness, enhancing patients' motivation and compliance with CI use.

5. Conclusion

There were no significant differences in the speech perception in noise scores between FS4 and FS4-p. The FS4-p fine structure was rated higher subjectively than FS4 in the present study. Subjective evaluation may assist in the rehabilitation program of unilaterally deafened CI users potentially enhancing motivation, compliance, and, consequently, outcomes.

Acknowledgements

The authors would kindly like to acknowledge E. A. for statistical analyses; I. G. A. and U. D. for editing a version of this manuscript.

References

[1] Wilson, B.S., Finley, C.C., Lawson, D.T., Wolford, R.D., Eddington, D.K. and Rabinowitz, W.M. (1991) Better Speech Recognition with Cochlear Implants. *Nature*, **352**, 236-238. http://dx.doi.org/10.1038/352236a0

[2] Koch, D.B., Osberger, M.J., Segel, P. and Kessler, D.K. (2004) High Resolution and Conventional Sound Processing in the HiResolution Bionic Ear: Using Appropriate Outcome Measures to Assess Speech Recognition Ability. *Audiology & Neuro-Otology*, **9**, 214-223. http://dx.doi.org/10.1159/000078391

[3] Kiefer, J., Hohl, S., Sturzebecher, E., Pfennigdorff, T. and Gstoettner, W. (2001) Comparison of Speech Recognition with Different Speech Coding Strategies (SPEAK, CIS, and ACE) and Their Relationship to Telemetric Measures of Compound Action Potentials in the Nucleus CI 24M Cochlear Implant System. *Audiology*, **40**, 32-42. http://dx.doi.org/10.3109/00206090109073098

[4] Zierhofer, C.M. (2003) Electrical Nerve Stimulation Based on Channel Specific Sampling Sequences. US Patent No. 6594525.

[5] Müller, J., Brill, S., Hagen, R., Moeltner, A., Brockmeier, S.J., Stark, T., Helbig, S., Maurer, J., Zahnert, T., Zierhofer, C., Nopp, P. and Anderson, I. (2012) Clinical Trial Results with the MED-EL Fine Structure Processing Coding Strategy in Experienced Cochlear Implant Users. *ORL*, **74**, 185-198. http://dx.doi.org/10.1159/000337089

[6] Moore, B.C. (2008) The Role of Temporal Fine Structure Processing in Pitch Perception, Masking, and Speech Perception for Normal-Hearing and Hearing-Impaired People. *Journal of the Association for Research in Otolaryngology*, **9**, 399-406. http://dx.doi.org/10.1007/s10162-008-0143-x

[7] Lorens, A., Zgoda, M., Obrycka, A. and Skarzynski, H. (2010) Fine Structure Processing Improves Speech Perception as Well as Objective and Subjective Benefits in Pediatric MED-EL COMBI 40+ Users. *International Journal of Pediatric Otorhinolaryngology*, **74**, 1372-1378. http://dx.doi.org/10.1016/j.ijporl.2010.09.005

[8] Vermiere, K., Punte, A.K. and Van de Heyning, P. (2010) Better Speech Recognition in Noise with Fine Structure Processing Coding Strategy. *ORL*, **72**, 305-311. http://dx.doi.org/10.1159/000319748

[9] Arnoldner, C., Riss, D., Brunner, M., Durisin, M., Baumgartner, W.D. and Hamzavi, J.S. (2007) Speech and Music Perception with the New Fine Structure Speech Coding Strategy: Preliminary Results. *Acta Oto-Laryngologica*, **127**, 1298-1303. http://dx.doi.org/10.1080/00016480701275261

[10] Riss, D., Arnoldner, C., Baumgartner, W.D., Kaider, A. and Hamzavi, J.S. (2008) A New Fine Structure Speech Coding Strategy: Speech Perception at a Reduced Number of Channels. *Otology & Neurotology*, **29**, 784-788. http://dx.doi.org/10.1097/MAO.0b013e31817fe00f

[11] Riss, D., Hamzavi, J.S., Blineder, M., Honeder, C., Ehrenreich, I., Kaider, A., Baumgartner, W.D., Gstoettner, W. and Arnoldner, C. (2014) FS4, FS4-p and FSP: A 4-Month Crossover Study of Three Fine Structure Sound-Coding Strategies. *Ear & Hearing*. http://dx.doi.org/10.1097/AUD.0000000000000063

[12] Van de Heyning, P., Vermeire, K., Diebl, M., Nopp, P., Anderson, I. and De Ridder, D. (2008) Incapacitating Unilateral Tinnitus in Single-Sided Deafness Treated by Cochlear Implantation. *Annals of Otology, Rhinology & Laryngology*, **117**, 645-652. http://dx.doi.org/10.1177/000348940811700903

[13] Vermeire, K. and Van de Heyning, P. (2009) Binaural Hearing after Cochlear Implantation in Subjects with Unilateral Sensorineural Deafness and Tinnitus. *Audiology & Neuro-Otology*, **14**, 163-171. http://dx.doi.org/10.1159/000171478

[14] Buechner, A., Brendel, M., Lesinski-Schiedat, A., Wenzel, G., Frohne-Buechner, C., Jaeger, B. and Lenarz, T. (2010) Cochlear Implantation in Unilateral Deaf Subjects Associated with Ipsilateral Tinnitus. *Otology & Neurotology*, **31**, 1381-1385.

[15] Arndt, S., Aschendorff, A., Laszig, R., Beck, R., Schild, C., Kroeger, S., Ihorst, G. and Wesarg, T. (2010) Comparison of Pseudobinaural Hearing to Real Binaural Hearing Rehabilitation after Cochlear Implantation in Patients with Unilateral Deafness and Tinnitus. *Otology & Neurotology*, **32**, 39-47. http://dx.doi.org/10.1097/MAO.0b013e3181fcf271

[16] Stelzig, Y., Jacob, R. and Mueller, J. (2011) Preliminary Speech Recognition Results after Cochlear Implantation in Patients with Unilateral Hearing Loss: A Case Series. *Journal of Medical Case Reports*, **5**, 343. http://dx.doi.org/10.1186/1752-1947-5-343

[17] Firszt, J.B., Holden, L.K., Reeder, R.M., Waltzman, S.B. and Arndt, S. (2012) Auditory Abilities after Cochlear Implantation in Adults with Unilateral Deafness: A Pilot Study. *Otology & Neurotology*, **33**, 1339-1346. http://dx.doi.org/10.1097/MAO.0b013e318268d52d

[18] Hansen, M.R., Gantz, B.J. and Dunn, C. (2013) Outcomes after Cochlear Implantation for Patients with Single-Sided Deafness, Including Those with Recalcitrant Meniere's Disease. *Otology & Neurotology*, **34**, 1681-1687. http://dx.doi.org/10.1097/MAO.0000000000000102

[19] Távora-Vieira, D., Marino, R., Krishnaswamy, J., Kuthubutheen, J. and Rajan, G.P. (2013) Cochlear Implantation for Unilateral Deafness with and without Tinnitus: A Case Series. *Laryngoscope*, **123**, 1251-1255. http://dx.doi.org/10.1002/lary.23764

[20] Boothroyd, A. (1968) Developments in Speech Audiometry. *Sound*, **2**, 3-10.

[21] Bench, J., Kowal, A. and Bamford, J. (1979) The BKB (Bamford-Kowal-Bench) Sentence Lists for Partially-Hearing Children. *British Journal of Audiology*, **13**, 108-112. http://dx.doi.org/10.3109/03005367909078884

[22] Vlastarakos, P.V., Nazos, K., Tavoulari, E.F. and Nikolopoulos, T.P. (2013) Cochlear Implantation for Single-Sided Deafness: The Outcomes. An Evidence-Based Approach. *European Archives of Oto-Rhino-Laryngology*, **271**, 2119-2126. http://dx.doi.org/10.1007/s00405-013-2746-z

[23] Schatzer, R., Krenmayr, A., Au, D.K. and Zierhofer, C. (2010) Temporal Fine Structure in Cochlear Implants: Preliminary Speech Perception Results in Cantonese Speaking Implant Users. *Acta Oto-Laryngologica*, **130**, 1031-1039. http://dx.doi.org/10.3109/00016481003591731

4

Cut Throat Injuries—A Retrospective Study at a Tertiary Referral Hospital

Suman Arasikere Panchappa*, Dhinakaran Natarajan, Thangaraj Karuppasamy, Alaguvadivel Jeyabalan, Radhakrishnan Kailasam Ramamoorthy, Sivasubramanian Thirani, Rajaganesh Kutuva Swamirao

Department of ENT, Madurai Medical College, Madurai, India
Email: *rajsuman91@yahoo.com

Abstract

Objective: To analyze the socio demographic pattern, sex and age ratio, common causes, the most common site and extent of the injury in the patients with cut throat injury at our hospital. To compare the same with previous similar studies conducted at other centers in different parts of the world. Setting: Department of ENT, Government Rajaji Hospital, Madurai, India from January 2013 to June 2014. Methods: A total of 51 cases of cut throat injury were included in the study. Separate proforma was prepared to collect the patients' data. Structured questionnaire was offered. Results: 51 cases of cut throat injury patients were included in the study. Age varied from 4 years to 80 years. Out of 51 cases, there were 43 males, 7 females and one male child. Male to female ratio was 6.2:1. All the patients were belonging to lower socioeconomic status (Kuppusamy class 5). Amongst them 26 cases (50.98%) were due to homicidal attack; 13 cases (25.49%) due to suicidal attempt; 7 cases (13.72%) due to road traffic accident; 4 cases (7.84%) due to bull gore injury; 1 case (1.96%) due to accidental fall. Emergency tracheostomy was done in 16 cases (33.33%). An average hospital stay for most of the patients was less than 3 weeks. 2 victims (3.92%) died due to haemorhage, aspiration pnuemonia and septicemia. Conclusions: Our study found that the majority of the victims were males of age between 20 years to 40 years from poor socioeconomic status. Social commitment and political motivation, decrease in the poverty, individual awareness, increase in economic growth, and literacy rate will prevent the cut throat injuries. Early and improved management will reduce the mortality and morbidity.

Keywords

Cut Throat Injury, Treatment, Outcome

*Corresponding author.

1. Introduction

Penetrating neck trauma involves a sharp object penetrating the skin and violating the platysma layer of the neck. This includes gunshot wounds, stab or puncture wounds, and impalement injuries. Penetrating neck injuries, like any trauma, may be classified as intentional or non intentional. It can also be classified as homicidal, accidental or suicidal. The objects causing these injuries can be divided into stabbing instruments (e.g., knives, cutting instruments, razors, blades, broken glass pieces, broken bottles, puncturing objects, impaling objects) and shooting instruments (e.g., missiles, projectiles). Wounding instruments have specific characteristics that affect surgical findings. For example, stab wounds typically have a 10% higher rate of negative exploration than injuries from projectiles. The object's mass and shape will determine the extent of a penetrating injury.

Globally, cut throat injuries account for approximately 5% to 10% of all traumatic injuries with multiple structures being injured in 30% of patients. However, in developing countries the incidence is increasing at a fast rate partly because of increasing conflict over limited resources, poor socioeconomic status, poverty, unemployment, easy access to firearms, alcohol and substance misuse and increased crime rates [1]-[3].

According to Roon and Christensen's classification, neck injuries are divided into three anatomical zones.

Zone I is defined as the area from the clavicles to the inferior margin of cricoid cartilage. Structures within this zone include the vertebral and proximal carotid arteries, major thoracic vessels, superior mediastinum, lungs, esophagus, trachea, thoracic duct and spinal cord.

Zone II extends from the inferior margin of the cricoid cartilage to the angle of the mandible. The carotid and vertebral arteries, jugular veins, esophagus, trachea, larynx and spinal cord are found in this zone.

Zone III is located between the angle of the mandible and the base of the skull. It includes the carotid and vertebral arteries, pharynx and spinal cord [1].

The location of the injury suggests which structures may be involved. Injuries to the larynx and trachea can be asymptomatic or may cause hoarseness, laryngeal stridor, subcutaneous emphysema or dyspnea secondary to airway compression or aspiration of blood. Injury to the great vessels presents with visible external blood loss, neck hematoma, bruit, pulselessness, distal ischaemia, hypotension and in varying degrees of shock. Following the cut throat, hemorrhage, shock and asphyxia from aspirated blood are the commonest causes of death. Immediate measures will save lives in vast majority.

Cut throat injuries pose a great challenge because multiple vital organs for phonation, deglutition, vascular and neurological structures vulnerable to injuries are present in the small, confined unprotected area. Many of these are close to the skin and easily vulnerable to injury. Injuries to the neck can be both complex and challenging to treat them. The management of these injuries requires a multidisciplinary approach requiring the close association of the otolaryngologists, the vascular surgeons, the anesthetists and the psychiatrists [4].

2. Aims and Objectives

1) To study the socio demographic pattern of cut throat injuries at our hospital.
2) The most common causes for cut throat injury.
3) Site and depth of the injury.
4) Treatment received at our hospital and outcome.

3. Methods and Materials

The study was conducted at Government Rajaji Hospital, Madurai, India. Our hospital is the highest referral unit for south Tamilnadu province, India. This is a 2518 bedded hospital. On an average the total number of trauma cases per year is around 23,840. It encompasses a total population of twenty-five million. The study period was 18 months from Jan 2013 to Jun 2014. The type of study is a retrospective study.

A total of 51 cases of cut throat injury were included in the study irrespective of their age and sex who attended ENT department and also patients referred from general surgery and trauma departments. The data regarding the study population were collected from the trauma department and from the registers of operation theatres and complied in a proforma. The study population were selected by purposive sampling from those patients who were admitted to this hospital and matches the inclusion criteria. All the data pertinent to the patients kept confidential.

Data were categorized according to the socio demographic pattern of the patient, cause for the injury, site of the neck injury (according to the defined zone of the neck), type and extent of the injury, presentation at time of admission, delay in the hospital arrival and duration of the hospital stay, records of mortality, treatment and outcome. The Kuppusamy classification was opted to know the socio economic status. The Kuppusamy classification includes education, occupation and monthly family income. A score of 26 - 29 is upper, 16 - 25 is upper middle, 11 - 15 is middle, 5 - 10 is lower upper and 0 - 5 is lower socioeconomic class. The accumulated data were compiled and analyzed by standard statistical method and then presented in the following **Tables 1-9**.

The evaluation of a patient with cut throat injury should start with advanced trauma life support (ATLS), which begins with a primary survey giving importance to airway, breathing, and circulation (ABC) [5]. After patients vitals are stable, they undergo a secondary survey which includes a complete history and a thorough physical examination. These steps help to identify the likely injury complex and to direct further treatment or diagnostic testing.

The patients with superficial cut injuries, their wound was closed in layers under aseptic precautions. For those patients who had their larynx or trachea or pharynx severed were taken to operation theatre for repair and reconstruction under tetanus toxoid and broad spectrum antibiotic coverage. In such cases emergency tracheastomy was done. Defect in the laryngeal cartilage was reconstructed by 3-0 prolene. The mucous membrane, muscles, thyroid gland and soft tissues were approximated by 3-0 vicryl. Skin was closed with 3-0 prolene.

Table 1. Sex distribution of the patients (n = 51).

Sex	No.	%
Male	44	86.27%
Female	7	13.27%
Total	51	100%

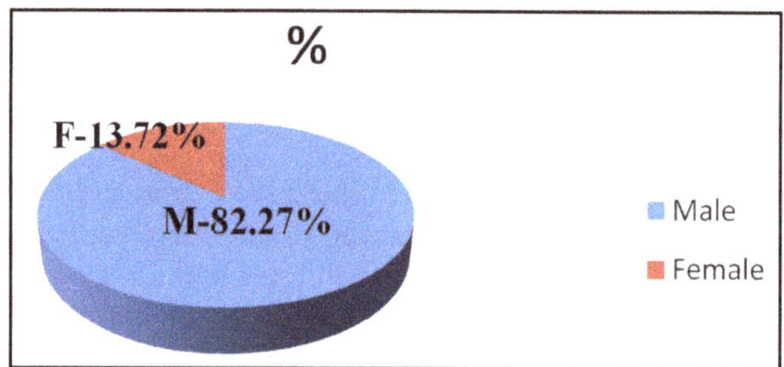

Table 2. Age distribution of the patients.

Age in years	Male	Female	Total
0 - 20	5	1	6
20 - 40	27	3	30
40 - 60	7	2	9
60 - 80	5	1	6
Total	44	7	51

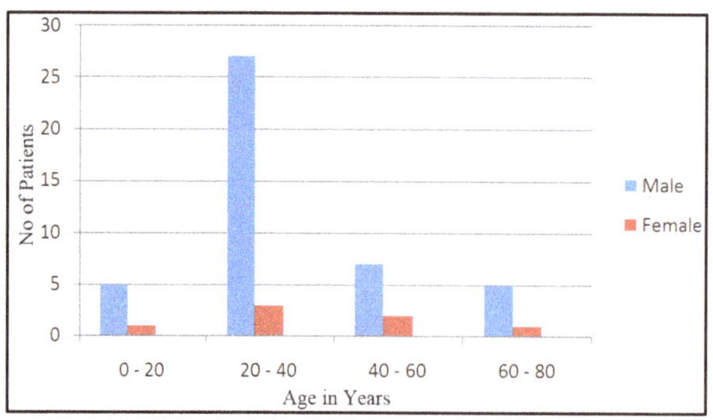

Table 3. Habitat of the patients.

Habitat	No.	%
Rural	43	84.31%
Urban	8	15.68%
Total	51	100%

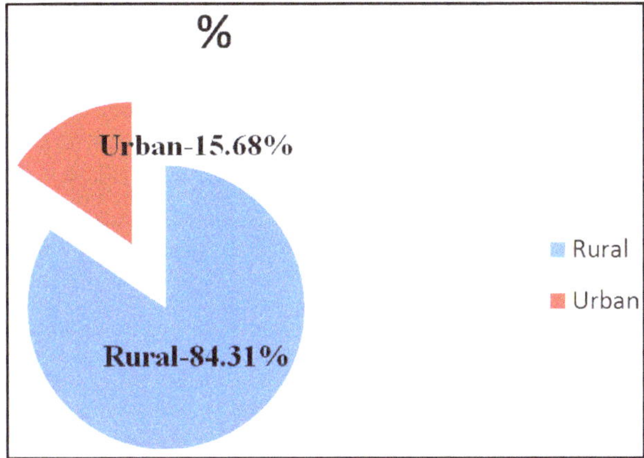

Table 4. Mode of injury of the cut throat patients.

Mode of injury	No.	%	Male	Female
Homicidal	26	50.98%	23	3
Suicidal	13	25.49%	11	2
RTA	7	13.72%	5	2
Bull gore injury	4	7.84%	4	0
Accidental fall	1	1.96%	1	0
Total	51	100%	44	7

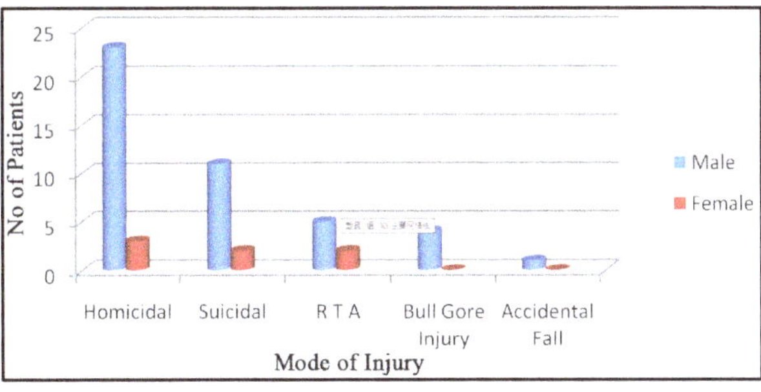

Table 5. Anatomical sites (zones) of injury of the patients.

Anatomical sites (zones)	No.	%
Zone I	5	9.80%
Zone II	32	62.74%
Zone III	14	27.45%
Total	51	100%

Table 6. Presentation of the cut throat patients.

Presentation	No.	%
Open wound & bleeding	19	37.25%
Respiratory distress	16	31.37%
Inadequate wound management	6	11.76%
Proper wound management	6	11.76%
Severe cut injury in shock	4	7.84%
Total	51	100%

Table 7. Injury of structures of the neck.

Injury of structures of the neck	No.	%
Skin, soft tissue & small vessels	51	100%
Laryngeal injury	12	23.52%
Hypopharynx	4	7.84%
Throid & thyroid vessels	8	15.68%
Trachea	1	1.96%
Carotid vessels	2	3.92%

Table 8. Time of delay in hospital arrival of patients.

Time of delay in hospital arrival	No.	%
<6 hrs	8	15.68%
6 - 12 hrs	28	54.90%
13 - 24 hrs	9	17.64%
>24 hrs	6	11.76%
Total	51	100%

Table 9. Treatment provided for cut throat patients.

Treatment provided for cut throat patients	No.	%
Simple wound closure	35	68.62%
Laryngeal repair	12	23.52%
Laryngeal & hypopharyngeal repair	16	31.37%
Tracheostomy	16	31.37%
Tracheal reconstruction	1	1.96%
Blood transfusion	5	9.80%
Psychiatric consultation	13	25.49%

Ryles tube was placed for hypopharyngeal repair. On an average hospital stay was less than three weeks.

4. Results and Analysis

A total 51 cases of cut throat injury were included in the study, in that males were 44 (84.3%), females were 7 (13.72%). and one male child (1.96%). Male to female ratio was 6.2:1. Age ranged from 4 years to 80 years (mean 25.2). Majority of the patients were young adults aged between 20 to 40 years. 43 (84.31%) cases were from rural community. The most common cause of cut throat in our study was homicide (50.98%), followed by suicidal (25.49%), road traffic accident (13.72%), bull gore injury (7.84%) and accidental fall (1.96%). According to the anatomical site, 32 (62.74%) cases had injury in Zone II, 14 (27.45%) cases in Zone III and 5 (9.80%) cases in Zone I. 16 (31.37%) cases had emergency tracheostomy.

Majority of the patients were referred to our hospital after primary resuscitation at other hospitals. The most common presentation was with open wound and bleeding & 19 (37.25%) cases presented with this finding. Cut throat injury with respiratory distress were 16 (31.37%) cases. Referred patients with inadequate wound management at primary center were 6 cases (11.76%). 6 patients (11.76%) were referred to our hospital with proper wound management and 4 cases (7.84%) were with severe cut injury in shock.

Skin, soft tissue and small vessels were severed in all the cases (100%). 12 cases (23.52%) had laryngeal injury. Pharynx was injured in 4 cases (7.84%). Thyroid and thyroid vessels were injured in 8 cases (15.68%). Trachea was cut in one case (1.96%). Carotid vessel injury observed in 2 cases (3.92%). Study was done to know the time required to reach our hospital. Majority patients arrived in 6 hrs to 12 hrs following injury.

Treatment provided at our hospital was analyzed. Simple wound closure was done in 35 (68.62%) cases. Laryngeal repair was done in 12 (23.52%) cases. Laryngeal and hypopharyngeal repair done in 16 (31.37%) cases. Tracheostomy was done in 16 (31.37%) cases. Tracheal reconstruction done in 1 (1.96%) case. Blood transfusion given for 5 (9.80%) cases. Psychiatric consultation obtained for 13 (25.49%) cases.

The hospital stay was on an average less than three weeks. Two patients died .The cause of death in one patient was hemorrhagic shock and second patient died on post operative day one due to cardiopulmonary arrest. Most common causes of morbidity were wound infection, change of voice, dysphagia, tracheal stenosis and permanent tracheostomy.

5. Discussion

Penetrating neck injury constitutes 5% to 10% of all the trauma cases. Amongst these, 30% patients have multiple injuries in other parts of the body. According to the world Health Organization (WHO), every year over 5 million people around the world die as a result of injury. As per WHO, it is estimated that for every death 10 - 20 gets hospitalized and 50 - 100 receives emergency care, indicating the burden on the resources of the country. Management of cut throat injury is a challenging task as the most important organs like larynx, trachea, pharynx, carotids and nerves are present in a small confined area. Cut throat injuries are less commonly reported in the literature.

In our study we included 51 cases of cut throat injury. Males to female ratio was (6.2:1). Cut throat injury was common in males, who came from rural area. Most of them were unemployed and of low education level. The age group ranged from 4 years to 80 years. Most of them were young between the age group 20 to 40 years. Our results were similar to other previous studies. Male preponderance in this age group is due to their active participation in risky behaviors and their frequent involvement in interpersonal conflicts. This has great economic setback since these are people who are the major bread winners for the family. Their most productive years are lost in the sufferings and the injuries impose a considerable burden on their families and the society as a whole.

The most common cause was found to be homicide followed by suicidal attempt, road traffic accidents, bull gore injury and accidental fall in our study. Males dominated both in homicidal and suicidal cut throat injury. Study conducted in the western population shows suicidal cut throat to be the most common cause, in contrast to our study. But in developing countries homicide is the most common cause for cut throat. Bull fight is common in this part of India. Winning over the bull, depicts matador's bravery. Bull horn injuries have not been regularly documented in the history. Wound depth is dependent on the force of penetration of the bull's horn into the matador's body. They are usually penetrating and contusive [6].

The majority of injuries in our study were in Zone II and most of them had laryngeal injury which is in keeping with other studies [3]. The predominance of Zone II injuries in our study is attributable to the fact that unlike Zones I and III, Zone II is not protected by bony structures making it more vulnerable to injuries. Injuries in this zone are the easiest to expose in cut throat injury. Iseh K.R. *et al.* suggested that pharyngeal, hypopharyngeal and laryngeal mucosal lacerations should ideally be repaired early (within 24 hours) [7]-[9].

Most of the patient reached the hospital within 6 to 12 hrs following injury. Outcome was better for the patients who received timely primary care and who managed to reach the hospital at the earliest. Patients who had laryngeal and pharyngeal injury had tracheostomy done for airway management. For most of them tracheostomy tube removal was done by 10 to 12 days. Psychiatric support was obtained in the patients who attempted suicide to prevent further such episodes.

6. Conclusions

Incidence of cut throat injuries and associated morbidities & mortalities are not uncommon in present day life. The aim and objective of our study is to analyze the socio demographic pattern, causes or motives of the cut throat and its outcomes. The socio demographic data, motives of trauma, structures injured, treatment given at our hospital, complications and mortalities were analyzed. In conclusion according to our study homicide is the commonest cause of cut throat injury, in this part of India. Unemployed young adults of low socioeconomic class are mostly affected.

According to the results of our study it is supposed that the early appropriate measures could save lives in vast majority. Addressing the root causes of violence such as poverty, illiteracy, unemployment and substance abuse will reduce the incidence of cut throat injuries in our society. Providing the efficient emergency health care services for primary care and effective ambulance system for immediate transport of cut throat victims to hospital will decrease time delay in reaching the hospital. Stringent and appropriate measures by the government agencies for enforcement of law and order will reduce the burden of homicidal cut throat in near future [10] [11].

References

[1] Fagan, J.J. and Nicol, A.J. (2008) Neck Trauma. In: Gleeson, M., Ed., *Scott-Brown's Otorhinolaryngology, Head and Neck Surgery*, 7th Edition, Great Britain, Hodder Arnold, 1768.

[2] Penden, M., McGee, K. and Sharma, G. (2002) The Injury Chart Book: A Graphical Overview of the Global Burden of Injuries. World Health Organization, Geneva.

[3] Bhattacharjee, N., Arefin, S.M., Mazumder, S.M. and Khan, M.K. (1997) Cut Throat Injury: Retrospective Study of 26 Cases. *Bangladesh Medical Research Council Bulletin*, **23**, 87-90.

[4] Ladapo, A.A. (1979) Open Injuries of the Anterior Neck. *Ghana Medical Journal*, **18**, 182-186.

[5] Rao, B.K., Singh, V.K., Ray, S. and Mehra, M. (2004) Airway Management in Trauma. *Indian Journal of Critical Care Medicine*, **8**, 98-105.

[6] Lloyd, M.S. (2004) Matador versus Taurus: Bull Gore Injury. *Annals of the Royal College of Surgeons of England*, **86**, 3-5. http://dx.doi.org/10.1308/003588404772614597

[7] Iseh, K.R. and Obembe, A. (2011) Anterior Neck Injuries Presenting as Cut Throat Emergencies in a Tertiary Health Institution in North Western Nigeria. *Nigerian Medical Journal*, **20**, 475-478.

[8] Onotai, L.O. and Ibekwe, U. (2010) The Pattern of Cut Throat Injuries in the University of Port-Harcourt Teaching Hospital, Portharcourt. *Nigerian Medical Journal*, **19**, 264-266.

[9] Kendall, J.L., Anglin, D. and Demetriades, D. (1998) Penetrating Neck Trauma. *Emergency Medicine Clinics of North America*, **16**, 85-105. http://dx.doi.org/10.1016/S0733-8627(05)70350-3

[10] Aich, M., Alam, K., Talukder, D.C., Sarder, R., Fakir, A.Y. and Hossain, M. (2011) Cut Throat Injury: Review of 67 Cases. *Bangladesh Journal of Otorhinolaryngology*, **17**, 5-13. http://dx.doi.org/10.3329/bjo.v17i1.7616

[11] Kundu, R.K., Adhikary, B. and Naskar, S. (2013) A Clinical Study of Management and Outcome of 60 Cut Throat Injuries.

5

Complete Fusion of the Maxillamandibular: Report of a Rare Case and Review of the Literature

Hakim Chabbak, Amine Rafik*, Abdessamad Chlihi

National Center for Burns and Plastic Surgery, Casablanca, Morocco
Email: *Aminerafik8@gmail.com

Abstract

The maxillomandibular fusion is a very rare condition, with no more than forty cases described in the literature. Adhesions of bone and/or soft tissue between the mandible and maxilla manifest themselves in the inability to open the mouth added to impacts on mandibular growth, nutrition and speech. This condition can be isolated or, when congenital, associated with other anomalies such as cleft lip and palate, aglossia, or Van der Woude syndrome. In the present paper, we report a case of maxillomandibular fusion treated in our department at University Hospital, between February 2011 and June 2014. The case is a congenital maxillomandibular fusion in a two-year-old infant, associated with a syndrome of Van der Woude. We discuss the diagnostic and treatment difficulties on the anaesthetic and surgical levels and the action to be taken to avoid recurrence. To date, some classifications have been suggested in the literature, but there is no standard treatment protocol. Early treatment is necessary to allow freedom of the upper airway, and ensure proper nutrition and good growth of facial bones. The success of surgery is conditioned by an adequate physiotherapy follow-up likely to guarantee the non-recurrence of the lesion.

Keywords

Congenital Fusion, Maxillomandibular, Syngnathia

1. Introduction

The maxillomandibular fusion is a condition characterized by the presence of adhesions of osseous tissue and/or soft tissue between the mandible and maxilla. This condition may be congenital or acquired, isolated or asso-

*Corresponding author.

ciated with other abnormalities (temporomandibular ankylosis of the mandibular joint, cleft lip and palate, Van der Woude syndrome, etc.) [1]. Through this clinical case, we report diagnostic modalities of this rare disease, treatment difficulties (surgical and anaesthetic) and the action to be taken aiming at reducing the incidence of recurrence.

2. Case Report

E. Meriem is a 2-year-old infant admitted to the Plastic Surgery Service in university Hospital for a cleft lip and palate (CLP). The girl is an only child and there are no similar cases in the family. At the age of 7 months, she was hospitalized in another hospital to remedy the CLP but the occurrence of cardiac arrest at the anaesthetic induction, due to the impossibility of intubation, has discouraged the pursuance of the intervention.

At admission, clinical examination reveals a significant limitation of mouth opening with a 0.5-cm mandible, a CLP with fistulas of the lower lip including a Van der Woude syndrome. An X-ray CT highlighted the CLP but has provided no explanation for the limited opening of the mouth. The decision was made to remedy the cleft lip and perform an intraoral examination under anaesthesia. Indeed, it revealed the presence of bilateral maxillomandibular gingival adhesions explaining the mouth opening limitation. A section of these adhesions exposed a 2-cm mandible, which was maintained by the immediate postoperative establishment of a callus. Currently, 4 years later, the initial result was maintained through a regular physiotherapy follow-up (**Figure 1**).

3. Discussion

The maxillomandibular fusion is an extremely rare condition. A review of the literature is difficult because of the variety of classifications: "Congenital fusion of jaws", "Temporo Mandibular Joints Pseudoankylosis and even agnathia"... In 1936, Burket [2] reported the first case of "maxillomandibularsyngnathia" in a patient who also manifested a Temporo Mandibular Joints (TMJ) Pseudoankylosis, a gum fusion and a hemi-facial atrophy.

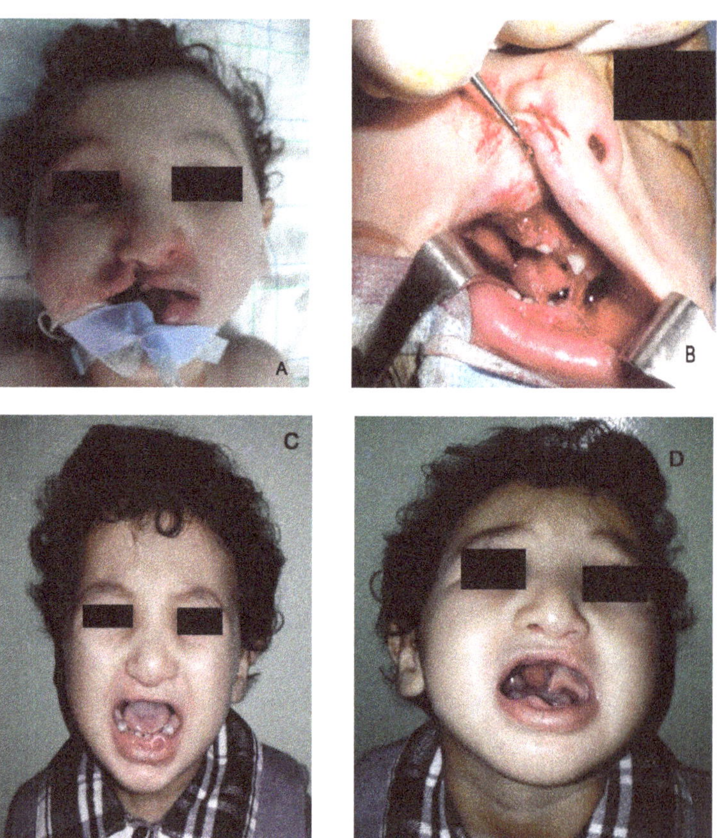

Figure 1. A and B: A 2-year-old child with a cleft palate and the maxillo-mandibular fusion; C and D: The result after 24 months.

In 2001, Laster *et al.* [3] stated 24 cases described in the literature. Hegab reported the last cases in 2012 [4]. Hence, forty reported cases.

The causes of congenital syngnathia are not well defined. Some have suggested a persistent oropharyngeal membrane, a constriction by amniotic bands in the area of the development of the first gill arch, violence, and the use of drugs such as high doses of vitamin A during pregnancy [5]. The diagnosis is made when the affected newborns develop respiratory difficulties, then nutrition difficulties, and it is the mouth opening limitation, which is the telltale sign. X-ray or CT can confirm the diagnosis when the fusion affects the bone. An MRI may be indicated when the fusion affects soft tissues. CT imaging gives more information and detects any skeletal dysmorphia [4] [5].

It is difficult to standardize the treatment because the disease is rare, and it is often part of a malformation syndrome [6]-[8]. In all cases, early treatment is essential. A long-term immobilisation would lead to the risk of ankylosis of Temporo Mandibular Joints, making a surgical treatment more complicated [9]. Early surgical release of adhesions is recommended to ensure a normal diet, prevent obstruction of the upper airway, allow normal mandibular function and ensure proper growth [9]. Early intervention is also important to reduce the risk of ankylosis of the ascending rami of mandible to the maxilla and zygomatic complex.

General anesthesia is often difficult. As in the first case where the infant presented problems during the induction that may be probably related to oesophageal intubation. Fiber optic laryngoscopes are required for endotracheal intubation, with careful handling because of the fragility of the mandibular bone with the risk of fracture [10]. Recurrence is a matter of course, along with the need for more interventions. Early, intense and regular physiotherapy follow up reduces this risk. However, it is difficult to establish especially in young patients.

4. Conclusions

The maxillomandibular fusion is a rare condition; however, the diagnosis must be carried out after the observation of respiration and nutrition difficulties in newborns, or a mouth opening limitation at an older age. CT or MRI then confirms the diagnosis.

Surgery and anesthesia are subtle and require a knowledgeable team. Early treatment is essential to limit the risk of ankylosis, and early intense and regular physiotherapy treatment reduces the risk of recurrence.

Conflict of Interest

No conflict.

References

[1] Daniels, J.S. (2004) Congenital Maxillomandibular Fusion: A Case Report and Review of the Literature. *Journal of Cranio-Maxillofacial Surgery*, **32**, 135-139. http://dx.doi.org/10.1016/j.jcms.2004.01.005

[2] Burket, L. (1936) Congenital Bony Ankylosis and Facial Hemiatrophy. *The Journal of the American Medical Association*, **106**,1719-1722.

[3] Laster, Z., Temkin, D., Zarfin, Y. and Kushnir, A. (2001) Complete Bony Fusion of the Mandible to the Zygomatic Complex and Maxillary Tuberosity: Case Report and Review. *International Journal of Oral and Maxillofacial Surgery*, **30**, 75-79. http://dx.doi.org/10.1054/ijom.2000.0009

[4] Hegab, A., ElMadawy, A. and Shawkat, W.M. (2012) Congenital Maxillomandibular Fusion: A Report of Three Cases. *International Journal of Oral and Maxillofacial Surgery*, **41**, 1248-1252. http://dx.doi.org/10.1016/j.ijom.2012.05.004

[5] Dawson, K.H., Gruss, J.S. and Myall, R.W. (1997) Congenital Bony Syngnathia: A Proposed Classification. *The Cleft Palate-Craniofacial Journal*, **34**, 141-146. http://dx.doi.org/10.1597/1545-1569(1997)034<0141:CBSAPC>2.3.CO;2

[6] Miskinyar, S.A. (1979) Congenital Mandibulo-Maxillary Fusion. *Plastic and Reconstructive Surgery*, **63**, 120-121. http://dx.doi.org/10.1097/00006534-197901000-00029

[7] Nwoku, A.L. and Kekere-Ekun, T.A. (1986) Congenital Ankylosis of the Mandible: Report of a Case Noted at Birth. *Journal of Maxillofacial Surgery*, **14**, 150-152. http://dx.doi.org/10.1016/S0301-0503(86)80281-8

[8] Rao, S., Oak, S., Wagh, M. and Kulkarni, B. (1997) Congenital Midline Palatomandibular Bony Fusion with a Mandibular Cleft and a Bifid Tongue. *British Journal of Plastic Surgery*, **50**, 139-141. http://dx.doi.org/10.1016/S0007-1226(97)91328-X

[9] Mortazavi, S.H. and Motamedi, M.H. (2007) Congenital Fusion of the Jaws. *Indian Journal of Pediatrics*, **74**, 416-418.

[10] Bozdag, S., Erdeve, O., Konas, E., Tuncbilek, G. and Dilmen, U. (2011) Management of Serious Isolated Gingival Synechia in a Newborn: Case Report and Review of the Literature. *International Journal of Oral and Maxillofacial Surgery*, **40**, 1428-1431. http://dx.doi.org/10.1016/j.ijom.2011.05.003

6

Large Foreign Body in the Nasal Cavity, Maxillary Sinus and Infratemporal Fossa—Atypical Presentation

Subrat Kumar Behera[1], Niranjan Mishra[2], Sharath Govindappa[1]

[1]Department of ENT, S.C.B. Medical College, Cuttack, India
[2]Department of OMFS, S.C.B. Medical College, Cuttack, India
Email: sharathg2006@gmail.com

Abstract

A 59-year-old male presented with complaints of trismus and discharge of altered blood from nose for 1 year. Patient had a history of facial trauma one year back. Nasal endoscopy and CT scan revealed a foreign body lodged in posterior half of both nasal cavity, left maxillary sinus and left infratemporal fossa penetrating the walls of maxillary sinus and nasal septum. Foreign body was removed by infratemporal fossa approach. This case has a rare location of a forgotten foreign body with atypical presentation.

Keywords

Foreign Body, Nose and Paranasal Sinuses, Infratemporal Fossa, Trismus

1. Introduction

In day-to-day practice, patients frequently present with lodgment of foreign bodies in the nasal cavities. Foreign bodies in the paranasal sinuses (PNS) are not common. Sharma *et al.* [1] reported a case of wooden foreign body in the periorbita of right eye, extending into the right sphenoid and ethmoidal sinuses. Mathews *et al.* [2] reported the base of a wristwatch in the left maxillary sinus and pterygopalatine fossa. Dutta *et al.* [3] reported a splinter (part of a bullet) in the right maxillary sinus. In this case, the patient had a 8 cm wooden foreign body lodged in posterior half of both nasal cavities, left maxillary sinus and left infra temporal fossa having to pierce the walls of maxillary sinus and nasal septum. The reason behind reporting this case is rarity of foreign body location and its atypical presentation.

2. Case Report

A 59-year-old male presented with complaints of trismus since 1 year and altered blood discharge from both nostrils also from 1 year (**Figure 1**). Patient had history of fall from tree and a penetrating injury to the left temporal area, which was sutured and the patient had speedy recovery.

On general physical examination, the patient was apparently healthy. The medical history was not significant and routine haematological investigations were within normal limits. A clinical intraoral examination revealed decreased mouth opening with normal healthy oral mucosa. On examination of nose, anterior rhinoscopy was normal. Nasal endoscopy revealed a blackish brown foreign body in posterior half of both nasal cavities (**Figure 2**).

Patient underwent CT scan (**Figure 3**, **Figure 4**) it revealed a non-metallic foreign body in the posterior part of nasal cavity, left maxillary sinus and left infratemporal fossa, piercing the walls of maxillary sinus nasal septum abutting near the posterior end of inferior turbinates.

Under general anaesthesia the foreign body was removed by infratemporal fossa approach. Using Al-Kayat Bramley's incision and zygomatic arch osteotomy foreign body was accessed and removed in single piece (**Figure 5**, **Figure 6**). Postoperative intravenous antibiotics and anti-inflamatory drugs were given.

Patient recovered well with 4 finger mouth opening at 2 weeks.

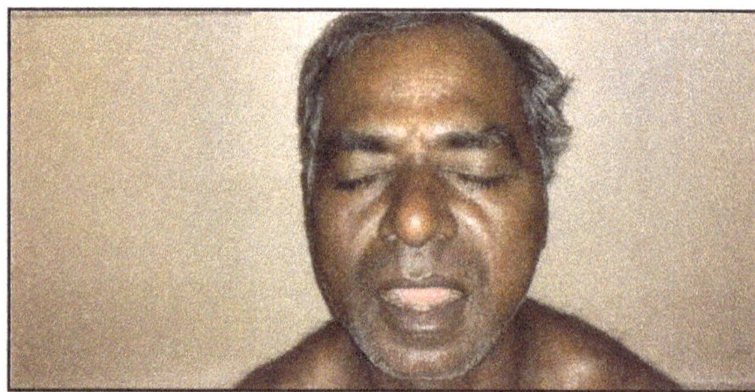

Figure 1. Trismus.

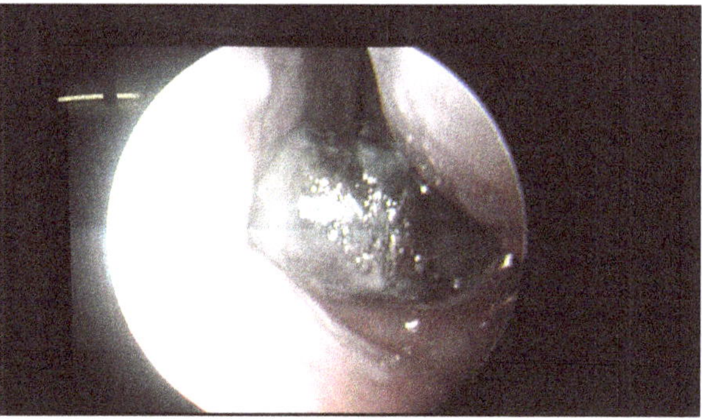

Figure 2. Nasal endoscopy showing foreign body.

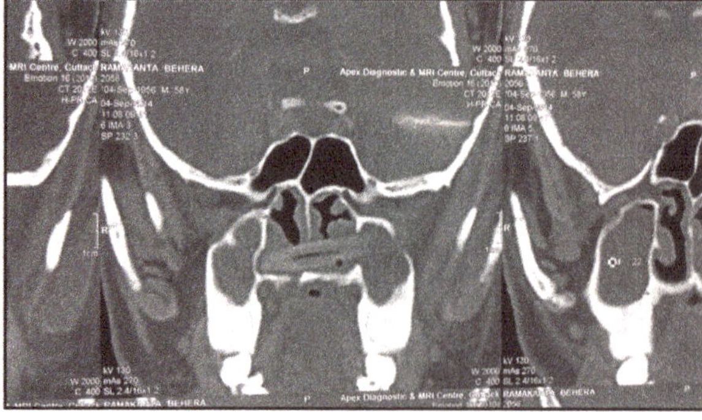

Figure 3. CT scan showing foreign body in nasal cavity.

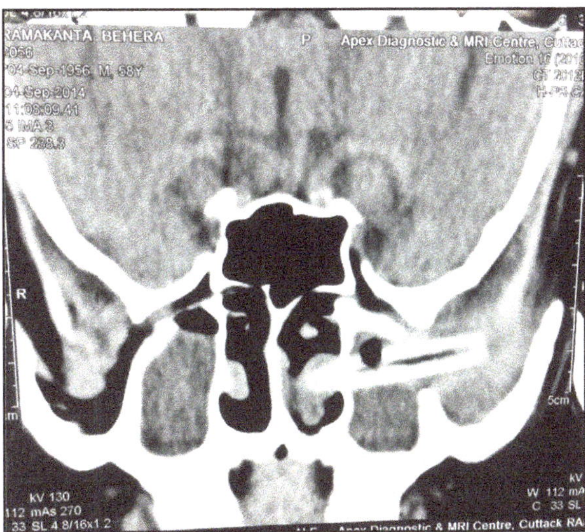

Figure 4. CT scan showing foreign body in maxillary sinus and infratemporal fossa.

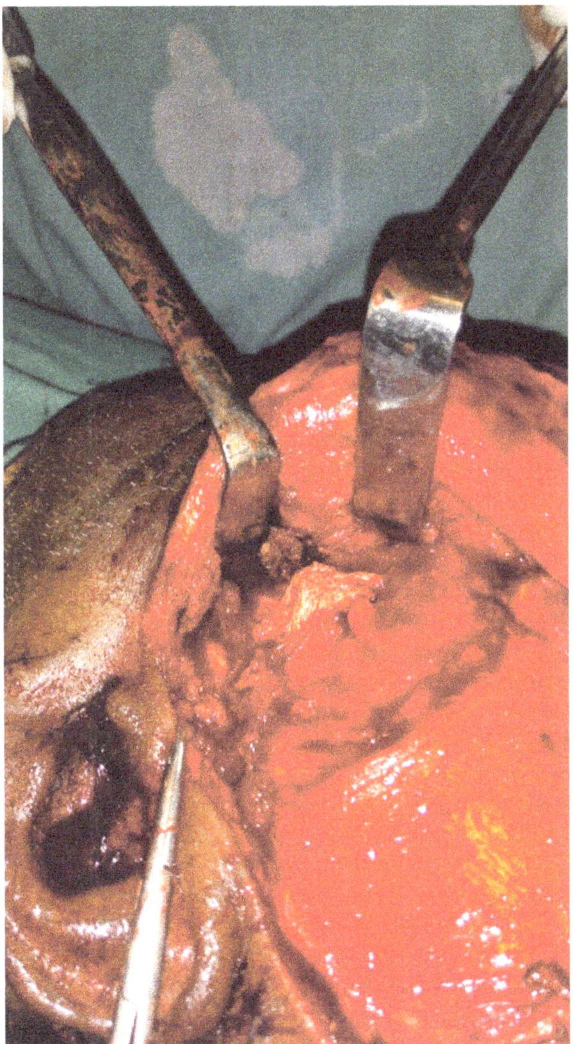

Figure 5. Intra operative picture of foreign body.

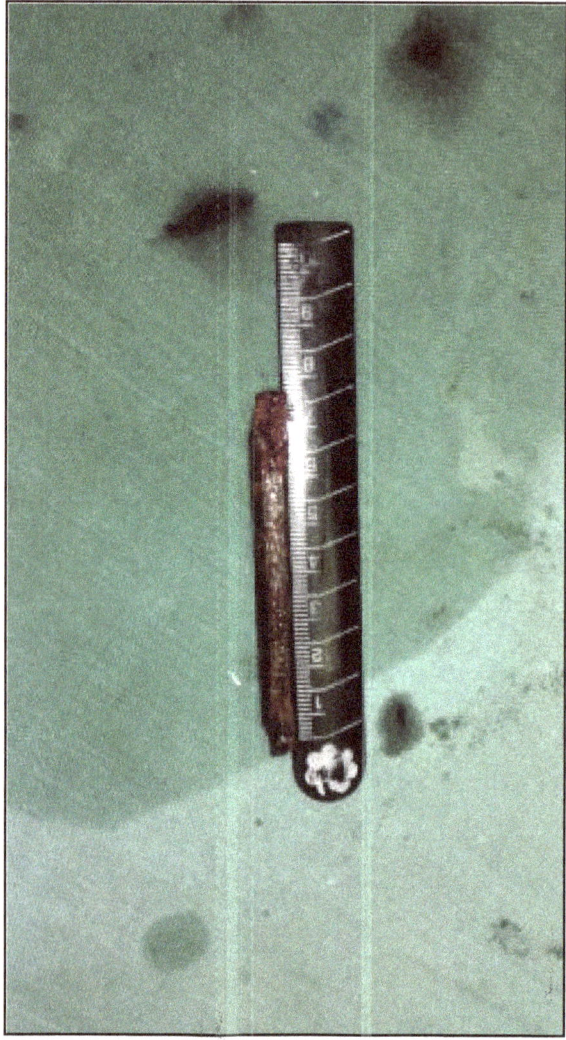

Figure 6. 8 cm foreign body removed in single piece.

3. Discussion

Foreign bodies in the PNS are not common. They are usually traumatic and in some cases iatrogenic. In most of the case reports pertaining to the foreign body infratemporal fossa the foreign body had found its way into the region following trauma and the main clinical symptom being trismus [4] [5]. Keeping in view the other important organs like eye and brain in the immediate vicinity of the space and its potential communicating portals with these organs via the anatomical foraminas, the foreign body in such a location with its potential to cause inflammatory reaction and tendency to migrate is always a potential threat for causing serious complications like proptosis with threat to vision and various intracranial complication [6]. Here we have a foreign body lodged in nasal cavity left maxillary sinus and left infratemporal fossa.

Foreign bodies in the PNS include splinters [1], gun pellets, woods [7], etc. Radio-opaque foreign bodies can easily be detected by X-ray of PNS anteroposterior and lateral views. X-ray of PNS anteroposterior view is better than occipeto-mental view as it helps better in assessing the actual position of the foreign bodies. CT scan and magnetic resonance imaging (MRI) may be necessary in some cases especially radio opaque foreign bodies.

Foreign bodies in the nose and PNS should be removed as early as possible. A retained foreign body can lead to sinusitis, cutaneous fistula and foreign body granuloma formation.

Caldwell-Luc approach is the usual procedure for removal of foreign bodies from maxillary sinuses. Endoscopic approach has the advantage of better visualization and illumination. In this case the foreign body was big measuring 8cm impacted in the nasal cavity maxillary sinus and infra temporal fossa. In order to remove the foreign body in one piece and prevent detainment of parts of foreign body an infratemporal fossa approach was used, which was also the route of entry of the foreign body.

4. Conclusion

A variety of foreign bodies ranging from wooden objects to bullets can be found in the nose and PNS. They can vary in size, shape, and location. Sometimes they can be found accidentally. Foreign bodies should be considered in the differential diagnosis of trismus, especially in patients with recent past history of trauma in the region and the possibility of missing some parts of foreign body during the initial emergency salvage procedures for such cases of trauma. The route and method of removal is decided based on the size, shape, and location of the foreign body. Use of nasal endoscopes can be very helpful for this purpose.

References

[1] Sharma, R., Minhass, R. and Mohindroo, M. (2008) An Unusual Foreign Body in the Paranasal Sinuses. *Indian Journal of Otolaryngology and Head Neck Surgery*, **60**, 88-90. http://dx.doi.org/10.1007/s12070-008-0028-7

[2] Mathews, A., Nair, A., Tandon, S. and D'Souza, O. (2010) Penetrating Foreign Body in the Maxillary Sinus and Pterygopalatine Fossa: Report of a Rare Case. *Internet Journal of Head & Neck Surgery*, **4**, 9.

[3] Dutta, A., Awasthi, S.K. and Kaul, A. (2006) A Bullet in the Maxillary Sinus. *Indian Journal of Otolaryngology and Head Neck Surgery*, **58**, 307-309.

[4] Purohit, J.P., Kumar, G., Singh, P.N. and Ganesh, K. (1996) An Unusual Foreign Body in Infratemporal Fossa. *Indian Journal of Otolaryngology and Head Neck Surgery*, **48**, 323-324.

[5] Thakur, J.S., Chauhan, C.G.S., Diwana, V.K. and Chauhan, D.C. (2007) Trismus: An Unusual Presentation Following Road Accident. *Indian Journal of Plastic Surgery*, **40**, 202-204. http://dx.doi.org/10.4103/0970-0358.37769

[6] Grant, C.A. and Rubin, P.A.D. (2000) An Infratemporal Fossa Foreign Body Presents as an Infraorbital Mass. *Archives of Ophthalmology*, **118**, 993-995.

[7] Lineback, M. (1955) Wooden Foreign Bodies in the Paranasalsinuses. *Laryngoscope*, **65**, 270-275. http://dx.doi.org/10.1288/00005537-195504000-00005

7

Chondroma of Tongue: A Rare Case Report & Review of Literature

Anoop Attakkil, Vandana Thorawade, Mohan Jagade, Rajesh Kar, Kartik Parelkar, Dnyaneswar Rohe, Poonam Khairnar, Reshma Hanowate

Department of ENT, Grant Medical College & Sir J.J. Hospital, Mumbai, India
Email: fasttrack2317@gmail.com

Abstract

Chondromas are common benign cartilaginous tumours in the skeletal system usually found in extremities. Extra skeletal chondromas are relatively uncommon of which those in head and neck regions are rarely documented. Although the tongue is one of the most common sites of oral soft tissue chondroma, lingual chondromas are rare as evidenced by the fact that only 33 cases are identified in the review of literature till now. This report has the objective of presenting a rare case of lingual enchondroma in a 26-year-old male which was excised with no evidence of recovery during follow up. We have also tried to present a concise review of the relevant literature.

Keywords

Soft Tissue Chondroma, Tongue

1. Introduction

Chondromas are benign lesions of hyaline cartilage. They are common, and all age groups are affected. Chondromas usually are asymptomatic and frequently discovered incidentally during an unrelated radiographic examination. They usually arise in the medullary canal, where they are referred to as "enchondromas". Rarely, they arise on the surface of the bone, where they are referred to as "periosteal chondromas" or "juxtacortical chondromas".

Chondromas of soft parts commonly occur in the upper and lower extremities, especially in relation to the small joints of the hand and feet [1]. Only two of Chung and Enzinger's series of 104 cases occurred in the head (1 case) and neck (1 case) [1]. Extraskeletal chondromas of the oral cavity are very rare with only 46 cases identified in review of the literature in 2011 [2]. They are found primarily in the tongue, tonsils or beneath ill-fitting dentures and only infrequently in the buccal mucosa and soft palate [1]. These tumours usually present as no symptomatic, slow-growing, and well-defined nodules, affecting both sexes equally.

Though tongue is mentioned as the common site, a case of chondroma of tongue gains significance when we consider the fact that only 33 cases are reported in world literature [2]. In this paper we report a case of soft tissue chondroma arising from tongue and present a review of the literature.

2. Case Report

A 26-year-old policeman presented with complaints of mass over posterior part of tongue noticed since 15 years which was insidious in onset and gradually progressive. It was not associated with pain, dysphagia or odynophagia. The patient had no history of any significant medical or surgical illnesses in the past. He gave no history of addictions. Oral cavity examination revealed a smooth surfaced, pedunculated, swelling of size 2 × 1 × 1 cm slightly lateral to midline on the ventral surface, arising from junction of anterior two third & posterior one third of the tongue. It was non tender, hard in consistency, non pulsatile with dilated blood vessels seen over the same (**Figure 1**).

On MRI of tongue, one well defined exophytic polypoidal mass lesion measuring 2.2 × 1.6 × 1.3 cm was seen arising from the tongue at the junction of anterior two third & posterior one third. It showed hyperintense with hypointense foci on stir and heterogenous on t1w and t2w images. There was no post contrast enhancement noticed. No deep extension or involvement of extrinsic or intrinsic muscles was present (**Figure 2**).

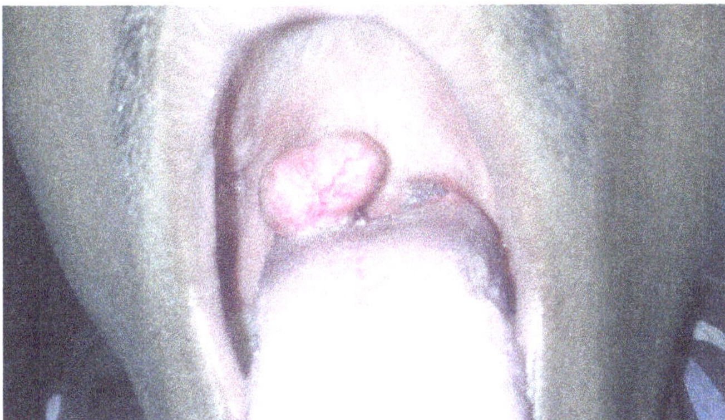

Figure 1. Chondroma on the tongue lying just lateral to midline.

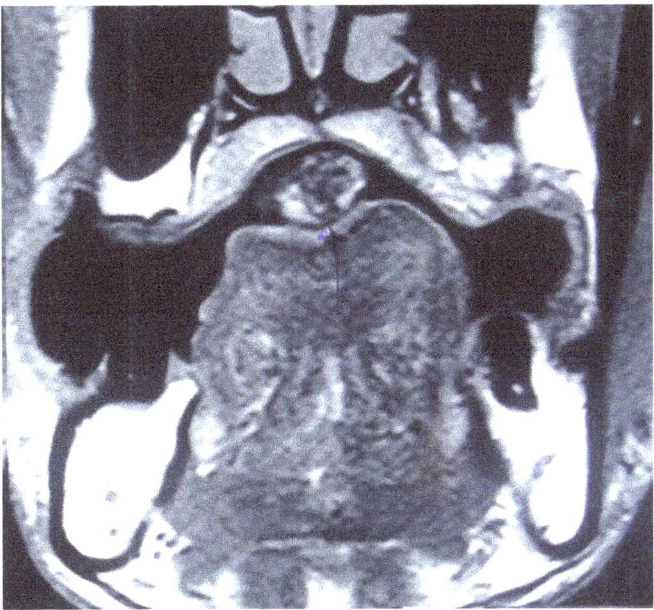

Figure 2. MRI of tongue showing the pedunculated lesion over tongue.

Under general anaesthesia, wide local excision of the tumour along with tongue tissue keeping 1 cm margin was done. Haemostasis was achieved with bipolar cauterisation and the specimen was sent for histopathological examination (**Figure 3**).

Histopathological examination showed the tumour was multinodular and greyish with slightly well-defined edges. Microscopic examination revealed, multiple nodules composed of spindle cells surrounded by inflammatory round cells and fibrosis. Some showed cartilaginous formation by chondrocytes confirming the diagnosis of chondroma (**Figure 4**).

Postoperative period was uneventful. Patient was followed up for 1 year with no evidence of recurrence.

3. Discussion

Tumours of the oral cavity and oropharynx may be either epithelial, mesenchymal, or haematolymphoid of which soft tissue chondromas are very rare. Soft tissue chondromas are usually diagnosed within the extremities, the fingers being frequently affected [3] [4]. Other sites reported include the dura, larynx, skin, and fallopian tube [3] [5]-[8].

Soft tissue chondromas of the oral cavity are rare; only 46 cases have been reported in the English literature [2]. The tongue was the most common site (33 of 46), followed by buccal mucosa (4 of 46), hard palate (4 of

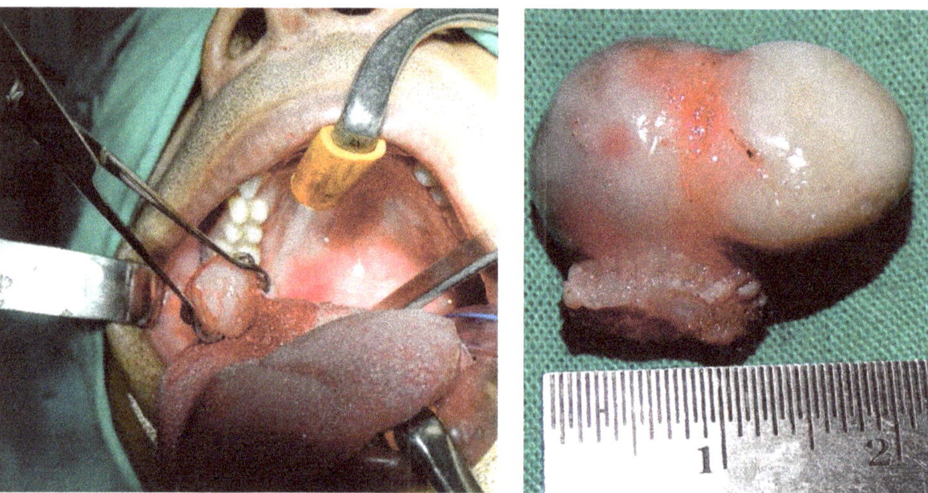

Figure 3. Intraoperative and post operative photographs showing the excision of 2 × 1 × 1 cm mass.

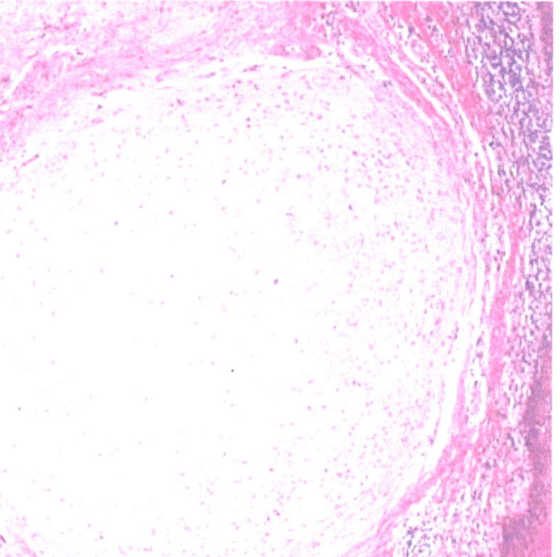

Figure 4. Microscopic appearance of the tumor (hematoxylin & eosin stain, 50× magnification).

46), gingiva (3 of 46), soft palate (1 of 46), and lip (1 of 46) [2]. Usually common in the middle age population with a slight higher incidence in females [2]. There are varied school of thoughts regarding the origin of chondromas in oral cavity. The "embryonic remnants theory" suggests that heterotopic cartilage remnants from the branchial arches get displaced during the development and get sequestered in the tongue [9] [10] which explains the increased incidence of the same in the tongue.

The "metaplastic theory" explains the lesions located on the lateral border, ventral surface or tip of the tongue, especially in an older age group more attractively. It suggests the factors like trauma, chronic irritation can stimulate metaplasia and subsequent development of tumours [11]-[15].

The high incidence of the recently described ectomesenchymal chondromyxoid tumours at the tongue may be explained by a possible pathogenetic mechanism involving the paraphysiologic cartilaginous tissue of the lingual septum (so-called "knorpelinsel") [16]. This theory may be used to explain the chondrosarcomas of the tongue also [17].

The origin of cartilage in our case is more in support of embryonic theory when we consider the presence of swelling from childhood and the site of tumour on the ventral surface of the tongue lateral to midline. Further there is no history of trauma or use of dentures in this case.

STCs are composed of lobules of mature, adult hyaline cartilage, with chondrocytic cells often growing in clusters [3] with a less incidence of calcification in the centre. Differential diagnosis include pleomorphic adenoma, tumours with primary cartilaginous differentiation (e.g., ectomesenchymal chondromyxoid tumour; extra skeletal myxoid and mesenchymal chondrosarcoma) or as a secondary metaplastic process (e.g., malignant nerve sheath tumours, oral malignant melanoma) [3] [16] [18]. Diagnosis is only confirmed after histopathological evaluation.

These tumours are usually benign with very low recurrence rate [3]. As evidenced in the literature, our patient underwent surgical excision and is on follow up with no evidence o recurrence.

4. Conclusion

To conclude, our case report presents one of the rare tumours of the tongue reported ever in the literature with a literature review and emphasizes on the proper histopathological evaluation of the tumours in head and neck region despite the benign nature.

References

[1] Barnes, L. (2000) Surgical Pathology of the Head and Neck. 2nd Edition, Vol. 2, CRC Press, Boca Raton, 953.

[2] Kawanoa, T., Yanamotoa, S., Kawasakia, G., Mizunoa, A., Fujita, S. and Ikedab, T. (2011) Soft Tissue Chondroma of the Hard Palate: A Case Report. *Asian Journal of Oral and Maxillofacial Surgery*, **23**, 92-95. http://dx.doi.org/10.1016/j.ajoms.2011.01.002

[3] Nayler, S. and Heim, S. (2002) Soft Tissue Condroma. Tumors of Soft Tissue and Bone. In: Fletcher, D.M., Unni, K.K. and Mertens, F., Eds., *WHO Classification of Tumours* (*Chondro-Osseous Tumours*), WHO, Lyon, 180-181.

[4] Dahlin, D.C. and Salvador, A.H. (1974) Cartilaginous Tumors of the Soft Tissues of the Hands and Feet. *Mayo Clinic Proceedings*, **49**, 721-726.

[5] Brownlee, R.D., Sevick, R.J., Rewcastle, N.B. and Tranmer, B.I. (1997) Radiologic-Pathologic Correlation. Intracranial Chondroma. *The American Journal of Neuroradiology*, **18**, 889-893.

[6] Devaney, K.O., Ferlito, A. and Silver, C.E. (1995) Cartilaginous Tumors of the Larynx. *Annals of Otology, Rhinology and Laryngology*, **104**, 251-255. http://dx.doi.org/10.1177/000348949510400313

[7] Ando, K., Goto, Y., Hirabayashi, N., Matsumoto, Y. and Ohashi, M. (1995) Cutaneous Cartilaginous Tumor. *Dermatologic Surgery*, **21**, 339-341. http://dx.doi.org/10.1111/j.1524-4725.1995.tb00186.x

[8] Han, J.Y., Han, H.S., Kim, Y.B., Kim, J.M. and Chu, Y.C. (2002) Extraskeletal Chondroma of the Fallopian Tube. *Journal of Korean Medical Science*, **17**, 276-278. http://dx.doi.org/10.3346/jkms.2002.17.2.276

[9] Weitzner, S., Stimson, P.G. and McClendon, J.L. (1987) Cartilaginous Choristoma of the Tongue. *Journal of Oral and Maxillofacial Surgery*, **45**, 185-187. http://dx.doi.org/10.1016/0278-2391(87)90412-5

[10] Moore, K., Worthington, P. and Campbell, R.L. (1990) Firm Mass of the Tongue. *Journal of Oral and Maxillofacial Surgery*, **48**, 1206-1210. http://dx.doi.org/10.1016/0278-2391(90)90539-E

[11] Toida, M., Sugiyama, T. and Kato, Y. (2003) Cartilaginous Choristoma of the Tongue. *Journal of Oral and Maxillofacial Surgery*, **61**, 393-396. http://dx.doi.org/10.1053/joms.2003.50065

[12] Cutright, D.E. (1972) Osseous and Chondromatous Metaplasia Caused by Dentures. *Oral Surgery, Oral Medicine, Oral Pathology and Oral Radiology*, **34**, 625-633. http://dx.doi.org/10.1016/0030-4220(72)90346-5

[13] Magnusson, B.C., Engstrom, H. and Kahnberg, K.E. (1986) Metaplastic Formation of Bone and Chondroid in Flabby Ridges. *British Journal of Oral and Maxillofacial Surgery*, **24**, 300-305. http://dx.doi.org/10.1016/0266-4356(86)90097-5

[14] Takeda, Y. (1987) Cartilaginous Metapalasia of the Human Aponeurosis Linguae: Histologic and Ultrasutructural Study. *Journal of Oral Medicine*, **42**, 35-37.

[15] Lloyd, S., Lloyd, J. and Dhillon, R. (2001) Chondroid Metaplasia in a Fibroepithelial Polyp of the Tongue. *Journal of Laryngology & Otology*, **115**, 681-682. http://dx.doi.org/10.1258/0022215011908630

[16] de Visscher, J.G.A.M., Kibbelaar, R.E. and van der Waal, I. (2003) Ectomesenchymal Chondromyxoid Tumor of the Anterior Tongue. Report of Two Cases. *Oral Oncology*, **39**, 83-86. http://dx.doi.org/10.1016/S1368-8375(01)00117-8

[17] Roy, J.J., Klein, H.Z. and Tipton, D.L. (1970) Osteochondroma of the Tongue. *Archives of Pathology*, **89**, 565-568.

[18] Rosemberg, A.E. and Heim, S. (2002) Extraskeletal Osteosarcoma. Tumors of Soft Tissue and Bone. In: Fletcher, D.M., Unni, K.K. and Mertens, F., Eds., *WHO Classification of Tumors* (*Chondro-Osseous Tumours*), WHO, Lyon, 182-183.

8

Linear Stapler in Total Laryngectomy

Carolina Durao[1], Sofia Decq Motta[1], Ana Hebe[2], Ricardo Pacheco[2], Pedro Montalvão[2], Miguel Magalhães[2]

[1]Otolaryngology Department, Hospital Prof. Doutor Fernando Fonseca, Amadora, Portugal
[2]Otolaryngology Department, Portuguese Oncology Institute of Lisbon, Francisco Gentil, Portugal
Email: carolinapinheirodurao@gmail.com

Abstract

Introduction: Stapler application for pharyngeal closure after total laryngectomy allows rapid watertight closure. We intend to report the experience of the Portuguese Oncology Institute of Lisbon, Francisco Gentil (IPOLFG). Material and Methods: Retrospective study of patients submitted to total laryngectomy using linear stapler device treated in IPOLFG from 2005 to 2010. Results: 108 patients were studied. The majority of patients were male, aged from 60 to 69 years old, and had smoking and alcohol habits. The average length of hospital stay was 13.1 days. Post-operative complications occurred as follows: wound infection in 6.5%, cervical hematoma in 4.6% and pharyngocutaneous fistula in 11.1% of cases. Conclusions: The mechanical suture of the pharynx in total laryngectomy is a simple and quick method. It does not increase the incidence of post-operative complications. It seems to be a very safe method, as long as its limits regarding the location and extent of tumour are respected.

Keywords

Pharyngeal Closure, Total Laryngectomy, Linear Stapler

1. Introduction

Since the first total laryngectomy performed in 1873 by Theodor Billroth [1] there has been great progress. Nowadays some controversies still exist, namely, regarding the ideal method for closure of the pharyngeal defect created after total laryngectomy.

The requirements for pharyngoesophageal closure are absence of tension on wound edges and the possibility to preserve of viability of the mucosa, in order to create a waterproof barrier that contains pharyngeal secretions [2]. Closure of the pharynx is one of the most important surgical steps and requires special attention from the surgeon. The efficacy of this closure influences postoperative recovery and may be determinant in the occurrence of post-operative complications, particularly pharyngocutaneous fistula.

Originally, hand suture closure of the pharynx was the only method available. But in recent decades, the closure of the pharynx with linear stapler during total laryngectomy has been popularized.

In the Portuguese Oncology Institute of Lisbon, Francisco Gentil (IPOLFG) the use of linear stapler for pharynx closure is performed with closed technique and exclusively on endolaryngeal tumours. We believe that this technique, if applied to such cases, allows a safe oncologic surgery. It should not be applied to larynx tumours where it is not possible to guarantee adequate tumour-free surgical margins [2]-[5].

When the resection of the larynx is performed as usual, it implies opening the pharynx and contaminating the surgical field with pharyngeal secretions. Alternatively, with linear stapler closed technique, the larynx is detached from the pharynx only when the closure of the pharynx is complete. This converts a surgery with a septic time into an aseptic intervention and might reduce postoperative complications [5].

Currently several authors advocate linear stapler closure numerous advantages comparing to the manual closure [2] [4]-[7].

It has been reported that hand suture closure is associated with an increase of operative time, and tissue necrosis [2] [6]. Necrosis is most likely induced by repeated manipulation of the mucosa by surgical instruments, or by the ischaemia induced by suture's wires. Conversely, the linear stapling machine allows a secure, haemostatic closure, with little tissue injury or inflammation [6].

Some even suggest that the linear stapler is associated with a lower rate of post-operative complications, namely pharyngocutaneous fistula, especially in previously irradiated patients or in those who undergo organ preservation protocols with chemotherapy associated with radiotherapy [4].

We also consider the fact that there is less variability among surgeons in pharyngeal closure with linear stapler than with manual closure [2]. Linear stapler allows that the pharynx closure depends more on local tissue factors, rather than on individual manual closure technique.

In order to clarify some of these aspects, the aim of this study is to report the experience of the Portuguese Oncology Institute of Lisbon, Francisco Gentil (IPOLFG) with the use of linear stapler for closure of the pharynx.

2. Material and Methods

We conducted a retrospective study of patients from IPOLFG, who, in the period from 2005 to 2012, underwent total laryngectomy for squamous cell carcinoma and closure of the pharynx with linear stapler. We included patients previously submitted to radiotherapy alone or combined with chemotherapy and patients with tracheotomy prior to surgery.

The population was characterized epidemiologically. Initial therapeutic approach and concomitant surgical procedures were characterized. Post-operative in-hospital stay, beginning of oral feeding and rate of surgical complications were evaluated.

The decision regarding the type of pharynx closure was made based on pre-operative endoscopy and computed tomography. In some cases it was complemented with suspension laryngoscopy under general anaesthesia and peri-operative exploration of the pharynx and tongue base. Mechanical suture was applied exclusively in endolaryngeal tumours with indication for total laryngectomy. Cases in which there was extralaryngeal tumour involvement, or when it was not possible to ensure adequate surgical margins were excluded.

Mechanical linear suture was applied with a stapling machine that enables application of two parallel rows of titanium staples. Firstly, the instrument approximates the edges of the tissue to suture. Then, when the trigger is activated, it fires staples. In theory, this double row of staples ensures the formation of an impermeable barrier between the neopharynx and the remaining cervical tissues. The model available at the IPOLFG is TX 60, which performs a linear suture of 60 mm long, with titanium staples.

IPOLFG uses linear stapler for pharynx closure with closed technique. Initially, the larynx is separated from its muscular and neurovascular attachments. After that, transection of the trachea is done, as well as the separation between the larynx and cervical oesophagus, keeping the pharynx closed. At this stage, in which resection of the larynx is imminent, the epiglottis is fixed in anterior position in order to avoid being included in the suture line. It is important to ensure that the entire tumour is completely contained in the piece to remove and that the surgical margins are adequate. After this, the linear stapling machine is applied longitudinally between the pharynx and the larynx and the closest to the thyroid cartilage, in order to preserve as much as possible of healthy pharyngeal mucosa (**Figure 1**). When all these steps are completed, the trigger of the linear stapler may be securely activated, thus, creating a double suture line. At this stage, the pharynx is separated from the larynx without contaminating the operating field with pharyngeal secretions (**Figure 2**). After this, the linear stapling

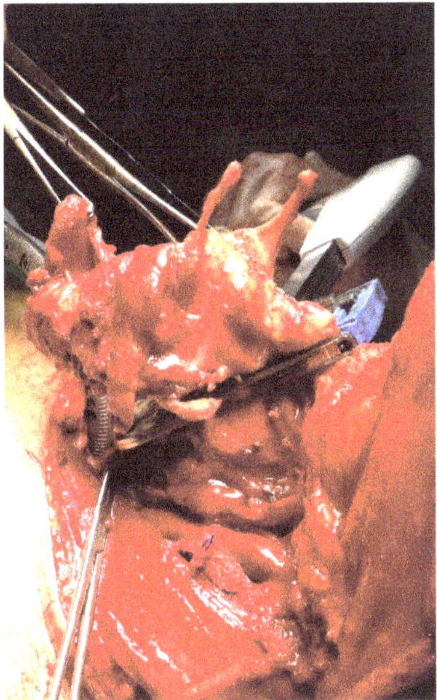

Figure 1. Linear stapler placed between larynx and the pharynx.

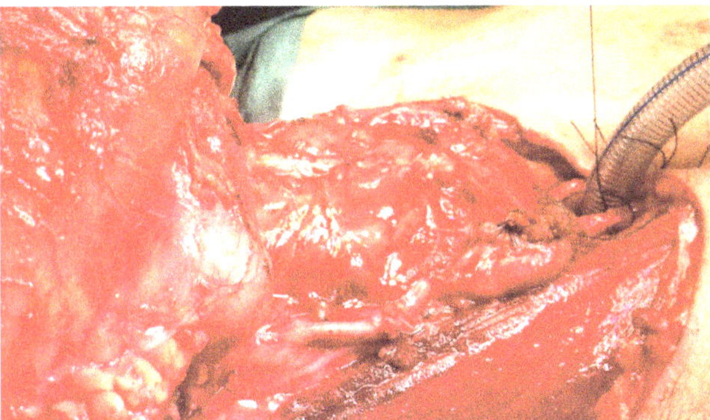

Figure 2. Mechanical suture of the pharynx.

machine is removed and the suture is inspected in order to confirm that it is securely watertight. The following steps are similar to those used in the conventional technique.

3. Results

A total of 474 total laryngectomies were performed from 2005 to 2010. Of these, 108 patients (22.6%) underwent closure of the pharynx with linear stapler. In the 108 patients, the predominant age group was 60 - 69 years old. There was male predominance (97.2%) and the majority had smoking habits (74%). Fifty (50%) had moderate to severe drinking habits. The most frequent presenting symptoms of laryngeal cancer were dyspnea and dysphonia. In 28.7% of cases, dyspnea led to emergency tracheotomy before surgery.

In our population, the initial treatment plan was surgery in 103 patients (95.4%). The remaining 4.6% were proposed to organ preservation protocol and, since they have not responded, salvage surgical treatment was performed. Of the 103 patients to whom surgery was proposed as initial treatment, 5 patients had radiotherapy and 1 patient had prior chemotherapy and radiotherapy for other tumours of the head and neck. In summary, surgery was carried out in 89.8% of cases without prior irradiation and with prior radiotherapy in 10.1% of cases.

Total laryngectomy with linear stapler was associated with bilateral neck dissection in 104 patients (96.3%). Voice prosthesis was applied in 10 patients (9.3%). Sporadically and whenever it was considered oncologically relevant, the emptying of the recurrential chain and/or a hemithyroidectomy was also performed. In one case, a myocutaneous flap of large pectoral was made.

Regarding the post-operative period, the average hospital stay was 13.1 days. Oral intake was started on average at the 12th post-operative day.

Five patients (4.6%) had post-operative cervical haematoma, twelve patients (11.1%) had salivary fistula and surgical wound infection occurred in 7 patients (6.5%). In one case there was a lymph fistula that motivated a revision surgery and ligation of the thoracic duct.

The vast majority of the salivary fistulae closed spontaneously (83.3%). The time for spontaneous closure ranged from 22 to 406 days. Of these 12 patients, only one patient had undergone radiotherapy prior to surgery.

Mean post-operative follow-up was 36.7 months (minimum 0.5 and maximum 87.9). In our series, 77.8% of patients were proposed for adjuvant radiotherapy, 5.5% received adjuvant chemoradiotherapy, and the remaining 16.7% did not carry out any adjuvant treatment. Most (90%) patients with voice prosthesis successfully performed speech rehabilitation. Sixteen patients reported dysphagia several months after surgery and radiotherapy. There was oesophageal stenosis requiring oesophageal dilatation in 87.5% of these cases. In 3 cases there was salivary fistula after surgery and radiotherapy.

Overall survival at 2 years was 80.9% and at 5 years was 50.4%.

4. Discussion

Demographic characteristics of our population are similar with the ones from the literature, confirming the predominance of cancer of the larynx in men between 50 and 70 years old with smoking and drinking habits. In 28.7% of the cases, dyspnea led to emergency tracheotomy before surgery. The surgery was performed in 89.8% of cases without prior irradiation.

The linear stapler technique employed at the Portuguese Oncology Institute of Lisbon, Francisco Gentil (IPOLFG) is very similar to the technique used in other centres. There are, however, some differences that will be listed. According to Bedrin *et al.* [2], the manual suture of pre-laryngeal muscles is unnecessary to reinforce the suture of the pharynx; the IPOLFG performs it routinely. Sofferman *et al.* [5] apply linear stapler with 2 shots from linear stapling machine, creating a double row of staples; in IPOLFG the suture is performed with only one shot. Altissimi *et al.* [7] perform traction of the epiglottis using endoscopy and a variant of the closed technique to ensure that the epiglottis is not trapped in the suture line, but in IPOLFG the retraction is made by palpation without direct visualization. Agrawal *et al.* [8] use a stapling machine of 90 mm long, on the other hand, in the IPOLFG we use one of 60 mm long. Despite these small differences in technique the percentage of surgical complications was similar to that of other centers.

Regarding the duration of surgery, all authors are unanimous in noting that the use of linear stapler appears to decrease the time of the intervention. Montoya *et al.* [6] sought to objectify this idea and compared the surgical time of total laryngectomy by manual suture with that of TL by linear stapler. It states a difference of 43 minutes between each technique. This may be beneficial for patients with high anaesthetic risk and may also reduce the costs.

The in-hospital stay and the start of oral feeding are conditioned by the existence of post-operative complications. In our series, the average hospital stay was 13.1 days and the average start of oral feeding was on the 12th post-operative day. Montoya *et al.* [6] state an average period of hospital stay of 13.5 days and Ortega of 12.4 days.

The occurrence of complications, especially of pharyngocutaneous fistula, depends on several factors, including the suture method used in closure of the pharynx. In our series, there was wound infection in 6.5% of cases, cervical haematoma in 4.6% of cases and pharyngocutaneous fistula in 11.1% of cases. It should be noted that voice prosthesis were not applied in any of these, and that only one patient had undergone radiotherapy prior to surgery. The percentage of patients with pharyngocutaneous fistula was similar to other centres. Ahumada *et al.* [9] studied 36 patients of whom 8.7% developed pharyngocutaneous fistula and Altissimi *et al.* [7] report a rate of 4.2% in a total of 70 patients with closure of the pharynx by linear stapler.

There are studies comparing the occurrence of pharyngocutaneous fistula between patients with closure of the pharynx by linear stapler and patients with closure of the pharynx by manual suture. They all report a lower percentage in the group subject to linear stapler with closed technique. Gonçalves *et al.* [4] report the occurrence of fistula in 36.7% of cases of manual suture and in 6.7% of cases of linear stapler. Montoya *et al.* [6] describe 27% of cases with pharyngocutaneous fistula in the group of manual sutures and 5% of cases in the group of linear stapler. In the future, it would be interesting to perform a similar comparison with patients of IPOLFG to ascertain whether there is a reduction of complications.

Finally, it is noted that the majority (90%) of patients in which voice prosthesis was placed conducted speech rehabilitation successfully and that the cases of dysphagia in our series occurred only after radiotherapy. It seems that this method of closure of the pharynx does not compromise the use of the voice prosthesis. Cases of dysphagia cannot be attributed exclusively to the method of linear stapler.

The advantages and details of the use of linear stapling machines for performing the closure of the pharynx have been listed. The biggest disadvantage of linear stapler by closed technique is not allowing visualization of the tumour during resection. Linear stapler was conducted only in cases where it was possible to ensure adequate surgical margins and complete tumour resection. The average 5-year survival is similar to other studies, for one can admit that the application of this type of suture in the pharynx did not adversely affect the prognosis of the patients. It seems that if we confine its application to endolaryngeal tumours this technique is safe and allows an adequate oncologic surgery [6].

5. Conclusion

The mechanical suture of the pharynx in total laryngectomy is a simple and fast method with low risk of contamination of the surgical site. It does not increase the incidence of post-operative complications. It seems to be a safe method provided that the limits of its indication, as to the location and tumour extension are respected.

Acknowledgements

The authors thank all the other members of the Otolaryngology Department of Portuguese Oncology Institute of Lisbon, Francisco Gentil (IPOLFG) for scientific assistance.

References

[1] Stell, P.M. (1975) The First Laryngectomy. *The Journal of Laryngology and Otology*, **89**, 353-358. http://dx.doi.org/10.1017/S0022215100080488

[2] Bedrin, L., Ginsburg, G., Horowitz, Z. and Talmi, Y.P. (2005) 25-Year Experience of Using a Linear Stapler in Laryngectomy. *Head & Neck*, **27**, 1073-1079. http://dx.doi.org/10.1007/s00405-009-0945-4

[3] Estibeiro, H. (2004) Total Laryngectomy, Surgery of the Larynx. N.P. Circulo Médico, 123-135.

[4] Gonçalves, A.J., Souza Jr., J.A., Menezes, M.B., Kavabata, N.K., *et al.* (2009) Pharyngocutaneous Fistulae Following Total Laryngectomy Comparison between Manual and Mechanical Sutures. *European Archives of Oto-Rhino-Laryngology*, **266**, 1793-1798. http://dx.doi.org/10.1007/s00405-009-0945-4

[5] Sofferman, R.A. and Voronetsky, I. (2000) Use of the Linear Stapler for Pharyngoesophageal Closure after Total Laryngectomy. *The Laryngoscope*, **110**, 1406-1409. http://dx.doi.org/10.1097/00005537-200008000-00035

[6] Montoya, F., Ruiz de Galarreta, J.C., Sánchez del Rey, A., Martínez Ibargüen, A., *et al.* (2002) Comparative Study between the Use of Manual versus Mechanical Sutures in the Closing of the Mucous Defect Following a Total Laryngectomy. *Acta Otorrinolaringológica Española*, **53**, 343-350.

[7] Altissimi, G. and Frenguelli, A. (2007) Linear Stapler Closure of the Pharynx during Total Laryngectomy: A 15-Year Experience (from Closed Technique to Semi-Closed Technique). *Acta Otorhinolaryngologica Itálica*, **27**, 118-122.

[8] Agrawal, A. and Schuller, E. (2000) Closed Laryngectomy Using the Automatic Linear Stapling Device. *The Laryngoscope*, **110**, 1402-1405. http://dx.doi.org/10.1097/00005537-200008000-00034

[9] Ahumada, N., Oliveira, C. and Takimoto, R. (2011) Stapler Device at the Closure of the Pharynx after Total Laryngectomy: 7 Years of Experience. *Revista Brasileira de Cirurgia da Cabeça e Pescoço*, **40**, 144-147.

9

A Rare Case of Facial Palsy Due to Mucormycosis

Vaishali Shah[1], H. Ganapathy[1], Ram Gopalakrishnan[2], N. Geetha[3]

[1]ENT Department, Apollo Main Hospital, Chennai, India
[2]Infectious Diseases Department, Apollo Main Hospital, Chennai, India
[3]Pathology Department, Apollo Main Hospital, Chennai, India
Email: drvaishalient@gmail.com

Abstract

A very uncommon instance of facial nerve palsy involving isolated temporal bone with associated uncontrolled diabetes mellitus has been noticed. A 53-year-old diabetic male presented himself with facial asymmetry, ear pain, and discharge in the right ear of one-month duration. Clinical examination revealed grade IV [House-Brackmann] right sided facial palsy, and otoscopy of small central perforation. Clinically acute otitis media with facial palsy diagnosis was made. There was minimal response to medical treatment. As per CT scan and audiometry findings, patient was subjected for exploratory mastoidectomy showing pale granulation tissue involving geniculate ganglion of facial nerve. The histopathology was suggestive of mucormycosis, an unusual presentation in middle ear. The patient was treated with injectable Amphotericin B. This case highlights a rare cause of isolated facial palsy and physicians should be aware of such atypical clinical presentation.

Keywords

Facial Palsy, Diabetes Mellitus, Mucormycosis

1. Introduction

The purpose of presenting this case report is to highlight the rare manifestation of mucormycosis causing facial nerve palsy. Many cases of mucormycosis [1]-[4] causing facial palsy have been reported in medical journals published in English literature. Very few publications [1] [2] have documented isolated tympanic bone involvement. Mucormycosis is an emerging fungal infection with a high rate of mortality. Mucormycosis is the term used to describe fungal infections caused by fungi in the order Mucorales, and species in the Mucor, genera rhizopus, absidia and cunninghamella are most often implicated [5]. This disease is often characterized by hyphae growing in and around vessels. Mucormycosis frequently involves the paranasal sinuses, brain, or lungs. While oral or cerebral mucormycosis is the most common type of the disease, this infection can also manifest in the gastrointestinal tract, skin, and in other organ systems. In rare cases, the temporal bone may be affected by mucormycosis.

2. Case Report

A 53-year-old diabetic male presented himself with facial asymmetry, ear pain, tinnitus and discharge in the right ear of one-month duration. At the onset of presentation, he had taken a conservative line of treatment for the same without any improvement. He was on oral antidiabetic treatment for the past 6 years. Clinical examination revealed absence of right nasolabial fold, deviation of angle of mouth to the left, inability to close the right eye, and asymmetry of face at rest (**Figure 1**). All these features suggested grade IV facial nerve palsy (House-Brackmann). Otoscopic examination revealed a small central perforation in the anteroinferior quadrant of the right tympanic membrane. Fistula sign was absent; and there was no evidence of meningitis.

Pure tone audiometry revealed sloping mixed hearing loss in the right ear and sensorineural hearing loss in the left. Culture and sensitivity of purulent discharge from the right ear showed insignificant growth of coagulase negative staphylococci. His fasting and postprandial blood sugar levels were 254 mg/dl and 375 mg/dl respectively. HbA1C was 11.7% suggesting uncontrolled diabetes mellitus. Serum creatinine was 0.9 mg. High resolution computed tomography of temporal bone revealed isodense opacification in the right mesotymapanum (**Figure 2**). Ossicles and external auditory canal were normal. A clinical diagnosis of acute otitis media with facial palsy was made.

Since there was no improvement with conservative line of treatment, the patient was subjected to exploratory mastoidectomy. Intra operatively, pale granulation tissue was seen lying in anterior epitympanum as well in the region close to geniculate ganglion. The white granular mass was removed in piecemeal exposing the facial nerve along the course of horizontal portion. The specimen was then sent for histopathological examination.

Histopathology examination revealed necrotizing subacute inflammation and associated osteomyelitis and aseptate hyphae suggesting mucormycosis (**Figure 3**). As per advice from infectious disease consultant the patient was started on injection Amphotericin B (1 mg/kg/day in dextrose drip over 22 hours) along with aggressive diabetic management with injectable insulin.

The course of Amphotericin B injection was continued for 24 days. Thereafter, the patient was put on a step down treatment with syrup Posaconazole 400 mg (10 ml) twice daily for 2 weeks. Post treatment clinical monitoring for seven months showed no deterioration in the condition of the patient. With treatment, partial improvement in eye closure and asymmetry of face was noticed (**Figure 4**), but grading of facial nerve palsy was same.

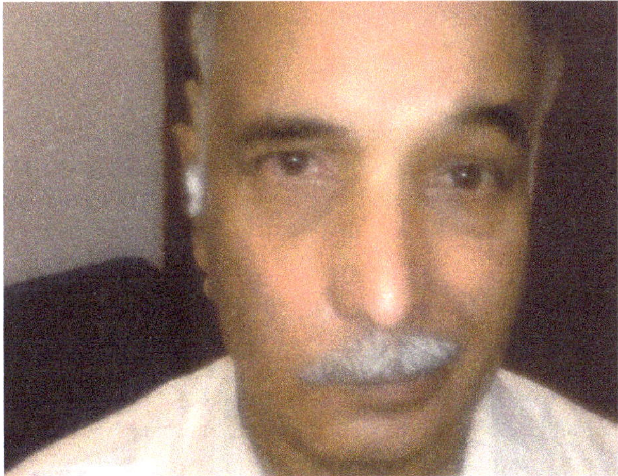

Figure 1. Preoperative clinical picture of patient showing facial asymmetry at rest, absence of right nasolabial fold and deviation of angle of mouth to left side.

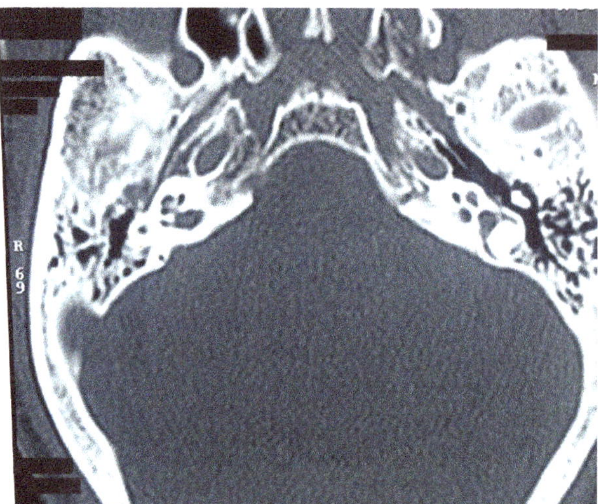

Figure 2. High Resolution CT Temporal bone axial view showing isodenseopacification of right sided mesotympanum, ossicles—intact, no bony erosion.

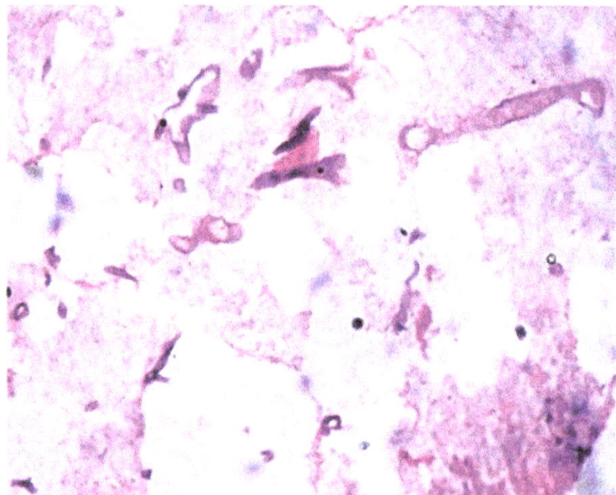

Figure 3. Histopathological slide with Hematoxilin & Eosin staining with 40× magnification showing aseptate hyphae.

3. Discussion

Mucormycosis is the second most common fungal infection in diabetic patients after aspergillosis [5]. Mucormycosis is caused by subclass of Zygomycetes fungi. Angioinvasive hyphae forms are responsible for tissue invasion and dissemination [5]. Factors associated with an increased risk of mucormycosis include diabetes mellitus, immunosuppression, metabolic acidosis and administration of high dose systemic corticosteroids in solid organs.

In head and neck region, mucormycosis normally manifests itself in the rhino-cerebral area. Very few cases have been reported in the tympanic bone; although rhino-cerebral involvement has been observed quite frequently [3] [4] [6]-[10]. Mucormycosis causing isolated facial nerve paralysis is extremely rare. We reviewed published reports of mucormycosis causing isolated facial paralysis and found only two cases. In one case, horizontal part of facial nerve and external auditory canal were involved [1]. In another case, site of lesion of facial nerve was not mentioned, but external auditory canal was found involved [2]. In our case, the horizontal portion of the facial nerve and the adjacent geniculate ganglion was found involved and external auditory canal was free from disease.

Many articles of mucormycosis spreading from nose or paranasal sinuses to temporal bone were identified

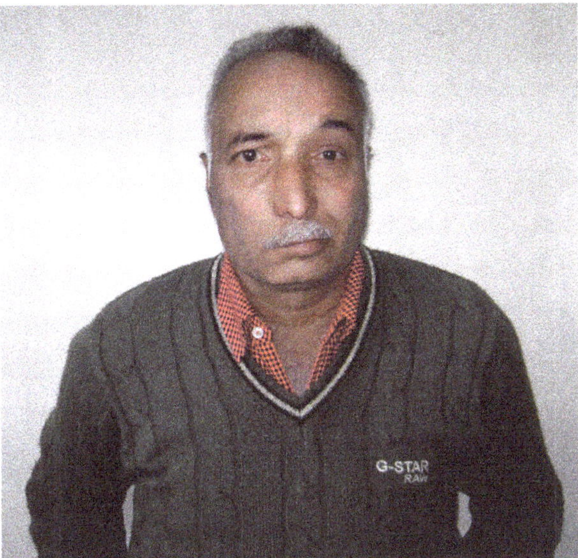

Figure 4. Postoperative clinical picture with slightly improved asymmetry of right-sided face.

while PubMed used as search engine. In two cases, it spread from nasopharynx [6] [7], and in the rest from the paranasal sinuses [3] [4] [8]-[10].

The clinical features of mucormycosis are dependent on the site of involvement. The common causes of facial palsy in diabetic patients include malignant otitis externa, acute on chronic otitis media, malignancy, diabetic neuritis, or Bell's palsy. Fungal infection causing facial palsy is very rare but should be kept in mind before diagnosing it as Bell's palsy. Prognosis of fungal infection is better than malignant otitis externa.

Incidence of Rhino-cerebral mucormycosis with concomitant diabetes mellitus is 60% - 81% [11]. Diabetic patients are less likely to improve completely. Recurrence of facial palsy is more common in diabetic patients.

Treatment of mucormycosis is universal. Injectable Amphotericin B is the only drug effective against mucormycosis. Recommended dose of amphotericin is 1 - 2 mg/kg/day [5]. Liposomal amphotericin B can be given in high dose of 10 mg/kg/day. It is to be given for 4 weeks or till there is an improvement. Response rate of Amphotericin B of 50% has been reported [5]. Posaconazole has been reported with 60% - 70% response rate. In our case, as the patient could not afford liposomal Amphotericin B, we gave plain amphotericin B for 4 weeks. Since the patient developed acute renal failure during the treatment, amphotericin was stopped for 12 days and patient was treated with intravenous fluid therapy and potassium supplementation.

Post treatment, the patient continued to show symptoms of grade IV House-Brackmann facial palsy. However, the facial nerve function showed partial improvement in the form of improved eye closure, reduced facial asymmetry at rest although the grading was the same. As per the reported findings in the literature, recovery after grade IV facial nerve paralysis will start from the fourth month onwards [12]. Diabetic patients however tend to show partial recovery only.

4. Conclusion

A rare case of facial palsy due to mucormycosis in a diabetic individual has been presented. Physicians should be aware of such atypical clinical presentation. This would facilitate implementation of an early appropriate medical and surgical treatment. Such a treatment regimen would aid disease recovery and better prognosis.

Acknowledgements

No competing financial interests exist.

Summary

- Rhino-cerebral involvements are common in mucormycosis involving head and neck regions;

- This case report highlights rare presentation of mucormycosis causing isolated facial palsy. Physicians should be aware of such atypical clinical presentation;
- Amphotericin B is the universal treatment for the mucormycosis.

References

[1] Yun, M.W., Lui, C.C. and Chen, W.J. (1994) Facial Paralysis Secondary to Tympanic Mucormycosis: Case Report. *American Journal of Otology*, **15**, 413-414.

[2] Olalla, I., Ortín, M., Hermida, G., Cortés, M.A., Richard, C., Iriondo, A., *et al.* (1996) Autologous Peripheral Blood Stem Cell Transplantation in a Patient with Previous Invasive Middle Ear Mucormycosis. *Bone Marrow Transplant*, **18**, 1183-1184.

[3] Shekar, V., Sikander, J., Rangdhol, V. and Naidu, M. (2015) Facial Nerve Paralysis: A Case Report of Rare Complication in Uncontrolled Diabetic Patient with Mucormycosis. *Journal of Natural Science, Biology and Medicine*, **6**, 226-228. http://dx.doi.org/10.4103/0976-9668.149195

[4] Sachdeva, K. (2013) Rhino-Oculo Cerebral Mucormycosis with Multiple Cranial Nerve Palsy in Diabetic Patient: Review of Six Cases. *Indian Journal of Otolaryngology and Head & Neck Surgery*, **65**, 375-379. http://dx.doi.org/10.1007/s12070-013-0659-1

[5] Kontoyiannis, D.P. and Lewis, R.E. (2006) Invasive Zygomycosis: Update on Pathogenesis, Clinical Manifestations, and Management. *Infectious Diseases Clinics of North America*, **20**, 581-607.

[6] Oo, M.M., Kutteh, L.A., Koc, O.N., Strauss, M. and Lazarus, H.M. (1998) Mucormycosis of Petrous Bone in an Allogeneic Stem Cell Transplant Recipient. *Clinical Infectious Diseases*, **27**, 1546-1547. http://dx.doi.org/10.1086/517749

[7] Gussen, R. and Canalis, R.F. (1982) Mucormycosis of the Temporal Bone. *Annals of Otology, Rhinology & Laryngology*, **91**, 27-32. http://dx.doi.org/10.1177/000348948209100108

[8] Nomiya, R., Nomiya, S. and Paparella, M.M. (2008) Mucormycosis of the Temporal Bone. *Otology and Neurotology*, **29**, 1041-1042. http://dx.doi.org/10.1097/MAO.0b013e31817d0200

[9] Hamilton, J.F., Bartkowski, H.B. and Rock, J.P. (2003) Management of CNS Mucormycosis in the Pediatric Patient. *Pediatric Neurosurgery*, **38**, 212-215. http://dx.doi.org/10.1159/000069101

[10] Buhl, M.R., Joseph, T.P., Snelling, B.E. and Buhl, L. (1992) Temporofacial Zygomycosis in a Pregnant Woman. *Infection*, **20**, 230-232. http://dx.doi.org/10.1007/BF02033066

[11] Gupta, S., Koirala, J. and Khardori, R. (2007) Infections in Diabetes Mellitus and Hyperglycemia. *Infectious Diseases Clinics of North America*, **21**, 617-638. http://dx.doi.org/10.1016/j.idc.2007.07.003

[12] Bibas, T., Jiang, D. and Gleeson, M.J. (2008) Disorders of the Facial Nerve. In: *Scott-Browne's Otorhinolaryngology, Head and Neck Surgery*, 7th Edition, Vol. 3, Chap. 241c, Hodder Arnold, Great Britain, 3870-3894.

10

Squamous Cell Carcinoma of the Middle Ear Mimicking CSOM with Intracranial Complications: A Diagnostic Dilemma

Anoop Attakkil, Vandana Thorawade, Mohan Jagade, Rajesh Kar, Kartik Parelkar, Poonam Khairnar, Reshma Hanowate, Devkumar Rangaraja

Department of ENT, Grant Medical College & Sir J.J. Hospital, Mumbai, India
Email: fasttrack2317@gmail.com

Abstract

Cancer of the external auditory canal (EAC) and middle ear (ME) is rare, accounting for less than 1% of all head-and-neck malignancies [1] [2] of which squamous cell carcinoma (SCC) is the most common. Even though squamous cell carcinoma [SCC] of the middle ear and chronic suppurative otitis media (CSOM) co-exist, no definitive correlation has been proven. Here we are presenting a case of squamous cell carcinoma of the middle ear who presented with headache, fever and vomiting with a background history of chronic suppurative otitis media since childhood. A provisional diagnosis of mastoid abscess with intracranial complications secondary to chronic suppurative otitis media was made and modified radical mastoidectomy was done but histology of the mastoid specimen revealed well differentiated keratinizing squamous cell carcinoma, which was treated with radical radiotherapy. Objective of this presentation is to bring attention to the coexistence of CSOM and squamous cell carcinoma ear and also the importance to detect these lesions at an early stage. This report also highlights the requirement of histopathological analysis in mastoidectomy and discusses the aetiology and management of squamous cell carcinoma of the middle ear with review of literature.

Keywords

Squamous Cell Carcinoma, Mastoid, Otitis Media

1. Introduction

Cancer of the external auditory canal (EAC), the middle ear (ME) and the mastoid is fortunately rare. Its incidence has been estimated as 1 case per every 5000 - 20,000 patients admitted to hospitals with otological diseases [3]-[5] or as 6 cases per million in the general population [6]. Squamous cell carcinoma accounts for the most common histologic type in this region, occurring in more than 80% of cases [7] [8].

The major etiological factor is chronic suppurative otitis media (CSOM) [9]-[12] although irradiation and inverted papilloma of the middle ear have also been reported to be additional risk factors [9] [10] [13]. The co-existence of CSOM with or without cholesteatoma along with malignancy makes the early detection difficult. Many patients present with non-specific signs of chronic inflammation and infection that cause difficulty in reaching a proper clinical diagnosis of this malignant type. Additionally, chronic infections, those often precede the malignancy result in a delay in diagnosis by causing decreased follow-up motivation. Despite the development of increasingly radical surgical procedures and the advances in radiotherapy these tumours retain a poor prognosis. Hence it is very important to detect these lesions very early.

We present a case of squamous cell carcinoma of the middle ear which presented mastoid abscess with intracranial complications which gains relevance in light of the above mentioned diagnostic and therapeutic challenges. Describing this report we would like to emphasise that early diagnosis of malignancy in such a case rests on a high index of suspicion. Our case report also highlights the importance of submission of all mastoid tissues removed at mastoidectomy of unsafe variety of otitis media, however typical the clinical presentation of the disease may be, for histological confirmation of provisional clinical diagnosis.

2. Case Report

A 65 years old female was referred from a peripheral hospital with complaints of right sided ear discharge since 10 years of duration. There was associated severe right sided otalgia, hearing loss, and vertigo. She complained of headache with fever since 2 weeks. She underwent ear surgery on right side 30 years back but details were not available. She was a known case of diabetes mellitus on treatment with oral antihypoglycaemics. On clinical examination, patient was febrile and cachexic with unaltered sensorium. There was pale granulation tissue admixed with discharge in the right ear. Post aural swelling was present with tenderness suggestive of mastoid abscess.

Computerised tomography of brain done at a peripheral hospital showed erosion of osteolytic/erosion involving right petrous temporalbone, mastoid air cells and sinus plate associated with soft tissue density lesion in right middle ear cavity, mastoid air cells, attic and external ear (**Figure 1**).

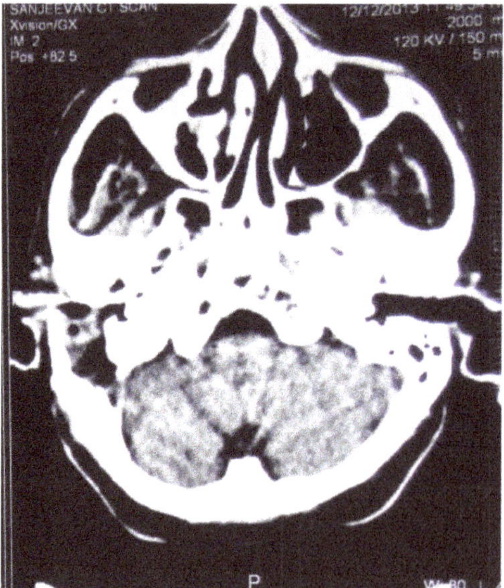

Figure 1. Computerised tomography of brain showing with soft tissue density lesion in right middle ear cavity, mastoid air cells, attic and external ear.

High resolution computerised tomography (HRCT) of temporal bone done shows peripherally enhancing collection in right mastoid and middle ear cavity with destruction of mastoid and tegmen tympani and sinus tympani involving right sigmoid sinus (**Figure 2**).

A diagnosis of left chronic suppurative otitis media, complicated by mastoid abscess and meningitis was made, to rule out an intracranial mass lesion.

Patient was posted for tympanomastoid exploration under GA which revealed purulent secretions mixed with keratinous debris and granulations eroding the dural plate and sinus plate. Granulations with bone fragments were removed but as it was invading the dura, disease clearance was not satisfactory (**Figure 3**). The specimen was sent for histopathological examination along with culture and sensitivity. Mastoid cavity was exteriorised and patient was started on intravenous third generation cephalosporins.

Histopathological examination of the specimen received 2.3 cms in aggregate revealed invasive well differentiated keratinising squamous cell carcinoma (**Figure 4**). Patient was reevaluated and commenced on palliative

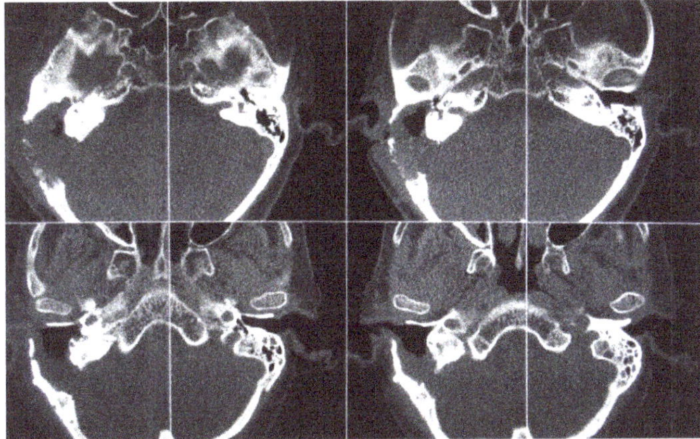

Figure 2. HRCT of temporal bone showing peripherally enhancing collection in right mastoid and middle ear cavity with destruction of mastoid and tegmen tympani and sinus tympani.

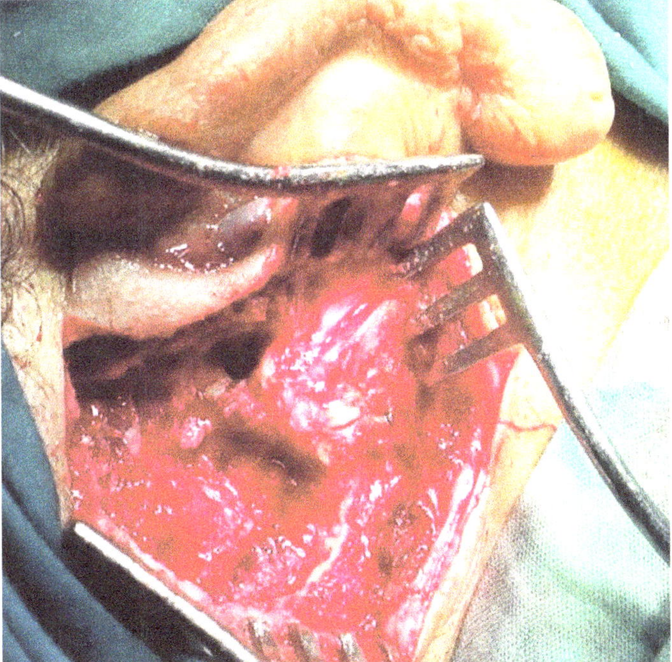

Figure 3. Intraoperative picture showing the keratinous debris, admixed with blood and discharge.

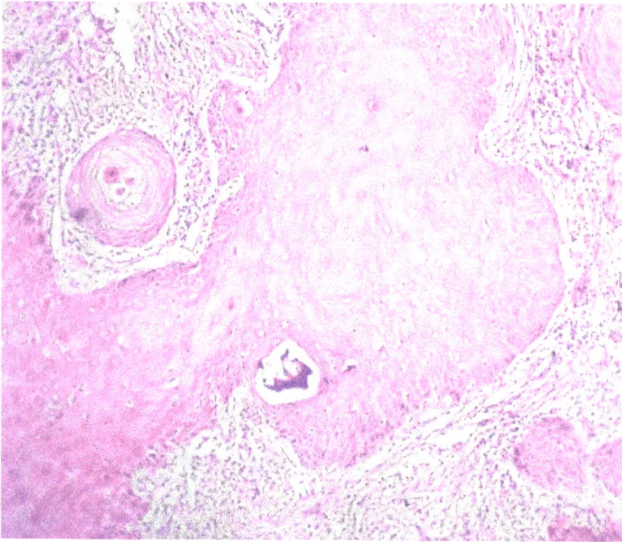

Figure 4. Microscopy showing well differentiated keratinising squamous cell carcinoma.

external beam radiotherapy with a direct lateral field encompassing the EAC, mastoid process with lower border at the angle of the jaw. She was discharged on completion of radiotherapy. Patient was evaluated for 6 months regularly and was subsequently lost for follow up.

3. Discussion

Squamous cell carcinoma of the middle ear and temporal bone is a rare malignancy but are associated with considerable morbidity and mortality, both owing to the disease processes themselves and the treatment modalities. Despite the diagnostic advances and therapeutic refinement in this field over the last half century, these malignancies still bear an ominous prognosis.

Squamous cell carcinoma accounts for 60% to 80% of all temporal bone malignancies followed by basal cell carcinoma [14]. The disease affect males and females equally, with an age range of 34 - 85 years and an average age of 60 years [15].

The rarity of the disease itself limits the performance of large risk assessment studies as a result of which the aetiology of these tumours is not well defined. It is frequently argued that chronic otitis media is a risk factor for temporal bone malignancy, especially squamous cell carcinoma [14].

The early symptoms of temporal bone carcinoma closely resemble those of chronic suppurative otitis media, including purulent foul-smelling otorrhoea, severe otalgia, bleeding, and pruritus [14]. Since the incidence of malignancy is rare, differentiating between a chronically draining ear with associated inflammation and a malignancy is usually difficult. Other presenting symptoms of malignancy include hearing loss, headaches, tinnitus, vertigo, and aural fullness. Cranial nerve palsies may occur. Spread into the glenoid fossa can result in trismus, and dural involvement can produce severe pain and headache [14].

In our case, patient presented with a classical presentation of chronic ear infection with mastoid abscess and meningitis for which she was immediately taken up for mastoidectomy and abscess drainage. In this case, the delay in diagnosis was obviously due to the nonspecificity of symptoms for which she was treated as a case of chronic inflammation of ear by the private otolaryngologist. Although the diagnosis is rare, early detection can have a considerable impact on outcome [14]. Chronic ear infections not responding to proper antibiotics, bloody or serosanguinous discharge should be evaluated with a suspicion of malignancy. There can be a secondary bacterial infection complicating the diagnosis. Facial nerve palsy, other cranial nerve palsies or headache should be treated considering a possibility of malignancy in such a background.

High-resolution computed tomographic (CT) scans show the bony anatomy of the temporal bone and demonstrate the extent of bony erosion [14]. But the presentation can resemble the intracranial complications of chronic suppurative otitis media that sometimes imaging studies may be less helpful in attaining diagnosis unless evaluated properly.

Although a history of chronic otitis media is found in 40% to 60% of patients with temporal bone malignancy, it is less clear what role chronic infection may have in the development of malignancy. On the contrary the chronic infections of ear are so common compared to the low frequency of malignancy Carcinoma may arise, in a manner similar to Marjolin's ulcers, from epithelium damaged by chronic otorrhoea or from bacterial toxins that can alter the normal mitotic activity of the epithelial cells. Some authors have found cholesteatoma associated with temporal bone malignancy, but a causal link has not been established [14].

The association of chronic suppurative otitis media with malignancy is not only important when we consider diagnosis but emphasis should be given to subject mastoid tissues removed at mastoidectomy for histopathological evaluation. However typical the presentation of the disease may be, it gains more significance when we consider the fact that early stage of diagnosis definitely make the prognosis better.

There is no universally accepted temporal bone malignancy staging system. The Pittsburgh system is based on radiographic findings and has been correlated successfully with both clinical outcome and histopathology examination of the involved temporal bones [14]. The University of Cincinnati system incorporates radiographic and intraoperative findings and has been successfully used as a guide for determining the extent of temporal bone resection required [14].

The treatment of the disease, surgery or radiotherapy or a combined approach is still controversial as a conclusive study is not yet published owing to the rarity of the disease. The classic surgeries include sleeve resection, lateral temporal bone resection, subtotal temporal bone resection, and total temporal bone resection. While some authors advocate total en bloc removal of the temporal bone surrounding the tumour and others argue for piecemeal removal of gross tumour with preservation of vital neurovascular structures followed by radiation therapy [14]. Mastoidectomy, lateral temporal bone resection (TBR) and subtotal TBR are more appropriate and these techniques showed similar survival in a retrospective review including 144 patients, with a five-year survival of 50%, 48.6% and 50%, respectively [16]. In a retrospective analysis, radical radiotherapy was proposed as the treatment of choice for patients with early stage squamous cell carcinoma of the external auditory canal and middle ear [17]. In addition, surgery, with negative surgical margins if possible, and radiotherapy was recommended in this study as the standard care for cases of advanced-stage disease.

The disparity in the studies itself shows that it is difficult to be certain about treatment results for mastoid squamous carcinoma from the literature. But in general, the treatment of squamous cell carcinoma of the temporal bone comprises surgical excision possibly followed by radiation. The prognosis of the disease remains usually bad owing to the late presentation which is even worse in cases with facial nerve paralysis, positive tumour margins, dural involvement, and regional lymph node involvement [14].

4. Conclusion

This case report highlights a rare and aggressive tumor which is associated with chronic suppurative otitis media which is in fact a very common disease that every practitioner encounters. Early diagnosis of malignancy in such a case rests on a high index of suspicion. Early diagnosis, detection and management are the simplest and most effective measures to increase patient survival in these cases. We have tried to highlight how closely the disease mimicked mastoid abscess and meningitis. Our case report also stresses on the significance of submission of mastoid tissues in each case of mastoidectomy for histopathological evaluation as the clinical evaluation and imaging may sometimes prove less useful in detection. Presenting this case, we expect the medical practitioners to have a prompt workup and evaluation for those cases of chronic inflammation of ear which are not responding to treatment.

References

[1] Arriaga, M., Hirsch, B.E., Kamerer, D.B. and Myers, E.N. (1989) Squamous Cell Carcinoma of the External Auditory Meatus (Canal). *Otolaryngology—Head and Neck Surgery*, **101**, 330-337.

[2] Arena, S. and Keen, M. (1988) Carcinoma of the Middle Ear and Temporal Bone. *American Journal of Otology*, **9**, 351-356.

[3] Ostfeld, E., Segal, M. and Czernobilsky, B. (1981) Malignant External Otitis: Early Histopathotogic Changes and Pathogenic Mechanism. *Laryngoscope*, **91**, 965-970. http://dx.doi.org/10.1288/00005537-198106000-00014

[4] Cohen, D., Friedman, P. and Eilon, A. (1987) Malignant External Otitis versus Acute External Otitis. *Journal of La-*

ryngology and Otology, **101**, 211-215. http://dx.doi.org/10.1017/S0022215100101550

[5] Cohen, D. and Friedman, P. (1987) The Diagnostic Criteria of Malignant External Otitis. *Journal of Laryngology and Otology*, **101**, 216-221. http://dx.doi.org/10.1017/S0022215100101562

[6] Babiatzki, A. and Sade, J. (1987) Malignant External Otitis. *Journal of Laryngology and Otology*, **101**, 205-210. http://dx.doi.org/10.1017/S0022215100101549

[7] Rodriguez Paramas, A., Gil Carrasco, R., Arenas Britez, O. and Yurrita Scola, B. (2004) Malignant Tumours of the External Auditory Canal and of the Middle Ear. *Acta Otorrinolaringológica Española*, **55**, 470-474.

[8] Yeung, P., Bridger, A., Smee, R., Baldwin, M. and Bridger, G.P. (2002) Malignancies of the External Auditory Canal and Temporal Bone: A Review. *ANZ Journal of Surgery*, **72**, 114-120. http://dx.doi.org/10.1046/j.1445-2197.2002.02313.x

[9] Martinez Subias, J., Dominquez Ugidos, L.J., Urpegui Garcia, A., Sancho Serrano, E., Royo Lopez, J., Millan Guevara, J. and Valles Verela, H. (1998) Middle Ear Carcinoma. *Acta Otorrinolaringológica Española*, **49**, 234-246.

[10] Maran, A.G.D. and Jacobson, I. (1990) Tumours of the Ear. In: Maran, A.G. and Stell, P.M., Eds., *Clinical Otolaryngology*, 3rd Edition, Blackwell Scientific Publications, Hoboken, 464-474.

[11] Newhart, H. (1917) Primary Carcinoma of the Middle Ear: Report of a Case. *Laryngoscope*, **27**, 543-555. http://dx.doi.org/10.1288/00005537-191707000-00002

[12] Pizzo, P.A., Freifeld, A.G., Meyer, J. and Walsh, T. (1993) Infection in the Cancer Patient. In: DeVita, V.T., Hellmann, S. and Rosenberg, S.A., Eds., *Cancer: Principle and Practices of Oncology*, 4th Edition, Vol. 62, 2292-2528.

[13] de Filippis, C., Marioni, G., Tregnaghi, A., Marino, F., Gaio, E. and Staffieri, A. (2002) Primary Inverted Papilloma of the Middle Ear and Mastoid. *Otology & Neurotology*, **23**, 555-559. http://dx.doi.org/10.1097/00129492-200207000-00027

[14] Decker, B.C. (2003) Glasscock-Shambaugh Surgery of the Ear. Vol. 1, 5th Edition, PMPH-USA, 743-754.

[15] World Health Organization (2005) Pathology and Genetics of Head and Neck Tumours IARC WHO Classification of Tumours Series Vol. 9 of World Health Organization Classification of Tumours. IARC Press, Lyon, 349.

[16] Prasad, S. and Janecka, I.P. (1994) Efficacy of Surgical Treatments for Squamous Cell Carcinoma of the Temporal Bone: A Literature Review. *Otolaryngology—Head and Neck Surgery*, **110**, 270-280. http://dx.doi.org/10.1016/S0194-5998(94)70769-3

[17] Ogawa, K., Nakamura, K., Hatano, K., *et al.* (2007) Treatment and Prognosis of Squamous Cell Carcinoma of the External Auditory Canal and Middle Ear: A Multi-Institutional Retrospective Review of 87 Patients. *International Journal of Radiation Oncology, Biology, Physics*, **68**, 1326-1334. http://dx.doi.org/10.1016/j.ijrobp.2007.01.052

11

Chordoma in Nasopharynx in a 70-Year-Old Female: A Rare Occurence

Bhaskar Mitra*, **Subhalakshmi Sengupta, Anshita Rai, Jay Mehta, Aruna Rai Quader, Subhendu Roy, Anita Borges**

Drs. Tribedi & Roy Diagnostic Laboratory, Kolkata, India
Email: *bhaskarmitra12@gmail.com

Abstract

The nasopharynx is an unusual site for extraosseous chordoma. The characteristic histology and immunohistochemistry confirmed the diagnosis. The behaviour of this tumour is locally aggressive. We report a case of nasopharyngeal chordoma in an elderly patient with literature review.

Keywords

Chordoma, Nasopharyngeal Tumours, Notochord

1. Introduction

Chordomas are rare, locally aggressive tumours that probably originate from embryonic remnants of the notochord. The sacrum is the commonest site followed by the base of the skull/clival region. Spheno-occipital chordomas giving rise to the formation of a nasopharyngeal mass have been described in literature [1]-[3]. When skull base chordomas occur at an extraosseous location (without lytic bone destruction), they may mimic other lesions of the nasopharynx.

It is important to consider extraosseous chordoma in the differential diagnosis of tumors in the nasopharynx because it requires a very different treatment plan and carries its own unique prognosis. We like to share our experience of a primary extraosseous chordoma involving the nasopharynx.

2. Case Report

A 70-year-old female, presented with persistent and profuse anterior rhinorrhea, for more than one year. The discharge was bilateral, had a bad odour and was associated with mild subjective hearing loss, nasal respiratory

*Corresponding author.

failure and closed rhinolalia.

Exploration by oropharyngoscopy revealed a mucosa covered soft mass, measuring 2.5 × 2 cms protruding from the soft palate into the central region of the posterior nasopharyngeal wall. The tumour was not indurated and showed no fluctuation or inflammatory signs. Otoscopy revealed bilateral seromucinous otitis.

A head and neck CT scan showed an ill defined heterogeneously enhancing soft tissue attenuating polypoid mass within the nasopharyngeal cavity (**Figure 1**). In the posterior aspect of the mass evidence of porous erosion is seen in anterior margin of the basi-sphenoid. The mass has occluded the posterior nasal air spaces and nasopharynx. The soft palate is thickened and inseparable from the mass superiorly. The pterygoid muscles and adjacent fat planes are maintained. No intrasphenoid or intracerebral extension of the mass was seen. The paranasal sinuses are well aerated and clear. Other routine investigations are within normal limits.

Pharyngoscopic excision biopsy was performed. On gross examination the lesion appeared soft, polypoid, multilobulated, semi translucent and grayish. Whole of it was processed. Microscopically it shows a tumour composed of nests of cells tending to be arranged in cords set in a pale matrix of mucopolysaccharide with a characteristic physaliphorous appearance (**Figures 2(A)-(C)**). Areas of necrosis not seen. The tumour cells do not show significant mitotic activity or nuclear anaplasia. Areas of congestion and hemorrhage are present. The overlying respiratory epithelium was unremarkable (**Figure 2(A)**). From the Haematoxyline and Eosin stained slides a provisional diagnosis of Chordoma was made. Immunohistochemistry was performed; the tumour cells were immunopositive for Cytokeratin, EMA [epithelial membrane antigen] and S-100 (**Figure 3**), confirming the diagnosis of nasopharyngeal chordoma.

Surgical excision of the lesion was performed through skull base approach. Imaging study helped to rule out any residual tumour by assessing the extent of tumour. Postoperative course being uneventful, the patient was discharged after 10 days and was monitored on an outpatient basis. The patient remains asymptomatic and without any abnormal findings reported on control imaging studies till date.

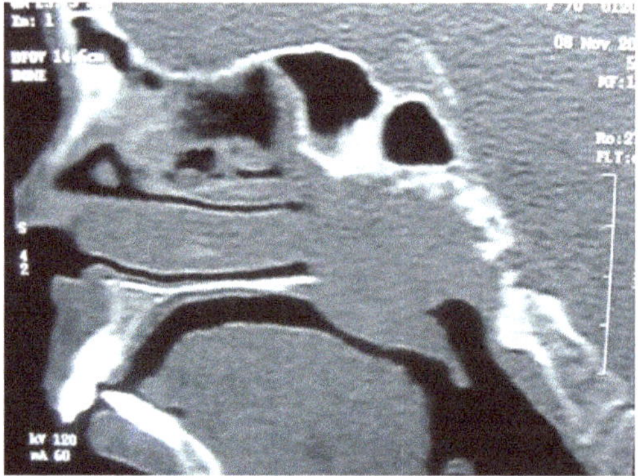

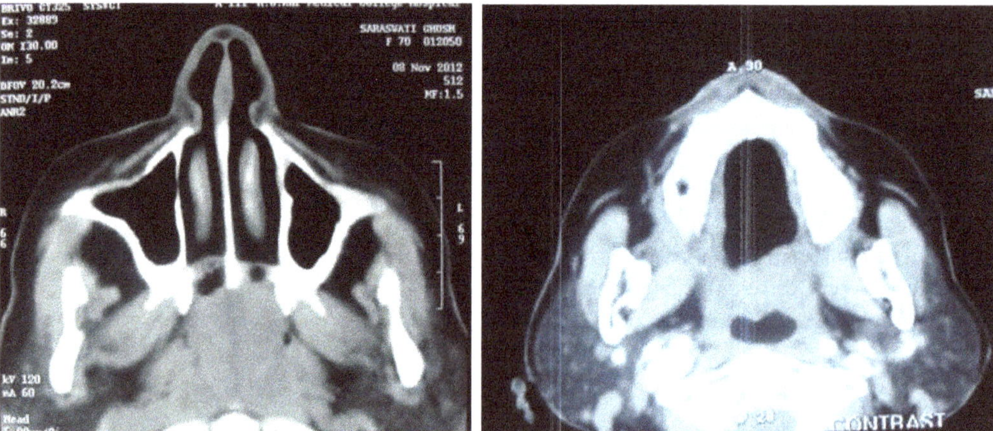

Figure 1. Coronal and sagital section CT scan showed (plain and contrast-enhanced) heterogeneously-enhancing soft tissue lobulated mass in the nasopharynx with evidence of bone erosion at the roof of nasopharynx (clival base).

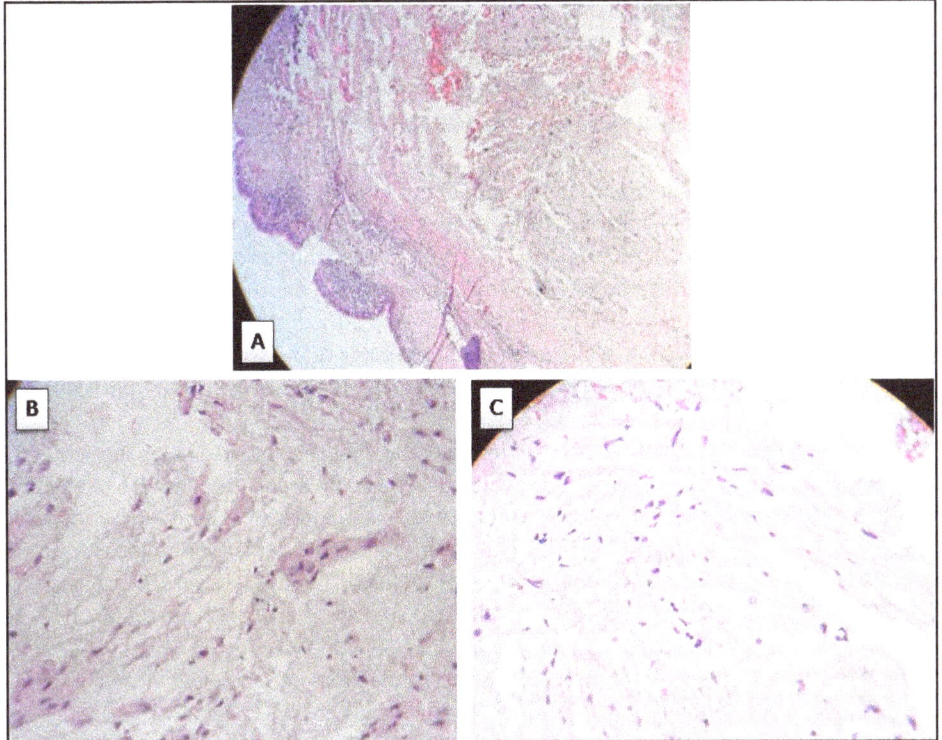

Figure 2. Tumour with overlying respiratory epithelium [(A), 10× H&E stain]. Nests of tumour cells tending to be arranged in cords set in a pale matrix of mucopolysaccharide with a characteristic physaliphorous appearance [(B) & (C), 40× H&E stain].

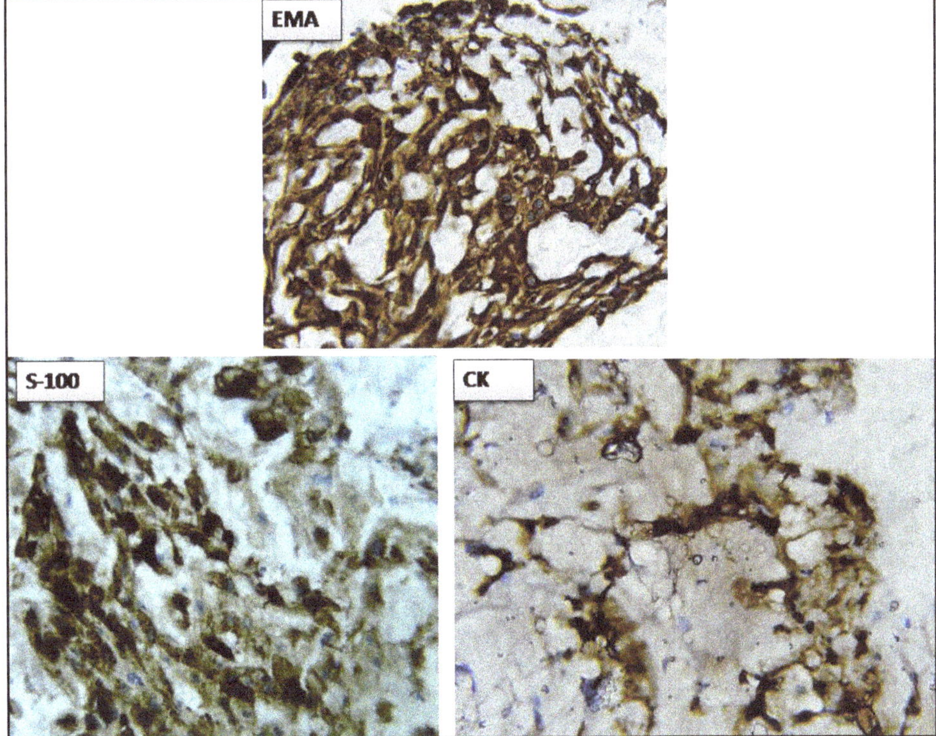

Figure 3. The tumour cells are immunopositive for Cytokeratin, EMA [epithelial membrane antigen] and S-100.

3. Discussion

Extraosseous nasopharyngeal chordoma is primarily a lesion of the nasopharyngeal soft tissues. Nasopharynx is an unusual site for chordoma. The histological features of this tumour were unlike that of a nasopharyngeal carcinoma or a lymphoma [4]-[6]. A small extraosseous chordoma may mimic a Tornwaldt cyst, a benign notochordal remnant entity.

Chordomas account for 1% of intracranial tumors and 4% of all primary bone tumors [7]-[10]. They may occur at any age but are usually seen in adults, with a peak prevalence in the 4th decade of life, but the age of our patient (seventh decade) is unusual. Chordomas have a 2:1 male predilection and affect whites more than blacks [11]-[13]. Intracranial chordomas constitute one-third of all chordomas and usually occur in the vicinity of the clivus, often in the region of the spheno-occipital synchondrosis [8] [9]. Although intracranial chordomas are generally slow growing, their intimate relation to critical structures and extremely high local recurrence rate have often resulted in high mortality rates in the past. However, recent advances in skull base surgery and radiation therapy now provide the opportunity for cure [14] [15].

Generally, chordomas grow slowly and produce symptoms insidiously. Symptoms of intracranial chordomas vary with the location and proximity of the lesion to critical structures and the sites of extension. The most common initial complaint is diplopia related to cranial nerve palsy and headache. Among cranial nerves, the abducent nerve is the most commonly affected [13]. Due to the extraosseous location of these lesions, the typical lytic changes in the clivus are absent; thus, the initial diagnosis is difficult. Intracranial extensions are also not found, though some amount of bone erosion is evident in the CT scan. The aggressive features of chordomas as evident in literature are lytic changes in the osseous structures, such as destruction of the superficial surface of the clivus and bones of the posterior sinonasal region, which are absent in our case. Our patient had a nasopharyngeal lesion with mass effect without any typical neurologic symptoms and cranial neuropathies as commonly seen in chordomas. Chordomas are thought to arise from physaliphorous cells as described by Virchow [16]. The notochord is a primitive cell line around which the skull base and axial skeleton develop. The major postoperative problem is tumor recurrence as a consequence of incomplete excision.

Both CT and MR imaging are used in the evaluation of chordoma. CT is ideal for evaluating the bony involvement, whereas MR imaging is useful for evaluating the surrounding soft tissues and extension into adjacent structures. MR imaging is considered the gold standard in pretreatment and post treatment evaluation of chordomas [11]. On CT, the typical appearance of an extraosseous chordoma is a lobular hypoattenuated soft-tissue mass with areas of dystrophic calcification and lytic changes of affected osseous structures. Scattered areas of hyperattenuation are consistent with descriptions in the literature of blood products and intratumoral hemorrhage in typical chordomas [11] [12].

Anterior tumor extension can involve the sphenoid sinus and, less commonly, the posterior ethmoid sinus, but extension to the paranasal sinuses is not seen in our case.

Surgical removal is a very effective treatment for intracranial chordomas. Longer survival rates have been associated with more extensive tumor removal [8]. With advances in imaging technology, presurgical evaluation can now provide more detailed knowledge of the lesion and suggest the best surgical approach. Local recurrence of intracranial chordomas is still common regardless of the mode of therapy [17].

4. Conclusion

Extraosseous nasopharyngeal chordomas are rare tumors with its own unique characteristics and should be considered in the differential diagnosis of nasopharyngeal lesions.

Acknowledgements

We would like to thank Dr. Ruby Sen for her kind assistance in this paper. The authors also gratefully acknowledge the assistance of the laboratory staffs of the Drs. Tribedi & Roy Diagnostic Laboratory.

Consent

Written informed consent was obtained from the patient for publication of this case report and accompanying images.

Competing Interest

There is no conflict of interest related to the work among the authors in this study.

Authors' Contribution

BM, SS and ARQ collected and analyzed the patient's data. SS and AR performed the gross examination.BM; ARQ & SR performed the histological examination and prepared the manuscript. JM & AB interpreted the Immunohistochemical slides and reviewed the case. ARQ & SR have supervised the work and final correction of the manuscript done by them. All the authors read and approved the final manuscript.

References

[1] Firooznia, H., Pinto, R., Lin, J., *et al.* (1976) Chordomas: Radiologic Evaluation of 20 Cases. *American Journal of Roentgenology*, **127**, 797-805. http://dx.doi.org/10.2214/ajr.127.5.797

[2] Omerod, R. (1960) A Case of Chordomas Presenting in the Nasopharynx. *Journal of Laryngology and Otology*, **74**, 245-254. http://dx.doi.org/10.1017/S0022215100056528

[3] Eisemann, M.L. (1980) Sphenooccipital Chordomas Presenting as a Nasopharyngeal Mass. A Case Report. *Annals of Otology, Rhinology & Laryngology*, **89**, 271-275. http://dx.doi.org/10.1177/000348948008900318

[4] King, A.D., Lei, K.I., Richards, P.S., *et al.* (2003) Non-Hodgkin's Lymphoma of the Nasopharynx: CT and MR Imaging. *Clinical Radiology*, **58**, 621-625. http://dx.doi.org/10.1016/S0009-9260(03)00182-X

[5] Weber, A.L., Al-Arayedh, S. and Rashid, A. (2003) Nasopharynx: Clinical, Pathologic and Radiologic Assessment. *Neuroimaging Clinics of North America*, **13**, 465-483. http://dx.doi.org/10.1016/S1052-5149(03)00041-8

[6] Urquhart, A. and Berg, R. (2001) Hodgkin's and Non-Hodgkin's Lymphoma of the Head and Neck. *Laryngoscope*, **111**, 1565-1569. http://dx.doi.org/10.1097/00005537-200109000-00013

[7] Erdem, E., Angtuaco, E., Hemert, R., *et al.* (2003) Comprehensive Review of Intracranial Chordoma. *Radiographics*, **23**, 995-1009. http://dx.doi.org/10.1148/rg.234025176

[8] DiFrancesco, L.M., Castillo, C.A.D. and Temple, W.J. (2006) Extra-Axial Chordoma. *Archives of Pathology & Laboratory Medicine*, **130**, 1871-1874.

[9] Masui, K., Kawai, S., Yonezawa, T., *et al.* (2006) Intradural Retroclival Chordoma without Bone Involvement. *Neurologia Medico-Chirurgica* (*Tokyo*), **46**, 552-555. http://dx.doi.org/10.1002/1097-0142(195211)5:6<1170::AID-CNCR2820050613>3.0.CO;2-C

[10] Dahlin, D.C. and MacCharty, C.S. (1952) Chordoma: A Study of 59 Cases. *Cancer*, **5**, 1170-1178. http://dx.doi.org/10.1002/1097-0142(195211)5:6<1170::AID-CNCR2820050613>3.0.CO;2-C

[11] Heffelfinger, M.J., Dahlin, D.C., MacCarty, C.S. and Beabout, J.W. (1973) Chordomas and Cartilaginous Tumors at the Skull Base. *Cancer*, **32**, 410-420. http://dx.doi.org/10.1002/1097-0142(197308)32:2<410::AID-CNCR2820320219>3.0.CO;2-S

[12] McMaster, M.L., Goldstein, A.M., Bromley, C.M., Ishibe, N. and Parry, D.M. (2001) Chordoma: Incidence and Survival Patterns in the United States, 1973-1995. *Cancer Causes Control*, **12**, 1-11. http://dx.doi.org/10.1023/A:1008947301735

[13] Mizerny, B.R. and Kost, K.M. (1995) Chordoma of the Cranial Base: The McGill Experience. *Journal of Otolaryngology*, **24**, 14-19.

[14] Raffel, C., Wright, D.C., Gutin, P.H. and Wilson, C.B. (1985) Cranial Chordomas: Clinical Presentation and Results of Operative and Radiation Therapy in Twenty-Six Patients. *Neurosurgery*, **17**, 703-710. http://dx.doi.org/10.1227/00006123-198511000-00002

[15] Al-Mefty, O. and Borba, L.A. (1997) Skull Base Chordomas: A Management Challenge. *Journal of Neurosurgery*, **86**, 182-189. http://dx.doi.org/10.3171/jns.1997.86.2.0182

[16] Ribbert, H. and Virchow, R. (1959) Chordoma. In: Windeyer, B.W., Ed., *Proceedings of the Royal Society of Medicine*, **52**, 1088-1100.

[17] Castro, J.R., Linstadt, D.E., Bahary, J.P., *et al.* (1994) Experience in Charged Particle Irradiation of Tumors of the Skull Base: 1977-1992. *International Journal of Radiation Oncology, Biology, Physics*, **29**, 647-655. http://dx.doi.org/10.1016/0360-3016(94)90550-9

12

Plexiform Neurofibroma of Nasal Tip

Rajanala Venkata Nataraj, Mohan Jagade, Kartik Parelkar, Reshma Hanawte, Arpita Singhal, Dev Rengaraja, Kiran Kulsange, Kartik Rao, Pallavi Gupta

Department of Ear, Nose & Throat and Head & Neck Surgery, Grant Government Medical College, Mumbai, India

Email: nataraj.rv@gmail.com

Abstract

Neurogenic tumor is the name given to any tumor that arises from the nerve tissue or its coverings. Neurogenic tumors of Sino-nasal cavity are a very rare entity. The most common types are Schwannomas and Neurofibromas and the plexiform subtype is one form of these neuroendocrine tumors. We report the case series of two such cases of a plexiform neurofibroma of the nasal tip, which were excised via an open rhinoplasty approach.

Keywords

Plexiform Neurofibroma, Schwannoma, Nasal Tip, External Nasal Deformity, Open Rhinoplasty

1. Introduction

The first reported cases of external nasal neurogenic tumors were reported by New and Devine in 1947 and Das Gupta *et al.* in 1969 [1] [2]. In these cases, the neuroendocrine tumors were found at alar cartilages and tip of the nose, respectively. In these articles, the terms Neurofibroma and Schwannomas were used synonymously as they were considered to be same clinical entity. In 2007, Rameh *et al.* published an article claiming to report the first case of Solitary Plexiform Neurofibroma of Nasal Tip, which was excised by the method of Open Rhinoplasty [3]. The rest of reported cases of neurogenic tumors of nasal tip have been proven to be Schwannomas.

We hereby report two cases of Solitary Plexiform Neurofibroma of Nasal Tip.

CASE-1. A 18 years old female presented to us, in 2014, with a slowly growing mass over nasal tip since past 9 years. There were no complaints of pain, nasal obstruction or epistaxis. Several courses of antibiotics were tried out with no visible effect. The patient didn't notice any other similar kind of swelling elsewhere on the body. There was no past history of trauma to nose or any form of surgical intervention. Family history was negative for similar complaints.

On examination, a soft, non tender 4 cm × 4 cm mass was seen over the tip and supratip area. The mass was non mobile and fixed to the alar cartilages. Anterior rhinoscopy and diagnostic nasal endoscopy were unremarkable. There was no evidence of café-au-lait spots and any other skin lesions (**Figure 1** and **Figure 2**).

MRI of the mass showed an ill defined mass over the nasal tip which was abutting the alar cartilages (**Figure 3**). The mass was the biopsied and histopathological report was suggestive of neurogenic tumor, most probably neurofibroma.

The patient was then planned for open rhinoplasty and excision of the mass. Intra-operatively a non encapsulated mass was seen adherent to the alar cartilages. Careful dissection was done and mass was excised, without damaging the alar cartilages (**Figure 4**). Immediate post operative pictures were taken which showed markedly improved facial aesthetics. Final histopathology report revealed Plexiform variety of Neurofibroma composed of spindled cells with wavy, darkstaining nuclei and scanty cytoplasm, in a background of wavy collagen fibres, myxoid stroma and mast cells (**Figure 5** & **Figure 6**). Unfortunately patient was lost to follow up, because of personal reasons.

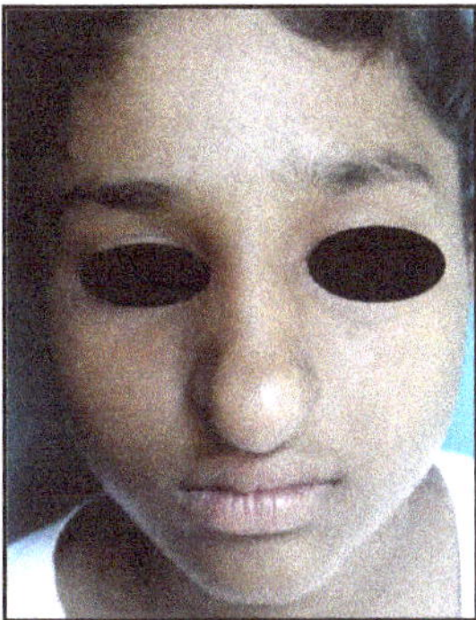

Figure 1. Frontal view.

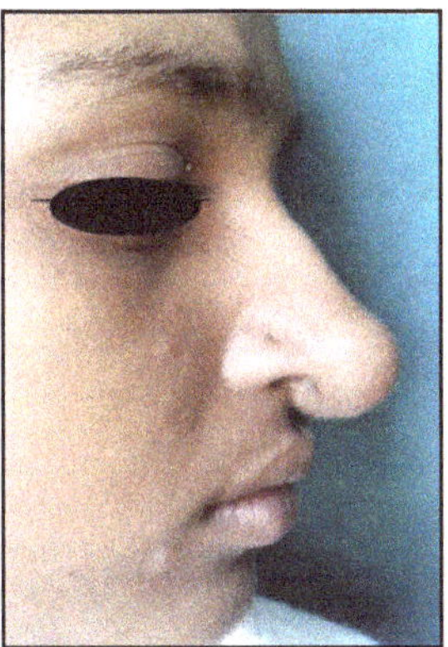

Figure 2. Lateral view.

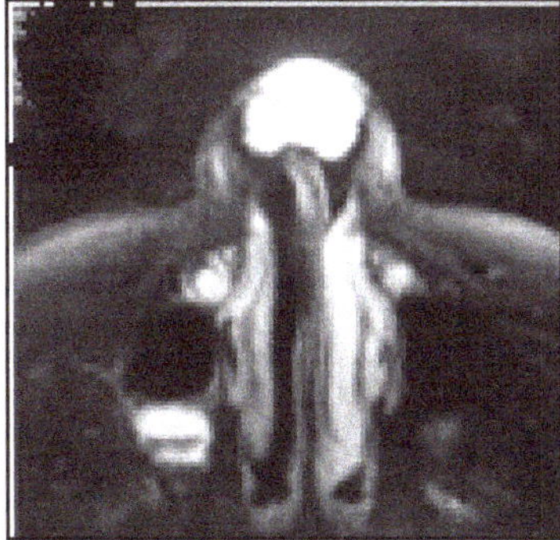

Figure 3. MRI showing hypodense mass lesion involving nasal tip.

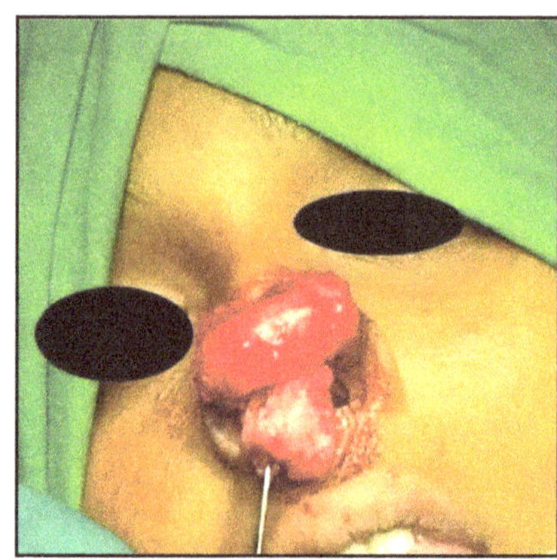

Figure 4. Intraoperative picture.

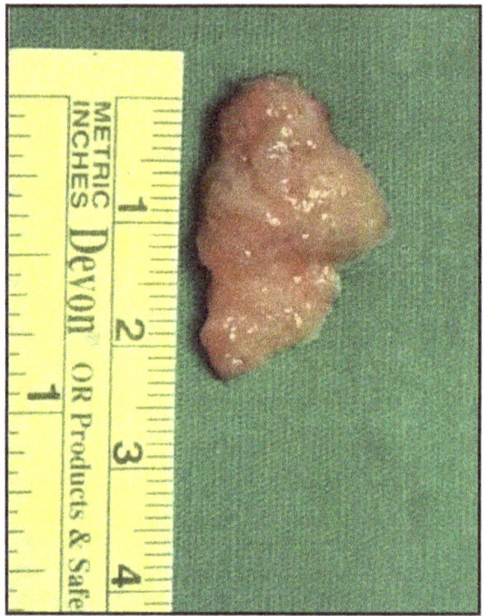

Figure 5. Resected specimen.

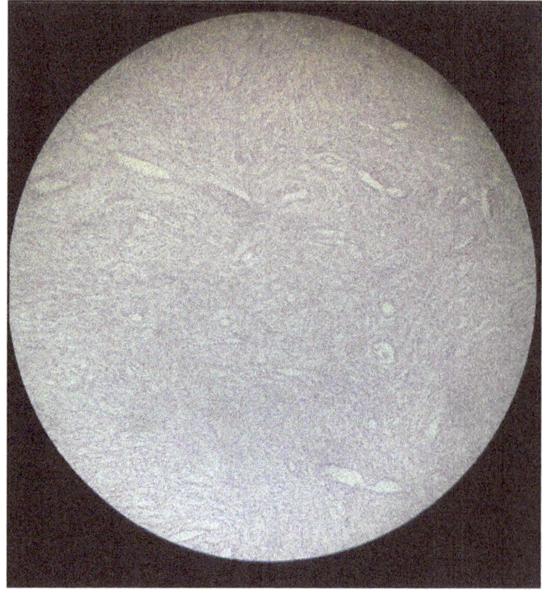

Figure 6. "Wavy" nuclei with bundles of collagen separated by a myxoid, degenerated stroma.

CASE-2. A 23 years old female presented to us in 1996, with complaints of progressive slow growing mass over nasal tip since 15 years. Initially the mass was limited to the nasal tip but had progressed to an extent where the nasal tip had attained a drooped appearance and had crossed the lower lip (**Figure 7** & **Figure 8**). This also led to functional complications in form of bilateral nasal obstruction. Upon palpation the mass was non-tender, firm in consistency and mobile. Alar cartilages were intact but flattened. Anterior rhinoscopy examination revealed columella which was shortened and bent upon itself, collapsed alar cartilages with markedly compromised external nares. Unfortunately the patient did not have enough financial support to undergo MRI at that point of time. The mass was biopsied and was reported as neuroendocrine tumor.

The mass was then excised through an Open Rhinoplasty approach. Post operatively, the aesthetic result was excellent and there was no recurrence even after 1 year (**Figure 9**).

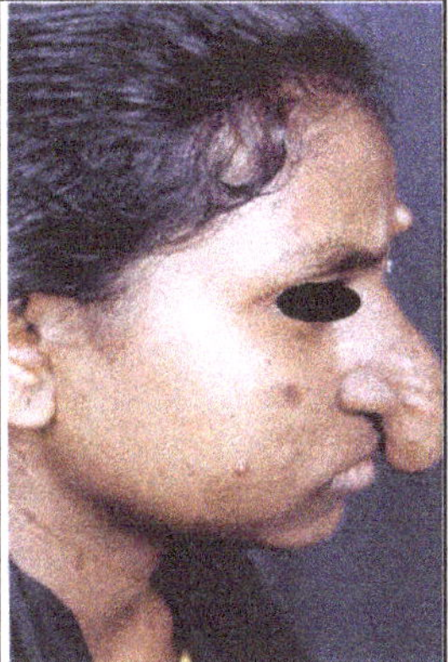

Figure 7. Lateral view.

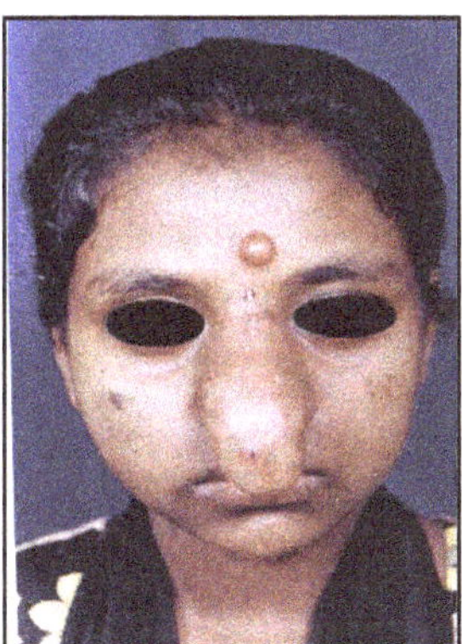

Figure 8. Frontal view.

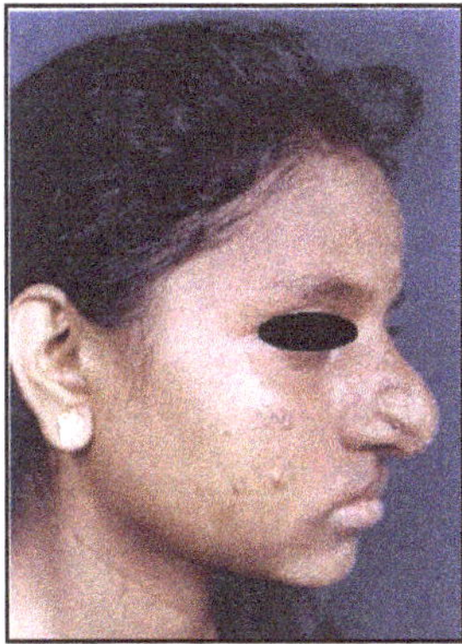

Figure 9. On 1 year follow up.

2. Discussion

Neuroendocrine tumors were first recognized as pathological entities by Verocay *et al.* in 1908 [4]. The benign types include two closely related tumors *viz* Neurilemoma (Schwannoma) and Neurofibroma. Ninety percent of these tumors are benign, around two-thirds being Schwannomas and one-third Neurofibromas [5]. Till late 1960s, these two terms were considered synonymous and were used interchangeably [1] [2]. However, later on, it was discovered that these two tumors have different cells of origin. Schwannomas tend to be encapsulated and contain a more homogenous population of differentiated neoplastic Schwann cells, whereas, Neurofibromas are not encapsulated and composed of a heterogenous cell population of Schwann cells, perineural hybrid cells and intraneural fibroblasts [6] [7]. It is a well established fact that Neurofibromas are associated with Neurofibromatosis or Von Recklinghausen's disease. But our patients didn't have any associated lesions suggestive of Neurofibromatosis.

DasGupta *et al.* stated that benign solitary tumors arising in peripheral nerves can develop in every possible anatomic location [2]. Around one third develop in the head and neck area [8]. Neuroendocrine tumors in head and neck area, particularly nose, usually arise from microscopic branches of various nerves, which makes it very difficult to pin point the nerve of origin.

Neuroendocrine tumors of sino-nasal origin are a very rare occurrence. But amongst the few cases reported, most of the cases were diagnosed as Schwannoma [3].

Radiographically, neurofibromas and schwannomas both show high signal on T2-weighted images and a capsule can be detected around the schwannomas [9]. But a definitive diagnosis, regarding nature of the lesion can only be obtained by histological examination of surgical specimen. Apart from differences in histological appearance, schwannomas show intense immunostaining for S-100, a neural crest marker antigen, while neurofibromas stain less intensely [10].

The only treatment option available is surgical excision. As schwannomas arise from the edge of a nerve and are encapsulated, they can enucleated easily without damaging the nerve [2]. On the other end of the spectrum, plexiform neurofibromas are non-encapsulated diffuse, which makes complete en bloc resection difficult. Furthermore, as the radiosensitivity of these tumors is very low, possibility of recurrence of these tumors is very likely. One favorable feature of such tumors, is that their risk of malignant degeneration is very low, and therefore, unnecessary wide unaesthetic excisions are often not necessary [2].

3. Conclusion

Neuroendocrine tumors of sinonasal tracts are rare. They often present as painless midline swellings and a high degree of suspicion is required for their diagnosis. Plexifrom neurofibroma is non encapsulated and diffuse, which makes it difficult to resect and increases the chances of local recurrence. But due to low rates of malignant transformation, aggressive disfiguring incisions are not required.

References

[1] New, G. and Devine, K. (1947) Neurogenic Tumors of Nose and Throat. *Archives of Otolaryngology*, **46**, 163-179. http://dx.doi.org/10.1001/archotol.1947.00690020172004

[2] DasGupta, T., Brasfield, R., Strong, E. and Hajdu, S. (1969) Benign Solitary Schwannoma (Neurilemomas). *Cancer*, **24**, 355-360. http://dx.doi.org/10.1002/1097-0142(196908)24:2<355::AID-CNCR2820240218>3.0.CO;2-2

[3] Rameh, C., Husseini, S., Tawil, A., Fuleihan, N. and Hadi, U. (2007) Solitary Plexiform Neurofibroma of the Nasal Tip: Case Report and Review of the Literature. *International Journal of Pediatric Otorhinolaryngology Extra*, **2**, 116-119. http://dx.doi.org/10.1016/j.pedex.2007.03.003

[4] Verocay, J. (1908) Multiple Geschwulste als Systemerkrankung am nervosen Apparate. Festschrift fur Chiari, Wien and Leipzig, 378.

[5] Hillstrom, R.P., Zarbo, R.J. and Jacobs, J.R. (1990) Nerve Sheath Tumors of the Paranasal Sinuses: Electron Microscopy and Histopathologic Diagnosis. *Otolaryngology Head and Neck Surgery*, **102**, 257-263.

[6] Berlucchi, M., Piazza, C., Blanzuoli, L., Battaglia, G. and Nicolai, P. (2000) Schwannoma of the Nasal Septum: A Case Report with Review of the Literature. *European Archives of Oto-Rhino-Laryngology*, **257**, 402-405. http://dx.doi.org/10.1007/s004050000242

[7] Ferner, R. and O'Doherty, M. (2000) Neurofibroma and Schwannoma. *Current Opinion in Neurology*, **15**, 679-684. http://dx.doi.org/10.1097/00019052-200212000-00004

[8] Wilson, J., McLaren, K., MdIntyre, M., von Haacke, N. and Maran, A. (1988) Nerve Sheath Tumors of the Head and Neck. *Ear, Nose & Throat Journal*, **67**, 103-110.

[9] Lemmerling, M., Moerman, M., Govaere, F., Praet, M., Kunnen, M. and Vermeersch, H. (1998) Schwannoma of the Tip of the Nose: MRI. *Neuroradiology*, **40**, 264-266. http://dx.doi.org/10.1007/s002340050582

[10] Donnelly, M., Al-Sader, M. and Blayney, A. (1992) View from Beneath: Pathology in Focus, Benign Nasal Schwannoma. *Journal of Laryngology and Otology*, **106**, 1011-1015. http://dx.doi.org/10.1017/S0022215100121644

13

Incidental Finding of an Elongated Styloid Process during Tonsillectomy Procedure

Loay Al-Ekri, Abdulkarim Alsaei

Department of ENT, Head & Neck Surgery, Salmaniya Medical Complex, Manama, Kingdom of Bahrain
Email: loayalekri@gmail.com, asaie@health.gov.bh

Abstract

Patients with recurrent throat pain, dysphagia, or facial pain symptoms might have Eagle's syndrome due to abnormal length of the styloid process or calcification of stylohyoid ligament complex. In adults, the styloid process is approximately 2.5 cm long. The etiology of this disease is not well understood, and usually asymptomatic. In some cases, the styloid tip, which is located between the external and internal carotid arteries, compresses the perivascular sympathetic fibers, resulting in a persistent pain. The disease can be diagnosed by physical examination through digital palpation of the styloid process in the tonsillar fossa or by radiographic workup that includes anterior-posterior and lateral skull films. We report a 33-year-old woman with an incidental finding of an elongated styloid process during a routine tonsillectomy procedure.

Keywords

Elongated Styloid Process, Eagle's Syndrome

1. Introduction

Styloid process (*Processus styloideus*) of the temporal bone is a cylindrical bony projection attached to base of the skull and situated immediately anterior to the stylomastoid foramen. It extends downwards, forwards and slightly medially. From its extremity, the stylohyoid ligament passes downwards and forwards to the lesser horns of the hyoid bone. The process is covered laterally by the parotid gland, and the facial nerve crosses its base, while the tip is situated between the internal and external carotid arteries, laterally from the pharyngeal wall and immediately behind the tonsil fossa. The anterior surface of the styloid gives origin to styloglossus muscle and its tip to stylohyoid muscle. On its deep surface, the process is separated from internal jugular vein by the origin of stylopharyngeus muscle [1].

Styloid process is derived from the second branchial arch of Reichert's cartilage and is part of the stylohyoid complex along with the lesser horns of hyoid bone and stylohyoid ligament. In adults, the styloid process is normally composed of dense connective tissue, but may retain its embryonic cartilage and the potential for ossification [2].

The length of the styloid process is usually 2 - 3 cm. When it is more than 3 cm, it is called as an elongated styloid process. This elongation was first described in 1937 by Eagle who defined "stylalgia" as pain associated with abnormal length of the styloid process and later called the Eagle's syndrome [3].

Elongation of the process may cause various clinical symptoms as neck and cervico-facial pain. Patients most often complain of pain, a sensation of foreign body or fish bone in the pharynx, and odynophagia. Clinically, hardness can occasionally be felt in the tonsillar fossa which is painful on palpation. If the styloid process causes pressure on the area of the carotid arteries, the symptoms are more complicated. The patient may record buzzing in the ears, headache around the orbit, or pain during head movement. [4]

The incidence of the elongated styloid process was determined around 4% - 7%, and revealed a female dominance. Out of these people, only 4% - 10% of them are symptomatic. The mean length of the styloid processes of the subjects reporting Eagle's syndrome was about 40 mm [5]. Some reports have described that it is the abnormal anterior angulation rather than elongation that is responsible for the symptoms [6].

2. Case Report

A 33-year-old Bahraini lady with a chronic history of recurrent attacks of tonsillo-pharyngitis and a persistent sensation of sore throat and odynophagia of more than 2 years' duration. There was no history of localized facial or neck pain, or foreign body sensation. She was booked for a routine tonsillectomy procedure. After a complete removal of both tonsils by cold dissection method and control of bleeding by electro cautery, an elongated apparent styloid process was noticed in the bed of the right tonsillar fossa, while the left side showed a slight bulge behind the superior constrictor muscle (**Figure 1**).

The patient was doing fine post operatively on intravenous hydration and medication and well tolerating her post tonsillectomy pain. She was kept in hospital for 3 days with no record of bleeding. About a week after the surgery, a regular follow up visit to ENT clinic showed an almost complete healing of both tonsillar fossae, with the apparent styloid process hidden behind the anterior pillar of the right side. Apart from the usual post Ty pain, the patient reported some localized symptoms of throat pain on the right side of the neck 'stylalgia'. On the following weeks of a routine follow-up visit, the patient reported no further symptoms of odynophagia, or cervico-facial pain.

Looking back through the patient's history of investigations, previous plain x-ray films have confirmed the diagnosis of a unilateral right sided elongated styloid process. It showed that the right styloid process was longer and thicker, measuring about 3.3 cm long, while the left one measured about 2.7 cm long (**Figure 2** and **Figure 3**).

3. Discussion

Eagle syndrome is characterized by recurrent pain in the head and neck region due to an elongated styloid process or calcified stylohyoid ligament. In his classic description, Eagle defined two clinical features caused by elongated styloid process. The classical stylohyoid syndrome which is almost invariable occurs after tonsillectomy.

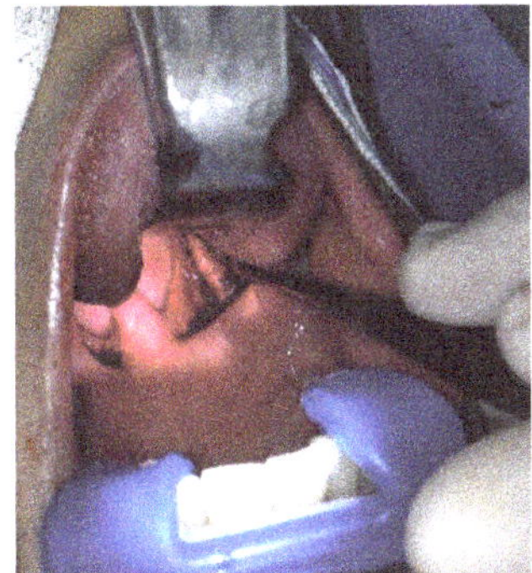
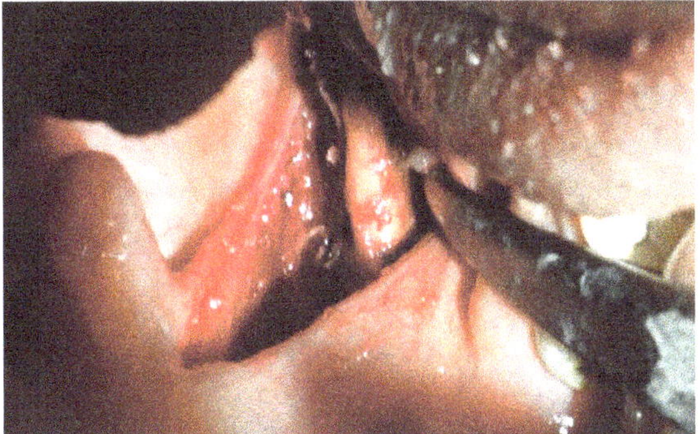

Figure 1. Intra-op pictures showing exposed elongated styloid process in the right tonsillar fossa.

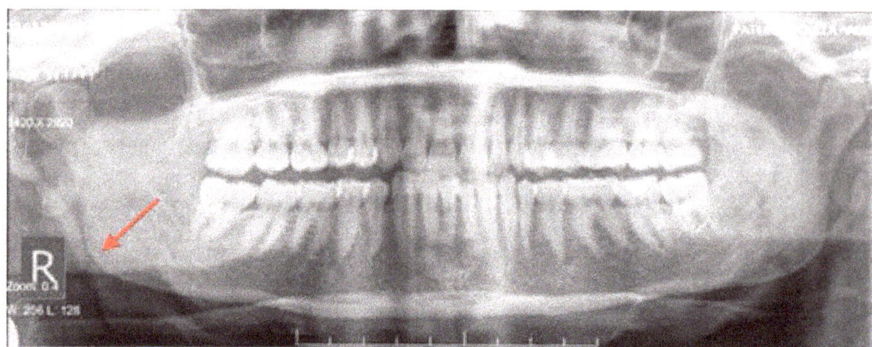

Figure 2. Orthopantomogram (OPG) showing a right-sided unilateral elongated styloid process (red arrow).

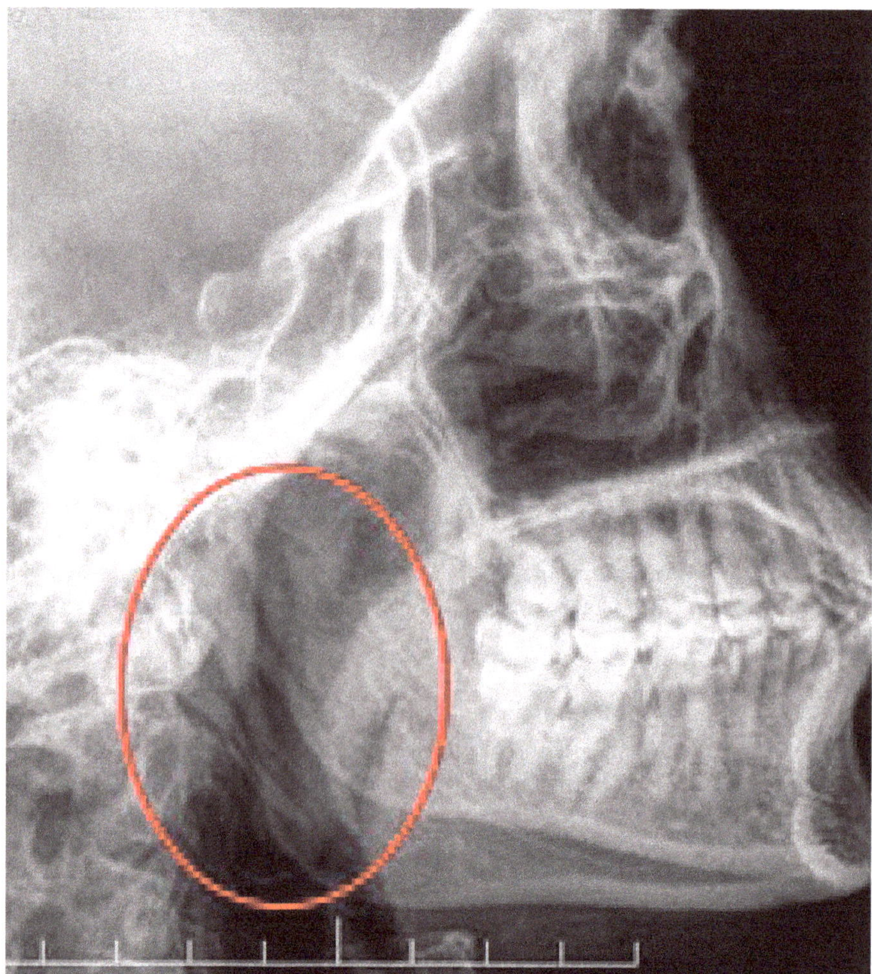

Figure 3. Lateral neck X-ray showing a unilateral elongated styloid process, the (red circle) clearly shows the difference in length between the two styloid processes.

It usually presents with a dull ache in the lateral pharyngeal wall and ipsilateral ear. This pain classically starts during the first week following tonsillectomy and remains at the same intensity level thereafter. The stylocarotid syndrome develops spontaneously, and is associated with cervical, ocular and facial pain, due to irritation of the area around the carotid artery [7] [8].

It is a rare condition and most of the patients may be asymptomatic; however, when these ossified structures exert pressure on the various structures in the head and neck, there can be a wide range of symptoms, including pharyngeal discomfort, painful neck movements, change in voice, painful tongue movements, increased secretion of saliva, otalgia, and headache [9].

Eagle also defined the length of a normal styloid process at 2.5 - 3.0 cm. The cause of this elongation of the styloid process is not well understood. It can be idiopathic, congenital (due to the persistence of cartilaginous elements of precursors of the styloid process), or acquired (due to the proliferation of osseous tissue at the insertion of the stylohyoid ligament).

An elongated styloid process occurs in about 4% of the general population, while only small percentages (between 4% and 10%) of these patients are symptomatic. In fact, the number of reported cases is underestimated because it is an incidental finding in radiographs. Diagnosis is supported by description of symptoms by patients, previous history of any cervical trauma and tonsillectomy, physical examination, and radiographs [10].

The symptoms have varied pathophysiological explanations, for example, symptoms may be due to: 1) fracture of the styloid process leading to granulation tissue and pressure on the surrounding structures; 2) compression of adjacent nerves, e.g., the glossopharyngeal, the lower branch of the trigeminal, or the chorda tympani; 3) degenerative and inflammatory changes at the tendinous portion of the stylohyoid insertion; 4) irritation of the pharyngeal mucosa due to direct compression, or post-tonsillectomy scarring involving the cranial nerves V, VII, IX, and X; 5) impingement of the carotid vessels with irritation of the sympathetic nerves in the arterial sheath [11].

Radiographs of the skull, both antero-posterior and lateral views, can reveal the elongated styloid process, but the superimposition of various other structures often makes diagnosis difficult. The development of three-dimensional CT (3D CT) has made it easier to delineate the anatomy of the surrounding structures. 3D CT is of great help when surgical correction is planned [12].

Surgical resection of elongated styloid process is the primary treatment for Eagle's syndrome. Even though medical treatment using analgesic or local steroid injection is an option, the condition is not yet proven to be well treated or resolved. There are two surgical methods that have been suggested: transoral and external transcervical approaches. Transoral resection, as described by Eagle, is technically easier. The protuberance of styloid process is identified and overlying mucosa is incised. Dissection over the superior constrictor muscle is performed to expose the tip and skeletonization is done until its origin. The ligaments and muscle tendons attached to it are separated and the free process is resected using bone nibbler as near as possible to its base. Then, muscles and mucosa over the surgical bed are closed in layers. Surgical failure rate is around 20% by means of partial relief of or recurrence of symptoms and can be due to inadequate shortening leading to constant irritation [13].

In review of the literature, we did not come across a similar report of an incidental finding of elongated styloid process while performing tonsillectomy. In fact, this case had brought an interesting scientific debate and discussion in the department of otolaryngology, head and neck surgery in regards to what should have been done for this patient and others if such a finding was encountered during a routine tonsillectomy. Should the elongated styloid process be excised and removed from the bed of the tonsillar fossa at the same time, to minimize the risk of eagle syndrome? Or should we leave it untouched and follow up the patient over a period of time to observe for the development of stylalgia? It will be very interesting to hear from other people and listen to their experience in managing asymptomatic elongation of the styloid process.

Conflicts of Interest

The authors declare no conflicts of interest or funding sources.

Consent to Publish

The patient was verbally consented and agreed to write a case report about her condition and accepted to publish it for educational and scientific purposes.

References

[1] Gray, H. (1918) Anatomy of the Human Body, the Temporal Bone.

[2] Kolagi, S.I. (2010) Elongated Styloid Process—Report of Two Rare Cases. *International Journal of Anatomical Varia-*

tions, **3**, 100-102.

[3] Eagle, W.W. (1937) Elongated Styloid Process: Report of Two Cases. *Archives of Otolaryngology*, **25**, 584-587. http://dx.doi.org/10.1001/archotol.1937.00650010656008

[4] Sandev, S. and Sokler, K. (2000) Styloid Process Syndrome. *ActaStomat Croat*, **34**, 451-456.

[5] Balcioglu, H.A., Kilic, C., Akyol, M., Ozan, H. and Folia, K.G. (2009) Length of the Styloid Process and Anatomical Implications for Eagle's Syndrome. *Folia Morphologica*, **68**, 265-270.

[6] Yavuz, H., Caylakli, F., Yildirlm, T. and Ozluoglu, L.N. (2008) Angulation of the styloid Process in Eagle's Syndrome. *European Archives of Oto-Rhino-Laryngology*, **265**, 1393-1396. http://dx.doi.org/10.1007/s00405-008-0686-9

[7] Eagle, W.W. (1948) Elongated Styloid Process: Further Observations and a New Syndrome. *Archives of Otolaryngology*, **47**, 630-640. http://dx.doi.org/10.1001/archotol.1948.00690030654006

[8] Eagle, W.W. (1958) Elongated Styloid Process, Symptoms and Treatment. *JAMA Otolaryngology—Head & Neck Surgery*, **67**, 172-176. http://dx.doi.org/10.1001/archotol.1958.00730010178007

[9] Rechtweg, J.S. and Wax, M.K. (1998) Eagle's Syndrome: A Review. *American Journal of Otolaryngology*, **19**, 316-321. http://dx.doi.org/10.1016/S0196-0709(98)90005-9

[10] Sadaksharam, J. and Singh, K. (2012) Stylocarotid Syndrome: An Unusual Case Report. *Contemporary Clinical Dentisity*, **3**, 503-506. http://dx.doi.org/10.4103/0976-237X.107456

[11] Murtagh, R.D., Caracciolo, J.T. and Fernandez, G. (2001) CT Findings Associated with Eagle Syndrome. *American Journal of Neuroradiology*, **22**, 1401-1402.

[12] Raina, D., Gothi, R. and Rajan, S. (2009) Eagle Syndrome. *Indian Journal of Radiology Imaging*, **19**, 107-108. http://dx.doi.org/10.4103/0971-3026.50826

[13] Baharudin, A., Rohaida, I. and Khairudin, A. (2012) Transoral Surgical Resection of Bilateral Styloid Processes Elongation (Eagle's Syndrome). *Acta Informatica Medica*, **20**, 133-135. http://dx.doi.org/10.5455/aim.2012.20.133-135

14

The Treatment of Peripheral Vestibular Dysfunction Using Caloric Vestibular Stimulation in Patients with Cerebral Hypertensive Crisis

Yana Yuriyvna Gomza[1], Ralph Mösges[2*]

[1]Otorhinolaryngology Department, National O.O. Bogomolets Medical University, Kiev, Ukraine
[2]Institute of Medical Statistics, Informatics and Epidemiology, University Hospital of Cologne, Cologne, Germany
Email: [*]ralph@moesges.de

Abstract

Background: To verify the efficacy of caloric vestibular stimulation in patients with peripheral vestibular dysfunction after cerebral hypertensive crisis. Methods: Enrolled in the study were 60 patients with peripheral vestibular dysfunction caused by a cerebral hypertensive crisis, documented by vestibulometry. Thirty patients underwent standard treatment plus caloric vestibular stimulation, and 30 control group patients received standard treatment alone. Results: After the two-week treatment course, the sensation of vertigo was observed in 40.0% ± 8.9% of treatment group patients compared with 80.0% ± 7.3% of control group patients ($t = 3.46$; $p < 0.001$). Spontaneous vestibular somatic reactions were found in 46.7% ± 9.1% of the study treatment group in contrast to 86.7% ± 6.2% of the control group ($t = 3.63$; $p < 0.001$). Spontaneous nystagmus was seen in 40.0% ± 8.9% of treatment group patients compared with 93.3% ± 4.6% of control subjects ($t = 5.31$; $p < 0.001$). Spontaneous vestibular vegetative reactions were observed in 33.3% ± 8.6% of patients receiving study treatment in contrast to 93.3% ± 4.6% of control group patients ($t = 6.16$; $p < 0.001$). Also, 53.3% ± 9.1% of study treatment group patients showed asymmetry of labyrinths compared with 86.7% ± 6.2% of patients from the control group ($t = 3.03$; $p < 0.001$). Conclusion: Caloric vestibular stimulation was shown to be an effective treatment for peripheral vestibular dysfunction in patients with cerebral hypertensive crisis. During the 14-day treatment of cerebral hypertensive crisis, complete labyrinthine function recovery occurred in 46.7% of treatment group patients who underwent caloric vestibular stimulation as opposed to 13.3% of control group patients who received standard treatment alone.

[*]Corresponding author.

Keywords

Peripheral Vestibular Dysfunction, Cerebral Hypertensive Crisis, Labyrinthine Function

1. Introduction

Cerebral hypertensive crisis constitutes one of the most frequent cerebrovascular diseases, comprises 13% - 15% of all acute brain vascular disorders, and is found in two-thirds of patients with transient vascular disorders of the brain. Patients affected by it most often complain of headache accompanied by nausea, vomiting, and episodes of unconsciousness. Vestibular dysfunction in general is one of the earliest and most frequent manifestations, having different cerebrovascular pathologies. The early phylogenetic formation of the vestibular system makes it highly sensitive to external and pathogenic influences. Hearing impairment has also been observed in such patients. The inner ear consists of the hearing organ, the cochlea, which is joined topographically, anatomically, and functionally to the vestibular apparatus (vestibule and semicircular channels) [1]-[16].

Caloric vestibular stimulation (CVS) has traditionally been used as a tool for neurological diagnosis. It is a routine diagnostic technique applied in the neurological assessment of vestibular function and brain death [17]-[22]. However, CVS has also been applied effectively in the treatment of patients with certain neurological disorders [20] [22]-[32].

The aim of this randomized, controlled study was to verify the efficacy of CVS in patients with peripheral vestibular dysfunction after cerebral hypertensive crisis.

2. Material and Methods

Sixty patients with peripheral vestibular dysfunction after cerebral hypertensive crisis were randomized into two patient groups. The study treatment group results were compared with those of the control group. Patients received inpatient treatment with CVS in the Otorhinolaryngology Department and the Neurology Department of the National O.O. Bogomolets Medical University, Ukraine. The trial study was provided as a part of scientific work of the Otorhinolaryngology Department of Bogomolets National Medical University, registration number 0113U007334. The study took place from March 2012 to September 2013 and was approved by the local ethics committee. Each participant signed an informed consent form.

The study treatment group comprised 30 patients aged 29 to 57 years, the average age being 47 ± 1 years. Sixteen patients were female and 14 were male. The average duration of disease prior to study enrollment was 6 ± 1 days. The control group included 30 patients who were 29 to 59 years old, the average age being 47 ± 2 years. Nineteen patients were female and 11 were male. The average duration of disease prior to study enrollment was 6 ± 1 days. All patients were subjected to an obligatory general clinical examination which included endoscopy. Only patients with no history of pathological changes to otorhinolaryngological organs were included in the investigation. All examined patients exhibited increased arterial pressure during cerebral hypertensive crisis, with an average systolic arterial pressure level of 169 ± 6 mm Hg. Neurologists applied the following brain hemodynamic examination methods to determine the main diagnosis of cerebral hypertensive crisis: rheoencephalography, electroencephalography, transcranial Doppler ultrasonography, nuclear magnetic resonance (NMR) imaging of the brain, and brain spiral computer tomography.

Vestibulometric examinations were conducted in the Otorhinolaryngology Department at the National O.O. Bogomolets Medical University, Ukraine. Such examinations were repeated in the study treatment group of 30 patients two weeks after beginning CVS. Patients from both groups also received standard medical therapy for cerebral hypertensive crisis. The study treatment group results were compared with the results of 30 control group patients who did not receive CVS, but instead underwent only standard therapy for cerebral hypertensive crisis.

The CVS method included external ear channel irrigation using 60 ml of cold water at 25°C for 10 s once daily over a course of 10 days.

Instrumental methods, *i.e.*, the methods of vestibular examination, consisted of: walking tests (walking along a path; flanking walk), Fukuda writing test, Fukuda stepping test, past-pointing test, finger-nose test, cephalography (the method of evaluating the quantity evaluation of balance, when a stationary apparatus is fixed at the patient's head and registers imbalance by calculating the cephalography index (the higher the index, the higher the level of imbalance)), Barany's rotating chair test, vestibular illusion of counterrotation test, caloric test, and electronystagmography (the study of spontaneous, positional nystagmus).

The statistical analysis was carried out using the statistics program SPSS 16.0. The results for the sensation of vertigo, spontaneous vestibular somatic reactions, spontaneous nystagmus, spontaneous vestibular vegetative reactions, and asymmetry of labyrinths were described using the following statistical parameters: mean, standard deviation, confidence interval 95%, median, 25th and 75th percentiles. The difference in the outcomes between the treatment groups was found to be significant using the Student's t-test ($p < 0.01$). The regressive analysis of the X and Y variables resulted in the linear dependency $Y \sim B*X$, where X and Y are the certain variables and B is the certain real number.

3. Results

Before treatment, the sensation of vertigo was recorded in 100% of the examined patients from both groups. Patients described the sensation of objects rotating around them or the sensation of their body rotating in one definite direction. During the antirotative vestibular illusion test, the average reaction period lasted 24 ± 3 s in the study treatment group and 25 ± 4 s in the control group. Under the vestibular illusion of counterrotation test, reaction period asymmetry was registered in 14 (46.6%) patients from the study treatment group and 15 (50.0%) from the control group.

The sensation of vertigo was noted after treatment in 12 (40.0%) patients from the study treatment group compared to 24 (80.0%) patients from the control group. The average reaction period under the antirotative vestibular illusion test lasted 18 ± 10 s in the study treatment group and 23 ± 9 s in the control group. Reaction period asymmetry under the vestibular illusion of counterrotation test persisted in 5 (16.6%) patients from the study treatment group and 10 (33.3%) from the control group.

Prior to treatment, all patients from both groups exhibited balance disturbances in the walking tests, Fukuda writing test, Fukuda stepping test, past-pointing test, finger-nose test, and in cephalography. During the Fukuda stepping test, imbalance manifesting as rectilinear body movement was observed in all patients, with the average value being 149 ± 14 cm in the study treatment group and 146 ± 16 cm in the control group. Imbalance in the form of body rotation was observed in all patients, with an average value of 92° ± 12° in the study treatment group and 91° ± 14° in the control group.

Spontaneous vestibular somatic reactions were observed in 14 (46.7%) patients after undergoing CVS as compared to 26 (86.7%) control group patients. The average pathologic deviation obtained in the Fukuda stepping test was 112 ± 12 cm in the study treatment group and 123 ± 12 cm in the control group. During this test, an abnormal body rotation angle was observed in the patients, with an average value of 45° ± 14° in the study treatment group and 62° ± 12° in the control group.

Before treatment, all patients from both groups showed significant vestibular somatic reactions, such as the appearance of spontaneous, positional nystagmus, which were recorded via electronystagmography. Visually determined spontaneous nystagmus was observed in 29 (96.6%) patients from the study treatment group. In 20 (66.6%) of these patients, it was horizontal and of the first stage of intensity, and in 9 (30.0%) patients the nystagmus was horizontal, of middle-level amplitude, and of the second stage of intensity. After conducting electronystagmography, spontaneous nystagmus was diagnosed in all patients from both groups. Positional nystagmus was also documented in all patients. Positional nystagmus combined with nonpermanent dizziness affected by moving or shaking the head was registered in 6 (20.0%) of the patients receiving study treatment. Irregular, unstable positional nystagmus was recorded in 24 (80.0%) study treatment patients.

Spontaneous and positional nystagmus was observed in 12 (40.0%) patients receiving study treatment compared to 28 (93.3%) control group patients after treatment.

Vestibular vegetative reactions were observed before treatment in all patients from both groups in all irritative tests: Barany's rotating chair test, vestibular illusion of counterrotation test, and caloric test. Spontaneous vestibular vegetative reactions were observed in 10 (33.3%) patients from the study treatment group after applying CVS and in 28 (93.3%) patients from the control group.

Before treatment, the reaction period asymmetry under Barany's test was documented in 15 (50.0%) patients from the study treatment group, with an average reaction period of 9 ± 1 s, and in 15 (50.0%) control group patients, with an average reaction period of 8 ± 1 s. After treatment, the reaction period asymmetry under Barany's test was registered in 8 (26.6%) patients from the study treatment group, with the average duration of Barany's reaction period being 16 ± 1 s, and in 12 (50.0%) patients from the control group, with the average duration of Barany's reaction period being 12 ± 1 s.

The most informative method of determining inner ear function was the caloric reflex test (*i.e.*, CVS) because it permitted examinations of the ears separately. Patients in the study treatment group received cold (25°C) and warm (39°C) irrigation courses of the external ear channels.

During the experimental nystagmus examination under load reactions in the caloric reflex test (*i.e.*, CVS), asymmetry of the labyrinths was shown to exist in all cases before treatment. Hyperreflection of the labyrinths was observed in 10 (33.3%) patients from the study treatment group and in 9 (30.0%) patients from the control group. Hyporeflection was seen in the other 20 (66.6%) study treatment patients and in 21 (70.0%) control group patients.

Labyrinthine function returned to normal after CVS. Asymmetry of the labyrinths was observed in 16 (53.3%) patients in the study treatment group and in 26 (86.7%) patients in the control group. Hyperreflection of the labyrinths was present in 5 (16.7%) patients from the study treatment group and in 8 (26.7%) patients from the control group. Hyporeflection was seen in another 11 (36.7%) treatment group patients and in 18 (60.0%) control group patients.

In patients with vestibular dysfunction after cerebral hypertensive crisis, the results from the vestibular apparatus function examination of patients who had undergone two weeks of CVS showed significant improvement in the indices of all vestibulometric tests compared to the results of the control group patients.

The sensation of vertigo, spontaneous vestibular somatic reactions, spontaneous nystagmus, spontaneous vestibular vegetative reactions, and asymmetry of the labyrinths were the main indices of vestibulometry, which was used to determine the vestibular function of the labyrinths (**Table 1**).

Thus, the sensation of vertigo was observed in 40.0% ± 8.9% of patients from the study treatment group compared to 80.0% ± 7.3% of patients from the control group ($t = 3.46$; $t > 3$; $p \leq 0.001$). Spontaneous vestibular somatic reactions were reported in 46.7% ± 9.1% of patients from the study treatment group compared to 86.7% ± 6.2% of control group patients ($t = 3.63$; $t > 3$; $p \leq 0.001$). Spontaneous nystagmus was documented in 40.0% ± 8.9% of patients from the study treatment group in comparison to 93.3% ± 4.6% of control group patients ($t = 5.31$; $t > 3$; $p \leq 0.001$). Spontaneous vestibular vegetative reactions were seen in 33.3% ± 8.6% of patients receiving the study treatment in contrast to 93.3% ± 4.6% of patients from the control group ($t = 6.16$; $t > 3$; $p \leq 0.001$). Asymmetry of the labyrinths was reported in 53.3% ± 9.1% of patients from the study treatment group compared to 86.7% ± 6.2% of patients from the control group ($t = 3.03$; $t > 3$; $p \leq 0.001$). Thus, an absence of inner ear dysfunction was documented in 46.7% ± 9.1% of study treatment group patients compared to 13.3% ± 6.2% of control group patients ($t = 3.03$; $t > 3$; $p \leq 0.001$).

4. Discussion

After analyzing the results, we agree with other authors about the effects of CVS in a wide range of contexts in

Table 1. Main indices of vestibulometry after two-week application of caloric vestibular stimulation or standard therapy.

Indices of vestibulometry	Percentage of patients with disorder, P		Disparity P1 - P2*	p1*	p2*	t*	p-value
	Study treatment group	Control group					
Sensation of vertigo	40.0	80.0	40.0	8.9	7.3	3.46	<0.001
Spontaneous vestibular somatic reactions	46.7	86.7	40.0	9.1	6.2	3.63	<0.001
Spontaneous nystagmus	40.0	93.3	53.3	8.9	4.6	5.31	<0.001
Spontaneous vestibular vegetative reactions	33.3	93.3	60.0	8.6	4.6	6.16	<0.001
Asymmetry of labyrinths	53.3	86.7	33.4	9.1	6.2	3.03	<0.001
Absence of inner ear dysfunction	**46.7**	**13.3**	**33.4**	**9.1**	**6.2**	**3.03**	**<0.001**

***P1:** Percentage of study treatment group of patients with vestibular dysfunction in cerebral hypertensive crisis after the two-week application of CVS. **P2:** Percentage of control group of patients with vestibular dysfunction in cerebral hypertensive crisis after the two-week application of standard therapy. **p1:** Mean error of P1. **p2:** Mean error of P2. **t:** Reliability criterion.

the cognitive and clinical neurosciences [20] [24]-[26] [29]-[35]. CVS represents a unique experimental method for use in neurophilosophical studies. Its reported phenomenological effects are of great interest for the study of brain activity, which is important to better understand the activation processes of brain structures [4] [20] [36]. However, after analyzing the results of treatment with CVS, we also observed the effective improvement of labyrinthine function in patients with vestibular dysfunction after cerebral hypertensive crisis: the vestibular apparatus (receptor organ) and the central vestibular pathway function were repaired. Labyrinthine asymmetry was present in 53.3% ± 9.1% of patients who had undergone CVS as opposed to 86.7% ± 6.2% of patients who had received standard therapy alone. The results of the investigation described here showed that CVS effectively improved labyrinthine function in patients with vestibular dysfunction after cerebral hypertensive crisis.

The mechanism by which peripheral labyrinthine function improved after CVS may be explained as the result of the activation of the entire vestibular apparatus, *i.e.*, the inverse response of the brain to the irritated peripheral receptors. It seems reasonable to presume that vestibular stimulation leads to the interaction between the somatosensory system and the vestibular apparatus [33] [34] [37]-[41]. It is necessary to mention that all this has given rise to considerable controversy, as it is a hypothesis and is still being studied. We agree with other authors who maintain that the routine application of CVS would provide, at least in theory, a more complete assessment of the inner ear and brain processes [20]. It would be of great interest and possibly open new perspectives in the field if investigators also applied this or other CVS methods in future studies.

5. Conclusion

Caloric vestibular stimulation was observed to be an effective treatment for peripheral vestibular dysfunction in patients with cerebral hypertensive crisis. This treatment method resulted in the complete recovery of labyrinthine function in almost half of all patients (46.7%) who received it. In contrast, only 4 out of 30 (13.3%) patients who underwent standard therapy experienced complete recovery of labyrinthine function. Our study results suggest that caloric vestibular stimulation should be prescribed to all patients with peripheral vestibular dysfunction after cerebral hypertensive crisis.

Acknowledgements

We would like to thank Gena Kittel and Marie-Josefine Joisten for their editorial assistance.

References

[1] Benoudiba, F., Toulgoat, F. and Sarrazin, J.L. (2013) The Vestibulocochlear Nerve (VIII). *Diagnostic and Interventional Imaging*, **94**, 1043-1050. http://dx.doi.org/10.1016/j.diii.2013.08.015.

[2] Fujita, N., Yamanaka, T. and Hosoi, H. (2002) Usefulness of MR Angiography in Cases of Central Vertigo. *Auris Nasus Larynx*, **29**, 247-252. http://dx.doi.org/10.1016/S0385-8146(02)00016-0.

[3] Gacek, R.R. (2008) A Place Principle for Vertigo. *Auris Nasus Larynx*, **35**, 1-10. http://dx.doi.org/10.1016/j.anl.2007.04.002.

[4] Goycoolea, M., Mena, I. and Neubauer, S. (2009) Is There a Difference in Activation or in Inhibition of Cortical Auditory Centers Depending on the Ear That Is Stimulated? *Acta Oto-Laryngologica*, **129**, 348-353. http://dx.doi.org/10.1080/00016480802495420.

[5] Kandel, E.R., Schwartz, J.H. and Jessell, T.M. (2000) Principles of Neuroscience. 4th Edition, McGraw-Hill, New York, 591-624.

[6] Koyuncu, M., Elhami, A.R., Alkan, H., Sahin, M., Basoglu, T. and Simsek, M. (2001) Investigation of the Vertebrobasilar Arterial System in Vertigo by Vestibulocochlear Test, SPECT and Angiography. *Auris Nasus Larynx*, **28**, 23-28. http://dx.doi.org/10.1016/S0385-8146(00)00068-7.

[7] Lamontagne, A., Paquet, N. and Fung, J. (2003) Postural Adjustments to Voluntary Head Monitoring during Standing Are Modified Following Stroke. *Clinical Biomechanics*, **18**, 832-842. http://dx.doi.org/10.1016/S0268-0033(03)00141-4.

[8] Lee, H. and Baloh, R.W. (2005) Sudden Deafness in Vertebrobasilar Ischemia: Clinical Features, Vascular Topographical Patterns and Long-Term Outcome. *Journal of the Neurological Sciences*, **228**, 99-104. http://dx.doi.org/10.1016/j.jns.2004.10.016.

[9] Lonsbury-Martin, B.L., Martin, G.K. and Coats, A.C. (1985) The Physiology of the Auditory and Vestibular Systems. In: Ballenger, J.J., Ed., *Diseases of the Nose, Throat, Ear, Head and Neck*, 13th Edition, Lea and Febiger, Philadelphia,

952-954.

[10] Mills, J.H., Khariwala, S.S. and Weber, P.C. (2006) Anatomy and Physiology of Hearing. In: Bailey, B.J., Johnson, J.T. and Newlands, S.D., Eds., *Head & Neck Surgery*: *Otolaryngology*, 4th Edition, Vol. 2, Lippincott Williams & Wilkins, Philadelphia, 1883-1903.

[11] Nakamichi, R., Yamazaki, M., Ikeda, M., Isoda, H., Kawai, H., Sone, M., *et al.* (2013) Establishing Normal Diameter Range of the Cochlear and Facial Nerves with 3D-CISS at 3T. *Magnetic Resonance in Medical Sciences*, **12**, 241-247. http://dx.doi.org/10.2463/mrms.2013-0004

[12] Pagarkar, W. and Davies, R. (2004) Dizziness. *Medicine*, **32**, 18-23. http://dx.doi.org/10.1383/medc.32.9.18.49908

[13] Pollak, L., Kushnir, M. and Stryjer, R. (2006) Diagnostic Value of Vestibular Evoked Myogenic Potentials in Cerebellar and Lower-Brainstem Strokes. *Neurophysiologie Clinique*, **36**, 227-233. http://dx.doi.org/10.1016/j.neucli.2006.08.014

[14] Sooy, C.D. and Boles, R. (1980) Neuroanatomy for the Otolaryngologist-Head Neck Surgeon. In: Paparella, M.M., Shunrick, D.A., Gluckman, J.L. and Meyerhoff, W.L., Eds., *Otolaryngology*, 2nd Edition, Vol. I, W.B. Saunders Company, Philadelphia, 151-154.

[15] Tóth, M. and Csillag, A. (2005) The Organ of Hearing and Equilibrium. In: Cillag, A., Ed., *Atlas of the Sensory Organs*: *Functional and Clinical Anatomy*, Humana Press, Totowa, 1-83. http://dx.doi.org/10.1385/1-59259-849-8:001

[16] Yamasoba, T., Kikuchi, S. and Higo, R. (2001) Deafness Associated with Vertebrobasilar Insufficiency. *Journal of the Neurological Sciences*, **187**, 69-75. http://dx.doi.org/10.1016/S0022-510X(01)00525-1

[17] Albernaz, P.L.M. and Ganança, M.M. (1972) The Use of Air in Vestibular Caloric Stimulation. *The Laryngoscope*, **82**, 2198-2203. http://dx.doi.org/10.1288/00005537-197212000-00008

[18] Fasold, O., Von Brevern, M., Kuhberg, M., Ploner, C.J., Villringer, A., Lempert, T. *et al.* (2002) Human Vestibular Cortex as Identified with Caloric Stimulation in Functional Magnetic Resonance Imaging. *Neuroimage*, **17**, 1384-1393. http://dx.doi.org/10.1006/nimg.2002.1241

[19] Fire, T.D., Tusa, R.J., Furman, J.M., Zee, D.S., Frohman, E., Baloh, R.W., *et al.* (2000) Assessment: Vestibular Testing Techniques in Adults and Children: Report of the Therapeutics and Technology Assessment. Subcommittee of the American Academy of Neurology. *Neurology*, **55**, 1431-1441. http://dx.doi.org/10.1212/WNL.55.10.1431

[20] Miller, S.M. and Ngo, T.T. (2007) Studies of Caloric Vestibular Stimulation: Implications for the Cognitive Neurosciences, the Clinical Neurosciences and Neurophilosophy. *Acta Neuropsychiatrica*, **19**, 183-203. http://dx.doi.org/10.1111/j.1601-5215.2007.00208.x

[21] (1995) Practice Parameters for Determining Brain Death in Adults (Summary Statement). The Quality Standards Subcommittee of the American Academy of Neurology. *Neurology*, **45**, 1012-1014.

[22] Webb, C. (1985) COWS Caloric Test. *Annals of Emergency Medicine*, **14**, 938. http://dx.doi.org/10.1016/S0196-0644(85)80671-5

[23] André, J.M., Martinet, N., Paysant, J., Beis, J.M. and Le Chapelain, L. (2001) Temporary Phantom Limbs Evoked by Vestibular Caloric Stimulation in Amputees. *Neuropsychiatry*, *Neuropsychology*, *and Behavioral Neurology*, **42**, 190-196.

[24] Bisiach, E., Rusconi, M.L. and Vallar, G. (1991) Remission of Somatoparaphrenic Delusion through Vestibular Stimulation. *Neuropsychologia*, **29**, 1029-1031. http://dx.doi.org/10.1016/0028-3932(91)90066-H

[25] Bottini, G., Paulesu, E., Gandola, M., Loffredo, S., Scarpa, P., Sterzi, R., *et al.* (2005) Left Caloric Vestibular Stimulation Ameliorates Right Hemianesthesia. *Neurology*, **65**, 1278-1283. http://dx.doi.org/10.1212/01.wnl.0000182398.14088.e8

[26] Cappa, S., Sterzi, R., Vallar, G. and Bisiach, E. (1987) Remission of Hemineglect and Anosognosia during Vestibular Stimulation. *Neuropsychologia*, **25**, 775-782. http://dx.doi.org/10.1016/0028-3932(87)90115-1

[27] Le Chapelain, L., Beis, J.M., Paysant, J. and André, J.M. (2001) Vestibular Caloric Stimulation Evokes Phantom Limb Illusions in Patients with Paraplegia. *Spinal Cord*, **39**, 85-87. http://dx.doi.org/10.1038/sj.sc.3101093

[28] Mueller-Jensen, A., Neunzig, H.P. and Emskötter, T. (1987) Outcome Prediction in Comatose Patients: Significance of Reflex Eye Movement Analysis. *Journal of Neurology*, *Neurosurgery & Psychiatry*, **50**, 389-392. http://dx.doi.org/10.1136/jnnp.50.4.389

[29] Ramachandran, V.S. and McGeoch, P.D. (2007) Can Vestibular Caloric Stimulation Be Used to Treat Apotemnophylia? *Medical Hypotheses*, **69**, 250-252. http://dx.doi.org/10.1016/j.mehy.2006.12.013

[30] Ramachandran, V.S., McGeoch, P.D. and Williams, L. (2007) Can Vestibular Caloric Stimulation Be Used to Treat Dejerine-Roussy Syndrome? *Medical Hypotheses*, **69**, 486-488. http://dx.doi.org/10.1016/j.mehy.2006.12.036

[31] Rode, G., Charles, N., Perenin, M.T., Vighetto, A., Trillet, M. and Aimard, G. (1992) Partial Remission of Hemiplegia and Somatoparaphrenia through Vestibular Stimulation in a Case of Unilateral Neglect. *Cortex*, **28**, 203-208.

http://dx.doi.org/10.1016/S0010-9452(13)80048-2

[32] Vallar, G., Sterzi, R., Bottini, G., Cappa, S. and Rusconi, M.L. (1990) Temporary Remission of Left Hemianesthesia after Vestibular Stimulation. A Sensory Neglect Phenomenon. *Cortex*, **26**, 123-131. http://dx.doi.org/10.1016/S0010-9452(13)80078-0

[33] Rossetti, Y. and Rode, G. (2002) Reducing Spatial Neglect by Visual and Other Sensory Manipulations: Noncognitive (Physiological) Routes to the Rehabilitation of a Cognitive Disorder. In: Karnath, H.O., Milner, D. and Vallar, G., Eds., *The Cognitive and Neural Bases of Spatial Neglect*, Oxford University Press, New York, 375-396. http://dx.doi.org/10.1093/acprof:oso/9780198508335.003.0027

[34] Rubens, A.B. (1985) Caloric Stimulation and Unilateral Visual Neglect. *Neurology*, **35**, 1019-1024. http://dx.doi.org/10.1212/WNL.35.7.1019

[35] Utz, K.S., Korluss, K., Schmidt, L., Rosenthal, A., Oppenlander, K., Keller, I., *et al.* (2011) Minor Adverse Effects of Galvanic Vestibular Stimulation in Persons with Stroke and Healthy Individuals. *Brain Injury*, **25**, 1058-1069. http://dx.doi.org/10.3109/02699052.2011.607789

[36] Neuman, A.C. (2005) Central Auditory System Plasticity and Aural Rehabilitation of Adults. *Journal of Rehabilitation Research & Development*, **42**, 169-186. http://dx.doi.org/10.1682/JRRD.2005.01.0020

[37] Bottini, G., Gandola, M., Sedda, A. and Ferrè, E.R. (2013) Caloric Vestibular Stimulation: Interaction between Somatosensory System and Vestibular Apparatus. *Frontiers in Integrative Neuroscience*, **7**, 66. http://dx.doi.org/10.3389/fnint.2013.00066

[38] Ferrè, E.R., Bottini, G. and Haggard, P. (2012) Vestibular Inputs Modulate Somatosensory Cortical Processing. *Brain Structure and Function*, **217**, 859-864. http://dx.doi.org/10.1007/s00429-012-0404-7

[39] Ferrè, E.R., Bottini, G. and Haggard, P. (2011) Vestibular Modulation of Somatosensory Perception. *European Journal of Neuroscience*, **34**, 1337-1344. http://dx.doi.org/10.1111/j.1460-9568.2011.07859.x

[40] Bottini, G., Paulesu, E., Sterzi, R., Warburton, E., Wise, R.J., Vallar, G., *et al.* (1995) Modulation of Conscious Experience by Peripheral Sensory Stimuli. *Nature*, **376**, 778-781. http://dx.doi.org/10.1038/376778a0

[41] Vallar, G., Bottini, G., Rusconi, M.L. and Sterzi, R. (1993) Exploring Somatosensory Hemineglect by Vestibular Stimulation. *Brain*, **116**, 71-86. http://dx.doi.org/10.1093/brain/116.1.71

15

Final Diagnosis of Pediatric Patients with Prolonged in Activated Partial Thromboplastin Time Preoperative Study

Noemí Aguirre[1], Francisca Córdova[2], Francisca Jaime[3], Ximena Fonseca[4], Pamela Zúñiga[5]

[1]Pediatrics Resident, Pontifical Catholic University of Chile, Santiago, Chile
[2]School of Medicine, Pontifical Catholic University of Chile, Santiago, Chile
[3]Pediatrician, Resident of Pediatric Gastroenterology and Nutrition, Pontifical Catholic University of Chile, Santiago, Chile
[4]Otorhinolaryngologist, Assistant Professor, Pediatrics Division, Medical School, Pontifical Catholic University of Chile, Santiago, Chile
[5]Hematologist-Oncologist, Assistant Professor, Pediatrics Division, Medical School, Pontifical Catholic University of Chile, Santiago, Chile
Email: noemi.a.rioseco@gmail.com

Abstract

Introduction: Activated partial thromboplastin time (aPTT) is one of the most used coagulation tests in preoperative evaluation. Incidental detection of a prolonged aPTT is a problem in primary care, in which the general pediatrician should be able to attend its initial management. Objective: To describe final diagnosis of patients with prolonged aPTT in preoperative study. Materials and Methods: This is a descriptive study of patients referred from otorhinolaryngology. Results: Totally, 508 adenoidectomies and/or tonsillectomies were performed in our center, 38 of which referred patients (7.5%) with prolonged aPTT, and 30 of which met inclusion criteria. The median age was 4 years. 56.6% of patients were males. 76.6% of patients normalized aPTT at the second follow-up. Among these, 73.9% showed a normal study, 4.3% ha2d lupus anticoagulant and in 21.7% Von Willebrand disease was detected. Among patients that persisted with prolonged aPTT, 42.8% had coagulant factors deficiency, 28.5% had lupus anticoagulant and in 28.5% of patients a diagnosis could not be achieved with the tests used in the present study. Multivariate analysis did not show correlation between final diagnosis and the variables measured. Conclusion: The presence of a prolonged aPTT in children under preoperative study is due to a pre-analytic factor in the majority of cases or to the presence of lupus anticoagulant, normalizing values on follow-up. We suggest that a new aPTT be performed on these patients, and only those that persist altered or present a symptoms and family history of coagulation disorders be referred to hematology.

Keywords

aPTT, Preoperative Study, Tonsillectomy, Adenoidectomy, Coagulopathy

1. Introduction

Activated partial thromboplastin time (aPTT) is one of the most used coagulation tests in the preoperative setting.

In this scenario, detection of an incidental prolonged aPTT is a concern in pediatric care, due to the fact that the test is commonly ordered without a history of bleeding [1], history that is difficult to obtain in younger patients that have not been exposed to hemorrhagic stress situations.

Among the pathologies that can cause a prolongation in the aPTT, there exist hereditary coagulopathies as isolated deficiencies in factors VIII, IX, XI, and XII and Von Willebrand disease with low VIII factor. There are also other acquired causes as the presence of heparin in the sample, being from treatment or contamination and the lupus anticoagulant (LA). This last one is caused by the presence of antiphospholipid antibodies, IgG and/or IgA immunoglobulins, which are present in almost 23% of apparently healthy children [2]-[4], most of all in the younger population [5] in which they are usually transitory in association with infections [4] [6] [7]. Duration in circulation of the lupus anticoagulant is not yet exactly known, but to be considered transitory, not related with autoimmune diseases as the antiphospholipid syndrome, it must be less than 12 weeks [6] [8]-[10].

To suspect the presence of LA, the aPTT study can be corrected by using a mix with normal plasma. This is done with a second aPTT with plasma from the patient, mixed with normal plasma from donors, in a 1:1 ratio. If there is a decrease in any coagulation factor, the new aPTT corrects to normal values. However, in the presence of LA, the aPTT will continue to be prolonged. To confirm this suspicion, there are various tests that can be used; in our institution, the test used is "dilute Russell viper venom".

There are few publications concerning this topic. Described groups reveal a prolonged aPTT in pediatric patients in preoperative study to be between 3% and 10% [11]-[15].

The present study will describe the final diagnosis of patients that have been found to have a prolonged aPTT, as an incidental finding in preoperative study for otorhinolaryngologic surgery. This will help guide general pediatricians in the course of action with this patient group, and will be the starting point for future investigations.

2. Objectives

2.1. Main Objective

To describe the final diagnosis of patients with prolonged aPTT in preoperative study.

2.2. Specific Objectives

1) To describe the distribution of patients with prolonged aPTT that resolve spontaneously on follow-up;
2) To describe the differences in this distribution based on:
a) Age and sex of patients;
b) Bleeding symptoms of the patient;
c) Family history of bleeding symptoms;
d) History of infection during the last month.

3. Patients and Methods

3.1. Study Design

The present study is descriptive and cross-sectional, with a prospective inclusion of patients by recruiting those that were seen in the ambulatory setting with preoperative study of otorhinolaryngologic (ORL) surgery at the Clinical Hospital of the Pontifical Catholic University of Chile with prolonged aPTT, between April 2013 and September 2014. aPTT is ordered routinely as part of the preoperative protocol for adenoidectomy with or without tonsillectomy. Inclusion and exclusion criteria are described in **Table 1**.

Patients that accepted inclusion were seen by a hematologist-oncologist (hemostasis specialist) (Pamela Z.) in ambulatory setting, signed an informed consent previously accepted by the ethics committee of our center and completed an internationally validated questionnaire of bleeding symptoms, attached in **Table 2** [16]. A bleeding score was calculated based on the questionnaire, being considered a significant result to have over 3 points in males and over 5 points in females. Tests used to assess the final diagnosis were those usually ordered for these patients (**Table 3**).

Table 1. Patient selection.

Inclusion criteria	Exclusion criteria
Patients < 18 years of age, and	Patients known to have a coagulopathy, or
Patients with aPTT over normal values in preoperative study for adenoidectomy and/or tonsillectomy, including tests not made in our laboratories, and	Patients known to have liver disease
Patients that had follow-up study done in our laboratories	

Table 2. Questionnaire.

General data

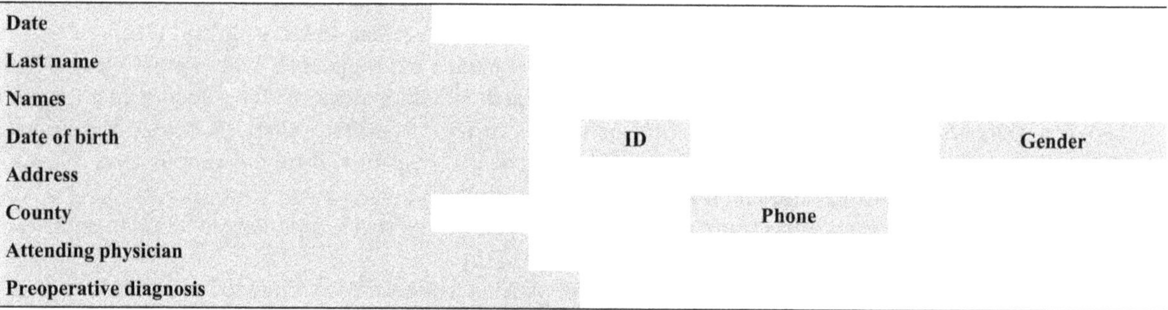

Date			
Last name			
Names			
Date of birth	**ID**		**Gender**
Address			
County		**Phone**	
Attending physician			
Preoperative diagnosis			

Bleeding score: Please assign a score for each symptom depending on its severity.

Symptoms	Score	
Epistaxis	0 = No or trivial 2 = Packing, cauterization	1 = Present 3 = Transfusion, replacement
Cutaneous symptoms	0 = No or trivial 2 = Hematomas	1 = Petechiae or bruises 3 = Medical consultation
Minor wounds	0 = No or trivial 2 = Medical consultation	1 = Present (1 - 5 episodes/year) 3 = Surgery/blood transfusion
Oral cavity bleeding	0 = No or trivial 2 = Medical attention	1 = Present 3 = Surgery/blood transfusion
Gastrointestinal bleeding	0 = No or trivial 2 = Medical Attention	1 = Present 3 = Surgery/blood transfusion
Muscle hematomas of hemarthrosis	0 = No or trivial 2 = Medical Attention	1 = Present 3 = Transfusion/intervention
Tooth extraction (most severe episode)	0 = No or trivial 2 = Suturing of packing	1 = Present 3 = Transfusion
Surgery (most severe episode)	0 = No or trivial 2 = Suturing or resurgery	1 = Present 3 = Transfusion
Menorrhagia	0 = No or trivial 2 = Consultation, pill use, iron therapy	1 = Present 3 = Transfusion, hysterectomy, dilatation-curettage, replacement therapy

Table 3. Tests ordered.

Lupus anticoagulant: in our center the test used is the Dilute Russell Viper Venom; includes aPTT and correction with normal plasma mix in 1:1 ratio.
Von Willebrand disease study.
Only in the cases that prolonged aPTT was corrected with normal plasma were factors XII, IX, and XI measured.

Do you have a family history of:
Hemofilia YES NO
Von Willebrand Disease YES NO
Bleeding symptoms YES NO
Other --
Have you had an infectious disease in the last month?
YES NO
Which? --

3.2. Statistical Analysis

Acquired data were input to an Excel database and were statistically analyzed with SPSS® version 20. Final diagnosis of the patient was considered a dependent variable whilst ages, sex, personal history of bleeding, family history of bleeding and infectious disease in the last 4 weeks were considered independent. For numerical variables median and range were calculated, and for categorical values percentage distribution was calculated. As to compare differences for numerical variables among the different groups in final diagnosis we used the Kruskal-Wallis test and for nominal variables we used chi square test. Furthermost a multinomial logistic regression was made.

4. Results

During the studied period (16 months), 508 adenoidectomies and/or tonsillectomies were performed at our center. 66 total patients (12.9%) were referred to our clinic from ORL, amongst which 38 (7.5%) had prolonged aPTT and were included (**Figure 1**).

The 28 remaining patients (5.5%) were referrals for prolonged bleeding time (20 patients), low partial thromboplast in time (7 patients) and thrombocytopenia (1 patient).

4 patients were excluded because of refusal to sign the informed consent, 2 patients did not complete the study and 2 patients were unreachable due to lack of assistance to follow-up.

Finally 30 patients with prolonged aPTT were followed, 3 of these had concomitant prolonged bleeding time, and 5 patients had concomitant low partial thromboplast in time. 73.3% had isolated prolonged aPTT.

Age median for prolonged aPTT patients was 4 years, 56.6% were male (**Table 4**).

Among the 30 recruited patients, 23 (76.6%) patients normalized aPTT at follow-up, 17 (73.9%) had normal follow-up study, 1 (4.3%) had lupus anticoagulant detected and 5 (21.7%) had Von Willebrand disease detected. (**Figure 2**).

Among patients that persisted with a prolonged aPTT, 3 patients (42.8%) had coagulation factors deficiency, 2 patients (28.5%) had lupus anticoagulant and in 2 patients (28.5%) a final diagnosis could not be achieved during this study.

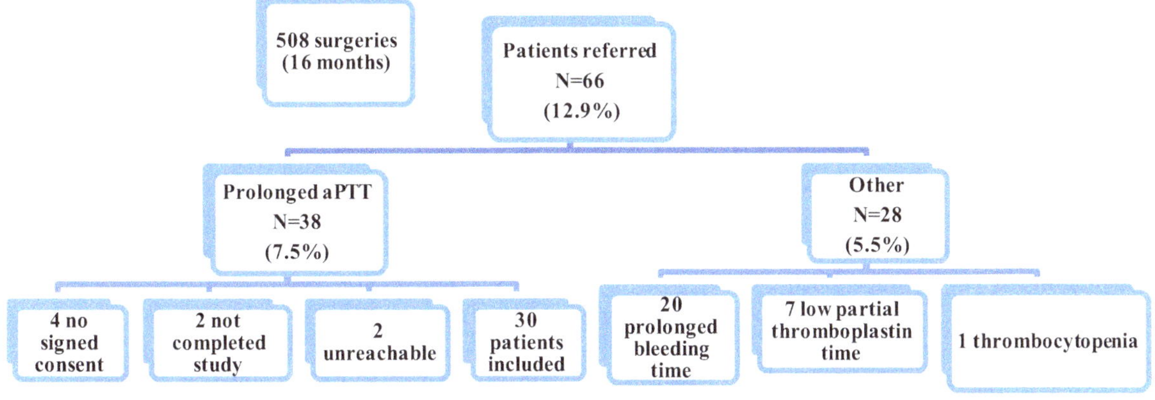

Figure 1. Distribution of patients. Shows how patients were recruited from referrals to the Otorhinolaryngology service, showing the number of excluded patients and the criteria for this exclusion. Additionally on the right branch we show other motives for referral due to altered hemostasis tests that were not the focus of the present study.

Table 4. Characterization of patients.

Variable	Normal N = 17	LA N = 3	Factor deficiency N = 3	vWD N = 5	No identifiable cause N = 2	Total N = 30
Male, N (%)	10 (58.8%)	2 (66.6%)	3 (100%)	2 (40%)	0 (0%)	17 (56.6%)
Age in years, median (range)	4.0 (3 - 12)	2.0 (2 - 7)	4.0 (1 - 6)	3.0 (2 - 5)	5.0 (4 - 6)	4.0 (1 - 12)
Bleeding score, median (range)	0 (0 - 2)	1 (0 - 4)	0 (0)	0 (0 - 1)	0 (0 - 1)	1 (0 - 4)
Family history of bleeding, N (%)	9 (52.9%)	0 (0%)	2 (66.6%)	3 (60%)	0 (0%)	14 (46.6%)
Infectious disease during the last month, N (%)	4 (23.5%)	1 (33.3%)	2 (66.6%)	0 (0%)	0 (0%)	7 (23.3%)

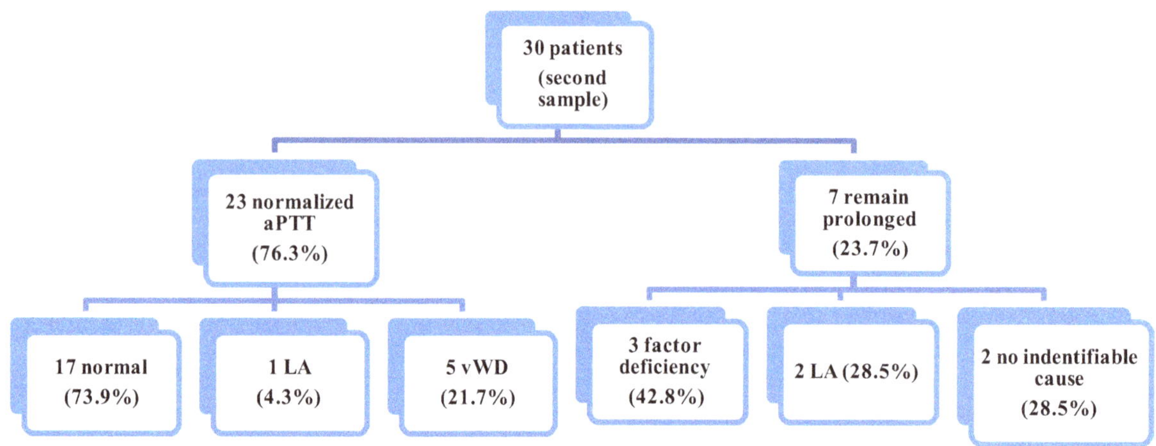

Figure 2. Results. Shows final diagnosis of patients after completing the tests included in our study.

Regarding the bleeding symptoms score, only 1 patient had a significant result and had lupus anticoagulant detected during further testing.

A family history of bleeding disorders was present in 52.9% of patients with normal follow-up tests, and in 66.6% of patients with coagulation factors deficiency, values that were not statistically different. However this history was not so clear due to confusion or ignorance of one or both parents.

During uni or multivariate analysis, there were no statistically significant differences amongst the variables analyzed (age, sex, bleeding score, family history of bleeding and history of infectious disease during the previous month) and the different final diagnosis of the patients.

5. Discussion

Tonsillectomy with or without adenoidectomy is the most frequent major surgical procedure in the pediatric patient [17].

A correct interpretation of coagulation tests when ordered is absolutely relevant given that the most frequent complication of this procedure is bleeding, being known to occur between 1% and 8% of total cases [17] [18]. It has been known that this risk is even greater amongst male patients, who in our study were the vast majority of patients referred for prolonged aPTT [17].

In our study, 7.5% of patients that had preoperative coagulation tests had a prolonged aPTT, figure that is within published ranges [11] [14] [15] [19].

Most of our patients normalized aPTT on second follow-up. This could be explained due to pre-analytic factors that were corrected, for example there are difficulties known regarding sample recovery from pediatric patients such as: anatomical conditions, or anxiety of the child, parent or caretaker. Another possibility is the presence of transitory LA, which correlates with the peak in prevalence of LA around 5 years of age reported by

Male *et al.*, corresponding with the age group analyzed in the present study [20] and the levels of LA reported as a cause of isolated prolonged aPTT in literature. These reports exceed the levels that we could confirm in our study (up to 53, 1% v/s 10% respectively) [2] [13] [14] [17] [21]. Looking back at the time interval between both samples obtained from our patients, most of these were retrieved after 3 months (average in weeks), which is greater than the time interval described for LA study in children [5] [6].

26.6% of the patients with prolonged aPTT were found to have a possible coagulation disorder that had not been identified previously (Von Willebrand disease or a coagulation factor deficiency), similar to available literature [14].

Prolonged aPTT due to coagulation factor deficiency was not common (10%), however it was higher if compared to published data [14] [17]. Every patient persisted with prolonged aPTT at follow-up. Frequency of vWD in our study was 16.6% (0,9% of all patients that had surgery), correlating with published data [14].

There are studies that show that a medical history of bleeding (family history or bleeding symptoms) has a better predictive value than coagulation tests for perioperative bleeding [18], however in pediatrics most of the patients have not been previously exposed to hemostatic stress to assign a greater value to personal history of bleeding; thus can be seen in the results of our study. Furthermore, there is a study that shows a frequency of 0.9% of positive clinical history in patients that have coagulation tests [13].

In the present study, no patient with probable coagulopathy (Von Willebrand disease or coagulation deficiency) had a significant bleeding score, this relates to the median age of 4 years. Given this fact, family history of bleeding gains importance, though not statistically significant, being present in 62.5% of these patients.

In light of present results, we think that if a prolonged aPTT is detected in preoperative study in an asymptomatic patient without family history, the test should be repeated in 12 weeks, taking pre-analytic factors into consideration. If the test to detect LA is available we recommend that it should be performed, and only those patients whose tests persist altered or those who have a positive personal or familiar history of bleeding be referred to a hematologist [2] [14] [22].

6. Conclusions

Prolonged aPTT in preoperative checkup is a frequent finding, being crucial a correct interpretation and course of action by the general pediatrician and the physician who performs the preoperative evaluation.

In children, the majority of cases are due to a pre-analytic factor or to the presence of lupus anticoagulant, normalizing values on follow-up testing.

It should be considered that mucocutaneous bleeding symptoms may not be present to orient a probable coagulopathy in this age group, which is why a family history of bleeding gains relevance.

We suggest repeating an aPTT in these children and referring to a hematologist those that persist with altered results or a family history of bleeding disorders.

7. Future Projections

To propose a management algorithm for children that are seen by general pediatricians due to a prolonged aPTT found incidentally, thus avoiding unnecessary referrals of these patients, which are costly and are not always available, furthermore avoiding high costs of specific exams on these children.

Additionally, this study could help future investigations in which the primary objective is to know if a relation between a prolonged aPTT and the presence of perioperative bleeding exists.

Acknowledgements

The authors wish to thank Rodrigo Donoso Martínez M. D. for his collaboration in translating the present study to the English language.

References

[1] Anjali, A. and Steven, W. (2008) Bleeding Disorders. *Pediatrics in Review*, **29**, 121-130. http://dx.doi.org/10.1542/pir.29-4-121

[2] Shah, M., O'Riordan, M. and Alexander, S. (2006) Evaluation of Prolonged aPTT Values in the Pediatric Population. *Clinical Pediatrics*, **45**, 347-353. http://dx.doi.org/10.1177/000992280604500407

[3] Edlinger, G., Gallistl, S. and Muntean, W. (1996) Lupus Anticoagulant and Factor XII Activity in Children with Prolonged PTT. *Thrombosis Research*, **83**, 403-404. http://dx.doi.org/10.1016/0049-3848(96)00150-8

[4] Katrin, F., Karl, L. and Philipp, V. (2005) Antiphospholipid Antibodies in Pediatric Patients with Prolonged Activated Partial Thromboplastin Time during Infection. *Immunobiology*, **210**, 799-805. http://dx.doi.org/10.1016/j.imbio.2005.10.012

[5] Shiomou, K., Galanakis, E., Tzoufi, M., Tsaousi, C. and Papadopoulou, Z.L. (2002) Transient Lupus Anticoagulant and Prolonged Activated Partial Thromboplastin Time Secondary to Epstein-Barr Virus Infection. *Scandinavian Journal of Infectious Diseases*, **34**, 67-69. http://dx.doi.org/10.1080/003655402753395229

[6] Mizumoto, H., Maihara, T., Hiejima, E., Shiota, M., Hata, A., Seto, S., Atsumi, T., Koike, T. and Hata, D. (2006) Transient Antiphospholipid Antibodies Associated with Acute Infections in Children: A Report of Three Cases and a Review of the Literature. *European Journal of Pediatrics*, **165**, 484-488. http://dx.doi.org/10.1007/s00431-006-0117-0

[7] Blank, M., Krause, I., Fridkin, M., Keller, N., Kopolovic, J., Goldberg, I., Tobar, N. and Shoenfeld, Y. (2002) Bacterial Induction of Autoantibodies to Beta2-Glycoprotein-I Accounts for the Infectious Etiology of Antiphospholipid Syndrome. *The Journal of Clinical Investigation*, **109**, 797-804. http://dx.doi.org/10.1172/JCI0212337

[8] Bermejo, A., Gonzalez, H., Abad, A., Figueroa, L., Muñoz, R., Marcos, M., Cebeira, M.J. and Alvarez, F.J. (2013) Anticoagulante lúpico en pediatria. Experiencia en nuestro centro. *Boletín de la sociedad de pediatría de asturias, cantabria, castilla y león*, **53**, 146-151.

[9] Lippi, G., Salvagno, G.L., Rugolotto, S., Chiaffoni, G.P., Padovani, E.M., Franchini, M. and Guidi, G.C. (2007) Routine Coagulation Tests in Newborn and Young Infants. *Journal of Thrombosis and Thrombolysis*, **24**, 153-155. http://dx.doi.org/10.1007/s11239-007-0046-4

[10] Hoyos López, M.C., Pascual Pérez, J.M., Blanco Quirós, A., Guerola Delgado, D., Valbuena Crespo, C. and Álvarez Guisasola, G. (1999) Anticoagulante lúpico en pediatria. Presentación de 4 casos. *Anales Españoles de Pediatria*, **51**, 637-642.

[11] Marioni, G. and de Filippi, C. (2009) Pediatric Otolaryngologic Manifestations of Bleeding Disorders. *International Journal of Pediatric Otorhinolaryngology*, **735**, S61-S64. http://dx.doi.org/10.1016/S0165-5876(09)70012-6

[12] Chng, W.J., Sum, C. and Kuperan, P. (2005) Causes of Isolated Prolonged Activated Partial Thromboplastin Time in an Acute Care General Hospital. *Singapore Medical Journal*, **46**, 450-246.

[13] Gabriel, P., Mazoit, X. and Ecoffey, C. (2000) Relationship between Clinical History, Coagulation Tests, and Perioperative Bleeding during Tonsillectomies in Pediatrics. *Journal of Clinical Anesthesia*, **12**, 288-291. http://dx.doi.org/10.1016/S0952-8180(00)00164-1

[14] Sandoval, C., Garcia, C., Visintainer, P., Ozkaynak, M.F. and Jayabose, S. (2003) The Usefulness of Preoperative Screening for Bleeding Disorders. *Clinical Pediatrics*, **42**, 247-250. http://dx.doi.org/10.1177/000992280304200308

[15] Asaf, T., Reuveni, H., Yermiahu, T., Leiberman, A., Gurman, G., Porat, A., Schlaeffer, P., Shifra, S. and Kapelushnik, J. (2001) The Need for Routine Pre-Operative Coagulation Screening Tests (Prothrombin Time PT/Partial Thromboplastin Time PTT) for Healthy Children Undergoing Elective Tonsillectomy and/or Adenoidectomy International. *International Journal of Pediatric Otorhinolaryngology*, **61**, 217-222. http://dx.doi.org/10.1016/S0165-5876(01)00574-2

[16] Rodeghiero, F., Castaman, G., Tosetto, A., Batlle, J., Baudo, F., Cappelletti, A., Casana, P., de Bosch, N., Eikenboom, J.C., Federici, A.B., Lethagen, S., Linari, S. and Srivastava, A. (2005) The Discriminant Power of Bleeding History for the Diagnosis of von Willebrand Disease Type 1: An Interntional, Multicenter Study. *Journal of Thrombosis and Haemostasis*, **3**, 2619-2626. http://dx.doi.org/10.1111/j.1538-7836.2005.01663.x

[17] Windfuhr, J.P. and Chen, Y.S. (2002) Incidence of Post-Tonsillectomy Hemorrhage in Children and Adults: A Study of 4848 Patients. *Ear, Nose & Throat Journal*, **81**, 626-628.

[18] Zagólski, O. (2010) Hemorragia postamigdalectomía: ¿tienen las pruebas de coagulación y el historial de coagulopatía un valor predictivo? *Acta Otorrinolaringológica Española*, **61**, 287-292. http://dx.doi.org/10.1016/j.otorri.2010.01.017

[19] Koshkareva, Y.A., Cohen, M., Gaughan, J.P., Callanan, V. and Szeremeta, W. (2012) Utility of Preoperative Hematologic Screening for Pediatric Adenotonsillectomy. *Ear, Nose Throat Journal*, **91**, 346-356.

[20] Li, J., Lai, X., Yan, C., Xu, A., Nie, L., Zhou, Y., Liao, C. and Ren, H. (2009) Age-Associated Developmental Changes in the Activated Partial Thromboplastin Time (aPTT) and Causes of Prolonged aPTT Values in Healthy Chinese Children. *Clinical Chemistry and Laboratory Medicine*, **47**, 1531-1537. http://dx.doi.org/10.1515/CCLM.2009.339

[21] Burk, C.D., Miller, L., Handler, S.D. and Cohen, A.R. (1992) Preoperative History and Coagulation Screening in Children Undergoing Tonsillectomy. *Pediatrics*, **89**, 691-695. http://dx.doi.org/10.1097/00132586-199212000-00035

[22] Genecov, D.G., Por, Y.C., Barcelo, C.R., Salyer, K.E., Mulne, A.F. and Morad, A.B. (2005) Preoperative Screening for Coagulopathy Using Prothrombin Time and Partial Thromboplastin Time in Patients Requiring Primary Cranial Vault. *Plastic and Reconstructive Surgery*, **116**, 389-394. http://dx.doi.org/10.1097/01.prs.0000172760.79803.68

16

Typical Aspects of the Granular Cell Tumor of the Oral Cavity

Paula Prieto-Oliveira[1], Sérgio Vitorino Cardoso[2], Florence Zumbaio Mistro[3], Sérgio Kignel[3], Suzana Cantanhede Orsini Machado de Sousa[4], Marco Túllio Brazão-Silva[5]

[1]Inter-Institutional Grad Program on Bioinformatics, University of São Paulo, São Paulo, Brazil
[2]Department of Oral Pathology, School of Dentistry, Federal University of Uberlândia, Uberlândia, Brazil
[3]Department of Semiology, School of Dentistry, Fundação Hermínio Ometto, Araras, Brazil
[4]Department of Oral Pathology, School of Dentistry, University of São Paulo, São Paulo, Brazil
[5]Department of Oral Diagnosis, School of Dentistry, School of Health Sciences, University of the State of Amazonas, Manaus, Brazil
Email: paulaprietoterra@yahoo.com.br, cardososv@gmail.com, florencemistro@uniararas.br, skignel@uol.com.br, scmsousa@usp.br, marcotullio@gmail.com

Abstract

Granular cell tumor (GCT) is a rare neoplasm that can occur in any part of the body, but mostly they are located intraorally. Its histogenetic origin remains controversial, but it probably arises from Schwann cells and is generally benign. The tumor is typically asymptomatic and appears as a nodule, with a relatively high predilection for the tongue. This article reports a case of a 72-year-old woman treated at the Center of Oral Diagnosis of the Fundação Hermínio Ometto Dental School. The patient presented with an asymptomatic nodule in the dorsal surface of the tongue for approximately 4 months. The patient was submitted to an excisional biopsy and histopatological examination revealed polyhedral cells with granular aspect. The immunohistochemical staining for S-100 presented strong reactivity, confirming the diagnosis of GCT. Finally, we made a concise discussion about the pathogenesis and fundamental clinico-pathological aspects of GCT making the differential diagnosis.

Keywords

Granular Cell Tumor, Mouth, Diagnosis

1. Introduction

Granular cell tumor (GCT) is a rare benign neoplasm of soft tissues which most often arises in head and neck regions (50% of cases). GCT arises at virtually any body site, but is mainly found in the subcutaneous tissue (32.6%), followed by oral cavity (28.1%), breast (15.9%), larynx (7.6%), gastrointestinal tract (4.7%) and bronchus (3.4%), perineum (2.4%) and miscellaneous sites (2.9%) [1]. Over half of head and neck lesions are found on the tongue. It is more common in females and adults, between 40 and 60 years. GCTs are thought to be of Schwann cell derivation and present a benign behavior in 98% of the cases [2] [3]. This article reports a case of benign GCT involving the tongue of a 72-year-old female patient, aiming to illustrate and discuss the presentation and origin of this disease.

2. Case Report

A 72-year-old faioderm woman presented at Center of Oral Diagnosis of Dental School of Hermínio Ometto Foundation complaining of an asymptomatic nodule on her tongue. It had been present for the past four months, and her medical history was irrelevant. Examination of the oral cavity evidenced a nodular lesion on the dorsum of the tongue, 1.5 cm in width, with a pinkish color and fibrous consistency. An excisional biopsy was performed, with clinical impression of focal fibrous hyperplasia (**Figure 1**).

The histopathological exam (**Figure 2**) revealed a lesion lined by a parakeratinized stratified squamous epithelium presenting parakerathosis and a mild acanthosis. In the lamina propria, there was a tumoral formation predominantly composed by large polyhedral cells showing a syncytial growth pattern, usually presenting eosinophilic cytoplasm and granular aspect, and variably amount of cytoplasmic hyaline globules. Nuclei were eccentrically located and presented a mild pleomorphism, mostly showing a vesicular appearance of chromatin. The cellular mass was intermingled with dense connective tissue and remnants of skeletal muscle fibers. Tumoral cells were PAS positive (diastase-resistant) and immunopositive for S-100. Surgical margins were free of tumoral cells. A conclusive diagnosis of GCT was rendered and the patient remains free of disease six months after surgical treatment.

3. Discussion

Despite the number of publications involving cases of GCT, its pathogenesis remains unclear. The first Brazilian case was reported in 1970 by Sequeira and colleagues using the term "myoblastoma" to describe a multicentric GCT involving bronchi, tongue and parotid [4]. Further this name was abolished due to S-100 and vimentin's positivity, as observed in the present case, favoring a neural origin of tumor cells. Other routine neural markers such p75 have also evidenced its nerve sheath differentiation [5]. On the other hand, the reason why these cells do not stain for S-100A6 protein, a form of S-100 protein found in other benign tumors of neural origin such schwannoma, neurofibroma, and palisaded encapsulated neuroma, needs to be clarified [6]. Besides the controversy

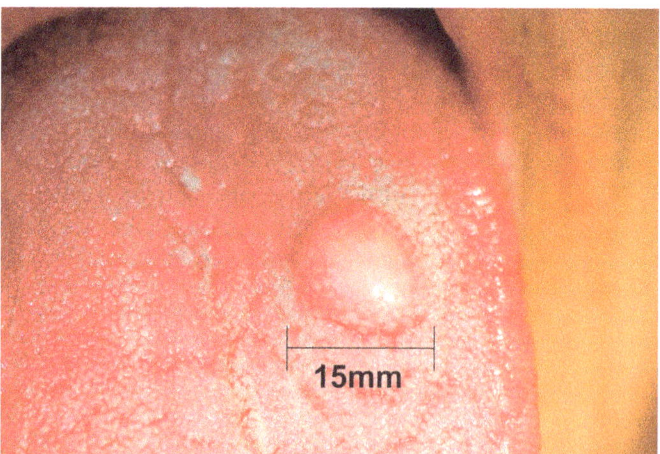

Figure 1. Clinical aspect of the lesion, showing the involvement of dorsum of tongue.

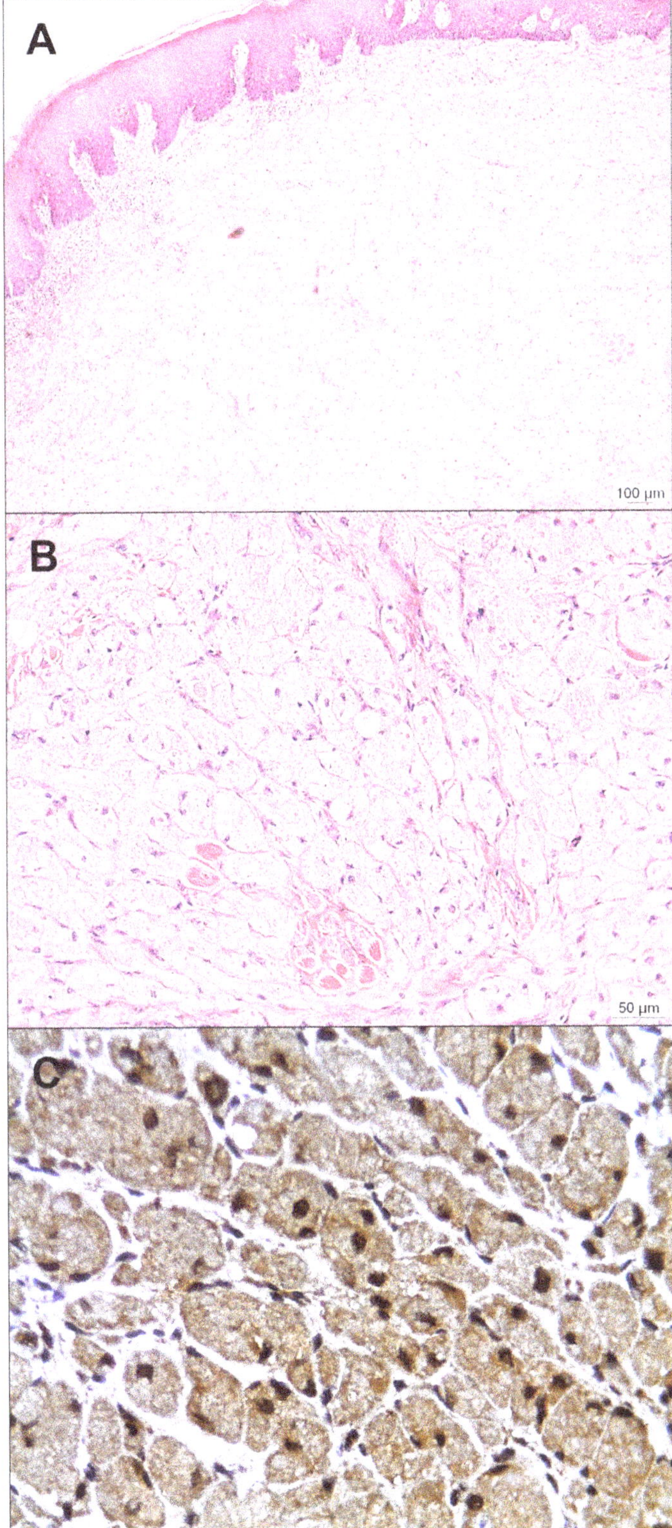

Figure 2. Histological aspects of the lesion. (A) The tumoral mass is seen next to the epithelium of tongue mucosa (hematoxylin-eosin). (B) Higher magnification showing the granular polyhedral cells containing eosinophilic granules intermingled with striated muscle fibers. (C) S-100 protein positivity of the tumor cells.

regarding its neural origin, some authors believe that small and well-circunscribed nodules as the present case represents the true neoplasm, and lesions showing infiltrative pattern with remote satellite nodules and larger and poorly circumscribed lesions may represents a diffuse process of metabolically induced granular change of local mesenchymal cells [7]. Thus, the pathogenesis of GCT still warrants new investigations.

Clinically, GCT of the oral cavity is usually a single, sessile and asymptomatic nodule, with less than 2 cm in diameter, with normal or slightly pale overlying mucosa. Approximately 10% to 20% of patients may present multiple lesions [2]. A study involving 68 cases of oral GCT reported a broad age range, between 7 and 82 years, with an average age of 38.3. There was a predominance of female patients (68%), and the tongue was the most affected site (80.8%). About tongue lesions, 48.5% of them were in dorsal surface, as seen in this report, while 27.9% were found in lateral border and 4.4% in ventral surface. Of the remaining cases, 5.9% were on lower lip, 4.4% on upper lip, 4.4% on buccal mucosa, 2.9% on soft palate, and 1.5% on floor of mouth [7].

The GCT cells may be round, oval, polygonal or slightly elongated. The edges tend to be inconspicuous, often giving a syncytial impression. The nucleus may range from small and hypercromatic to large and vesicular, with central or peripheral location. The cytoplasm is eosinophilic and presents fine granules. Ultrastructurally, the granularity of the cytoplasm seems to represent phagocytosed lysosomes containing infolded cell membranes [8]. The cells are arranged in islets, ribbons and sheets separated by fibrous septa. The granular cells can grow along the muscle fibers and sometimes seem to fuse with them. In some cases association with nerves, may be observed. Up to 70% of cases may present contact of tumoral cells with the overlying epithelium, and in 10% of GCT there is pseudoepitheliomatous hyperplasia, which may be misinterpreted as squamous cell carcinoma [7]. Finally, positivity for PAS, S-100 protein, and NSE are typical on GCT [1] [7].

Up to 2% of GCT behave aggressively and can metastasize. A classic study reported 39% of survival rate for malignant GCT at a median interval of 3 years and 29% of patients were alive with disease [9]. Six histologic features are used distinguishing benign, atypical, and malignant granular cell tumors: 1) necrosis; 2) spindling; 3) vesicular nuclei with large nucleoli; 4) increased mitotic activity (>2 mitoses/10 high-power fields at 200× magnification); 5) high nuclear to cytoplasmic (N:C) ratio; and 6) nuclearpleomorphism. GCT that met three or more of these criteria has been classified as histologically malignant, while the presence of one or two criteria defines an atypical GCT. The isolated presence of focal polymorphism can be observed in benign tumors [9]. On the other hand, the benign histopathological picture has been also reported in clinically malignant lesions, which highlights the importance of careful clinical examination. Features such as large size, rapid growth, invasion recurrence and nodal involvement have been used to define the malignant GCT regardless of its histopathological status [10].

Other lesions which may be confused with the GCT are the congenital epulis of the newborn and the polypoid S-100-negative GCT of the oral cavity. The former is a rare but well-recognized tumor of newborns with indolent behavior, mostly occurring as soft tissue swelling of the alveolar ridges, histologically presenting a degenerative process in the way of a granular cell component [11]. It may be separated from the GCT by location, patient age, absence of cytoplasmic hyaline globules, solid growth pattern, pericytic proliferation, attenuated overlying epithelium, and negativity for S-100 protein [12]. The latter is a rare lesion identified by its polypoid appearance, lack of staining for S-100 protein and NSE, slight atypia and mitotic activity, and lack of clear expression of most markers of differentiation, and should not be mistaken with a low-grade malignancy [13].

Treatment of GCT consists of surgical excision with safety margins [14]. Local recurrence is not expected, but can occur in up to 15% of cases, probably related to incomplete removal [15].

4. Conclusion

In spite of rarity of GCT, this lesion must be considered in diagnosis of lesions in the dorsum of the tongue. Histopathological analysis is necessary for diagnosis confirmation and evaluation of margins. The oral lesions generally affect the tongue and prognosis is excellent.

References

[1] Wang, B.Y., Zagzag, D. and Nonaka, D. (2009) Tumors of Nervous System. In: Barnes, L., Ed., *Surgical Pathology of the Head and Neck*, 3rd Edition, Informa Healthcare, New York, 669-771.

[2] Weiss, S.W. and Goldblum, J.R. (2001) Enzinger and Weiss's Soft Tissue Tumors. 4th Edition, Mosby, St Louis, 1622.

[3] Speight, P. (2005) Granular Cell Tumor. In: Eveson, J.W., Reichart, P. and Sidransky, D., Eds., *World Health Organization Classification of Tumors. Pathology and Genetics of Head and Neck Tumours*, IARC Press, Lyon, 185-186.

[4] Sequeira, O.F., Marcos-Martins, O., Hercules, H.C. and dos Santos, J.L. (1970) Mioblastoma múltiplo com localizacãoo brônquica, lingual e parotidiana. *Hospital* (*Rio J*), **77**, 1179-1195.

[5] Rejas, R.A., Campos, M.S., Cortes, A.R., Pinto, D.D. and de Sousa, S.C. (2011) The Neural Histogenetic Origin of the Oral Granular Cell Tumor: An Immunohistochemical Evidence. *Medicina Oral*, *Patologia Oral y Cirugia Bucal*, **16**, 6-10. http://dx.doi.org/10.4317/medoral.16.e6

[6] Fullen, D.R., Reed, J.A., Finnerty, B. and McNutt, N.S. (2001) S100A6 Preferentially Labels Type C Nevus Cells and Nevic Corpuscles: Additional Support for Schwannian Differentiation of Intradermal Nevi. *Journal of Cutaneous Pathology*, **28**, 393-399. http://dx.doi.org/10.1034/j.1600-0560.2001.028008393.x

[7] Vered, M., Carpenter, W.M. and Buchner, A. (2009) Granular Cell Tumor of the Oral Cavity: Updated Immunohistochemical Profile. *Journal of Oral Pathology Medicine*, **38**, 150-159. http://dx.doi.org/10.1111/j.1600-0714.2008.00725.x

[8] Mittal, K.R. and True, L.D. (1988) Origin of Granules in Granular Cell Tumor. Intracellular Myelin Formation with Autodigestion. *Archives of Pathology Laboratory*, **112**, 302-303.

[9] Fanburg-Smith, J.C., Meis-Kindblom, J., Fante, R. and Kindblom, L. (1998) Malignant Granular Cell Tumor of Soft Tissue: Diagnostic Criteria and Clinicopathologic Correlation. *American Journal of Surgical Pathology*, **22**, 779-794. http://dx.doi.org/10.1097/00000478-199807000-00001

[10] Choi, S.M., Hong, S.G., Kang, S.M., Chae, B.G., Kim, S.J., Park, P.K. and Park, H.S. (2014) A Case of Malignant Granular Cell Tumor in the Sigmoid Colon. *Clinical Endoscopy*, **47**, 197-200. http://dx.doi.org/10.5946/ce.2014.47.2.197

[11] Regezi, J.A., Sciubba, J.J. and Jordan, R.C.K. (2011) Oral Pathology: Clinical Pathologic Correlations. 6th Edition, Elsevier Saunders, St Louis, 388.

[12] Childers, E.L. and Fanburg-Smith, J.C. (2010) Congenital Epulis of the Newborn: 10 New Cases of a Rare Oral Tumor. *Annals of Diagnostic Pathology*, **15**, 157-161. http://dx.doi.org/10.1016/j.anndiagpath.2010.10.003

[13] Basile, J.R. and Woo, S.B. (2003) Polypoid S-100-Negative Granular Cell Tumor of the Oral Cavity: A Case Report and Review of Literature. *Oral Surgery*, *Oral Medicine*, *Oral Pathology*, *Oral Radiology*, *and Endodontology*, **96**, 70-76. http://dx.doi.org/10.1016/S1079-2104(03)00097-0

[14] Eguia, A., Uribarri, A., Gay-Escoda, C., Crovetto, M.A., Martínez-Conde, R. and Aguirre, J.M. (2006) Granular Cell Tumor: Report of 8 Intraoral Cases. *Medicina Oral*, *Patología Oral y Cirugía Bucal*, **11**, 425-428.

[15] Becelli, R., Perugini, M., Gasparini, G., Cassoni, A. and Fabiani, F. (2001) Abrikossoff's Tumor. *Journal of Craniofacial Surgery*, **12**, 78-81. http://dx.doi.org/10.1097/00001665-200101000-00013

17

Knowledge, Attitude and Awareness of Hazards Associated with Use of Cotton Bud in a Nigerian Community

Olajide Toye Gabriel[1*], Usman Aminu Mohammed[2], Eletta Adebisi Paul[2]

[1]Department of Ear, Nose and Throat Surgery, Federal Teaching Hospital, Ido Ekiti, Nigeria
[2]Department of Ear, Nose and Throat Surgery, Federal Medical Centre, Bida, Nigeria
Email: [*]toyeolajide@yahoo.co.uk, 2mausman@gmail.com, elettaadebisi@yahoo.com

Abstract

Background: Self-cleaning of ears with a cotton bud is a common practice, and the hazards associated with such action are well documented. The aim of this study is to find out the knowledge, attitude and awareness on the use of cotton buds among the people of Bida community. Design and Methodology: It is a community based cross sectional descriptive study carried out among people of Bida community. Subjects were selected by multistage sampling technique. Pre-tested semi-structured questionnaires were used to collect data from 278 young adults and adults' respondents. Results: There were a total number of 278 responses out of 290 respondents interviewed (M:F = 1:1.03). Age range was from 18 to 65 years with a mean of 29.64 ± 10.06 SD. The highest response was in the age group of 20 - 29 years. About 72.3% of the respondents had tertiary education, and 40.3% were civil servants. Majority (92.8%) of the respondents had indulged in the use of cotton buds to clean their ears. Most (57.8%) of those that had used cotton buds did so because of itching in the ears. Only 44.9% of respondents agreed that cotton buds could cause damage to the ears. Many (61.2%) believed that there was benefit of using cotton buds in cleaning the ears. Majority of the respondents (74.1%) had not got information on the danger of using cotton bud in cleaning their ears. Conclusion: From our data in this study, majority of the subjects had indulged in the use of cotton bud in cleaning their ears. And the commonest reason for using cotton buds is due to itching in the ears. Their Knowledge, attitude and awareness to the use of cotton buds are very poor with erroneous believe that there is benefit to its use. There is a need to increase awareness by public enlightenment and health education and to establish school health programme in our various schools.

Keywords

Knowledge, Awareness, Hazards, Cotton Bud, Nigerian Community

[*]Corresponding author.

1. Introduction

Cotton buds or cotton swabs consist of a small wad of cotton wrapped around one or both ends of a short rod, usually made of either wood, rolled paper, or plastic [1]. The cotton swab was invented in 1923 by Leo Gersternzang who observed his wife to have attached wads of cotton on toothpicks to clean his baby's ear [2]. Cleaning of ears with a cotton bud is a common practice which can traumatize the ear canal and such ear injuries are commonly seen in ENT practice [3] [4]. The primary reason (96%) given in one study for using cotton buds was to remove ear wax [5]. However, it is known that ear wax is produced in the outer part of the canal and migrates out with the epithelium toward the pinna. These objects are cheap and readily available from drug stores and super markets. Cotton bud tips are not only used by adults, but also commonly used in pediatric population either by children themselves or by parents [6]. Insertion of cotton buds inside ears is not only unnecessary but also potentially dangerous and has widely been condemned worldwide by otolaryngologists. This is due to well documented complications, including trauma, impacted ear wax, infection and retention of the cotton bud [7] [8]. Little studies have been conducted on the usage of cotton bud in Nigeria. We therefore decided to carry out this study in a community to find out their knowledge, attitude and awareness on the hazards of using cotton bud.

2. Design & Methodology

This is a community based descriptive study carried out among young adults and adults' residents of Bida, over a 4 weeks period between October and November, 2014. Bida is an urban settlement/town in the north central Nigeria, the capital city of the Nupe Kingdom and headquarter of Bida Local Government Area of Niger State. It is multicultural population comprising all the ethnic groups of Nigeria and people of all walks of life with an estimated population of about 185,553 people. All social classes in the society are well represented in the community. Subjects were selected from the social strata (market, schools/colleges and federal institutions) including the artisan by multistage sampling technique. Pre-tested semi-structured questionnaires were used as instrument of data collection and these were self administered. The questionnaires contained information on bio-data, knowledge, attitude and awareness of respondents towards usage of cotton bud, among others. It was not labeled in order to ensure confidentiality. Inclusion criteria were subjects that were 18 years and above and also having given consent to participate in the study. Approval to carry out the study was given by the ethical and research committee of the hospital. A simple descriptive analysis of the data obtained was carried out using SPSS version 15.0, and the results were presented in simple tables and charts.

3. Results

A total of 278 out of the 290 questionnaires that was administered were returned representing a 95.7% response rate. The male respondents were 137 (49.3%) while the female's was 141 (50.7%) given a male to female ratio of 1:1.03. Their age ranged was from 18 years to 65 years with a mean of 29.64 ± 10.06 SD. From **Table 1**, the highest response was in the age group of 20 - 29 years representing 51.1% of the respondents. Majority (50.4%) of the respondents were Nupe by tribe. One hundred and forty one (50.7%) were Christian, while 137 (49.3%) practice Islamic religion. Two hundred and one (72.3%) had tertiary education, 56 (20.1%) had secondary, 10 (3.6%) had primary while 11 (4.0%) had no formal education (**Figure 1**). One hundred and twelve (40.3%) of the respondents were civil servants, 99 (35.6%) were students, 32 (11.5%) engaged in business, 19 (6.8%) were farmer, 13 (4.7%) were artisan while 11 (4.0%) had no job. Two hundred and fifty eight (92.8%) of the respondents had used cotton bud in cleaning their ears, 17(6.1%) had never used it while 3 (1.1%) were not sure. Out of those that use cotton buds to clean their ears, majority (57.8%) of them used it because of itching in the ear (**Figure 2**). One hundred and thirty eight (53.5%) respondents used cotton buds on their own, 89 (34.5%) were introduced to it by their parents, 15 (5.8%) by health care provider, 12 (4.7%) by friends while 4 (1.6%) from their spouses. On whether the cotton bud can damage the ear, 123 (44.9%) of the respondents said yes, 77 (28.1%) said no while 74 (27.0%) were not sure. One hundred and seventy (61.2%) respondents believed that there is benefit from cleaning the ears with cotton bud, 61(21.9%) said there is no benefit of using it, while 47 (16.9%) were not sure if there is any benefit. Only Fifty eight (22.5%) of the respondents that uses cotton bud developed complications, 190 (73.6%) had no complication and 10 (3.9%) were not sure. Two hundred and six (74.1%) of the subjects had no information on the danger of using cotton buds in the ears, while only 72 (25.9%)

Table 1. Showing age, gender and socio-demographic characteristics of respondents. N = 278.

Category		Frequency (N)	Percent (%)
Age group (years)	10 - 19	21	7.6
	20 - 29	142	51.1
	30 - 39	69	24.8
	40 - 49	32	11.5
	50 - 59	6	2.2
	60 - 69	8	2.9
		278	**100.0**
Gender	Male	137	49.3
	Female	141	50.7
		278	**100.0**
Tribe	Yoruba	65	23.4
	Hausa	42	15.1
	Ibo	31	11.2
	Nupe	140	50.4
		278	**100.0**
Religion	Christianity	141	50.7
	Islam	137	49.3
		278	**100.0**
Education	Nil	11	4.0
	Primary	10	3.6
	Secondary	56	20.1
	Tertiary	201	72.3
		278	**100.0**

have information. Of those that had information, 51 (18.3%) of them got their information from health talk through the health workers in the hospital, 13 (4.7%) got information from their friends and neighbours, 7 (2.5%) through Radio/TV while only one (0.4%) subject had information from publications (**Table 2**).

4. Discussion

Cotton-bud-related injuries are a common reason for attendance at ear, nose and throat (ENT) referral clinics [3]. The response rate of 95.7% (278/290) from our subjects in this study was good and showed their willingness to take part in the study. This study also showed that Females' respondents were slightly higher than their male counterpart, in contrast to separate studies done by Hobson and Kumar *et al.* [4] [6], where they recorded male preponderance. However another study done by Lee *et al.* [8] did not showed any gender difference. The highest users of cotton buds in this study were in the age group 20 - 29 years. Similar findings were recorded in other studies [8] [9]. Despite the fact that majority of our respondents (72.3%) were literate, larger percentage (92.8%) of them had used cotton buds to clean their ears. This is similar to other studies [8] [10] [11]. There were various reasons why people clean their ears with cotton buds; in this study the commonest reason is to scratch itchy ear canals in 57.8% of the respondents. This is in contrast to other studies where most subjects used cotton buds to

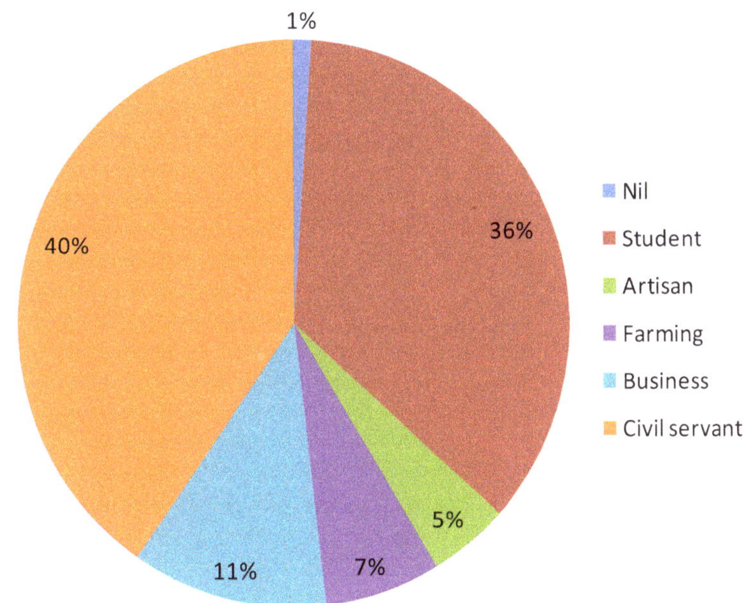

Figure 1. Occupation of respondents.

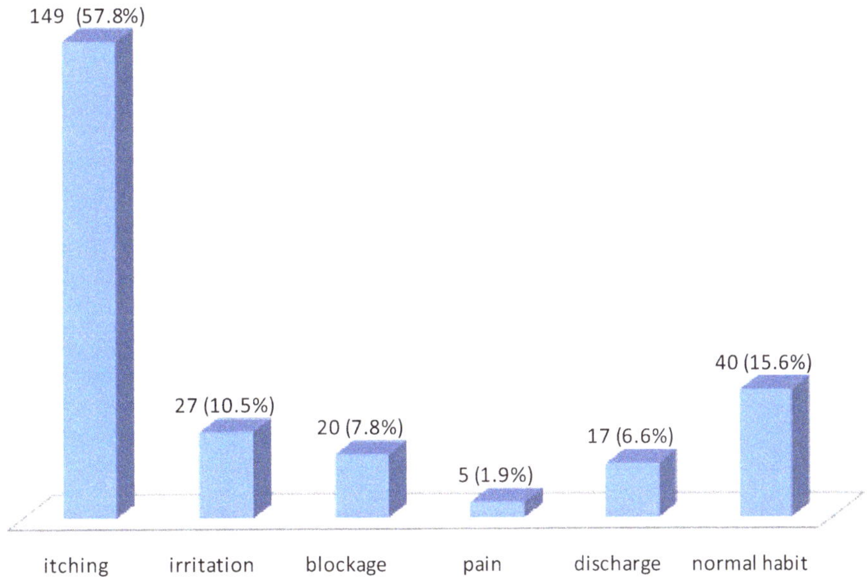

Figure 2. Reasons for cleaning ears with cotton buds.

remove wax in their ear canals [8]-[10]. The practice of using cotton bud to scratch ear canal is dangerous, as it can easily traumatize the ear canal and infection may eventually follows. Medical opinion should be sought from Otolaryngologist if ear itchiness persists, as this may be a symptom of otomycosis or eczema. Of worthy mention are those that make use of cotton bud as part of their normal/routine habit on daily basis not minding the consequences that followed it use. Majority (53.5%) of the respondents in this study used cotton buds on their own *ab initio*. however some of them imitate their parents, spouses and friends who also practiced the habit. About 5.8% claimed to have conceived the idea from health care workers. Hobson *et al.* also reported that only small numbers of his subjects were advised to use cotton bud by medical professionals [4]. This study also showed that majority (61.2%) of our respondents believed that there were benefits in using cotton bud hence only few (44.9%) them think that using cotton bud can cause damage to ears. Some of the respondents also claimed that apart from aesthetic appearance of cotton buds, the tip are softer and safer to use than the matches

Table 2. Showing the participants knowledge, attitude and awareness to the uses, damage, complications, benefits and source of information on the usage of cotton buds.

Category	Frequency (N)	Percent (%)
Uses cotton bud		
Yes	258	92.8
No	17	6.1
Not sure	3	1.1
Whether cotton bud can damage ear		
Yes	123	44.9
No	77	28.1
Not sure	74	27.1
Benefits of using cotton bud		
Yes	170	61.2
No	61	21.9
Not sure	47	16.9
Complications from use of cotton bud		
Yes	58	22.5
No	190	73.6
Not sure	10	3.9
Information on use of cotton bud		
No information	206	74.1
Had information	72	25.9
Health talk in the hospital	51 (18.3%)	
Friends/neighbour	13 (4.7%)	
Media (radio/TV)	7 (2.5%)	
Publication/journal	1 (0.4%)	

or broom stick which they noted to be sharp. In this study complication noted includes bruises with minor bleeding, otalgia and impaction of the cotton bud in the EAC leading to blockage. Otitis externa has been reported by overzealous use of cotton buds in some studies [8] [12]. Most (74.1%) of our respondents had never had information on the dangers of using cotton buds in the ears. This shows that the medical advice not to clean the ears is not widely known as also noted in a study done by Olaosun [10]. Of the few subjects that had the information, only 18.3% got their information in the hospital through health talk from health workers. It is glaring that awareness is very poor. Most of the subjects that use cotton buds were young adults, and this practice will continue as they teach their children to do this. There is need to create awareness among people in the community and in the schools through health education with emphasis that ear wax should not be removed with cotton buds. There is a natural mechanism where ear wax is removed from the ear canal.

5. Conclusion

In this study, majority (92.8%) of our participants indulged in the use of cotton buds in cleaning their ears. And the commonest reason for using cotton bud is due to itching in the ears. Their knowledge, attitude and awareness to the use of cotton buds are very poor with erroneous believe that there is benefit to its use. The medical advice not to clean the ears is not widely known. There is a need to increase awareness by public enlightenment and health education and to establish school health programme in our various schools.

References

[1] http://en.wikipedia.org/wiki/cotton_swab

[2] http://en.wikipedia.org/wiki/Leo_Gerstenzang

[3] Steele, B.D. and Brennan, P.O. (2002) A Prospective Survey of Patients with Presumed Accidental Ear Injury Presenting to a Paediatric Accident and Emergency Department. *Emergency Medicine Journal*, **19**, 226-228.

[4] Hobson, J.C. and Lavy, J.A. (2005) Use and Abuse of Cotton Buds. *Journal of the Royal Society of Medicine*, **98**, 360-361. http://dx.doi.org/10.1258/jrsm.98.8.360

[5] Nagala, S., Singh, P. and Tostevin, P. (2011) Extent of Cotton-Bud Use in Ears. *British Journal of General Practice*, **61**, 662-663. http://dx.doi.org/10.3399/bjgp11X606546

[6] Kumar, S. and Ahmed, S. (2008) Use of Cotton Buds and Its Complications. *Journal of Surgery Pakistan* (*International*), **13**, 137-138

[7] Raman, R. (1997) Should Cotton Buds Be Banned? *Tropical Doctor*, **27**, 250.

[8] Amutta, S.B., Yunusa, M.A., Iseh, K.R., Obembe, A., Egili, E., Aliyu, D. and Abdullahi, M. (2013) Sociodemographic Characteristics and Prevalence of Self Ear Cleaning in Sokoto Metropolis. *International Journal of Otolaryngology and Head & Neck Surgery*, **2**, 276-279.

[9] Lee, L.M., Govindaraju, R. and Hon, S.K. (2005) Cotton Bud and Ear Cleaning—A Loose Tip Cotton Bud? *Medical Journal of Malaysia*, **60**, 85-88.

[10] Olaosun, A.O. (2014) Self-Ear-Cleaning among Educated Young Adults in Nigeria. *Journal of Family Medicine and Primary Care*, **3**, 17-21. http://dx.doi.org/10.4103/2249-4863.130262

[11] Afolabi, A.O., Kodiya, A.M., Bakari, A. and Ahmad, B.M. (2009) Attitude of Self Ear Cleaning in Black Africans: Any Benefit? *East African Journal of Public Health*, **6**, 43-46. http://dx.doi.org/10.4314/eajph.v6i1.45743

[12] Nussinovitch, M., Rimon, A., Volovitz, B., Raveh, E., Prais, D. and Amir, J. (2004) Cotton-Tip Applicators as Aleading Cause of Otitis Externa. *International Journal of Pediatric Otorhinolaryngology*, **68**, 433-435. http://dx.doi.org/10.1016/j.ijporl.2003.11.014

18

Etiology Profile of the Patients Implanted in the Cochlear Implant Program

Saroj Mali, Divij Sonkhya, Mohnish Grover, Nishi Sonkhya*

Department of ENT, SMS Medical College and Hospital, Jaipur, India

Email: *drsonkhya@yahoo.co.in

Abstract

Hearing loss in children constitutes a considerable handicap because it is an invisible disability and compromises optimal development and personal achievement of a child. The period from birth to 5 years of life is critical for the development of speech and language; therefore, there is need for early identification and assessment of hearing loss and early rehabilitation in infants and children. Cochlear implants are the treatment of choice for patients with severe to profound sensorineural hearing loss. The goal of the present study was to investigate the different hearing impairment etiologies of patients implanted in cochlear implant program. The hospital based interventional study was conducted in the Department of Otorhinolaryngology, SMS Medical College, Jaipur from July 2011 to Dec. 2013. Present study included 60 prelingually deafened patients who attended ENT OPD and underwent cochlear implant. The most common cause of deafness in our study was acquired (56.66%), which predominantly included perinatal risk factors (64.70%), followed by prenatal risk factors (41.17%). The second common cause was hereditary (26.66%), followed by unknown (16.66%). Infection and ototoxic drug history were the most common risk factors in prenatal and postnatal group. The most common perinatal cause was low birth weight and prematurity.

Keywords

Hearing Impairment, Cochlear Implant, Congenital Sensorineural Hearing Loss, Familial Hearing Loss, Syndromic Hearing Loss

1. Introduction

Hearing loss in children constitutes a considerable handicap because it is an invisible disability and compromis-

*Corresponding author.

es optimal development and personal achievement of a child. Hearing loss in a child may develop from causes before birth (prenatal), during birth (perinatal) or thereafter (postnatal). Prenatal causes may pertain to the infant or the mother. An infant may be born with inner ear anomalies due to genetic or nongenetic causes. Anomalies affecting the inner ear may involve only the membranous labyrinth or both the membranous and bony labyrinths, which include Sheibe's dysplasia, Alexander's dysplasia, Bing-Siebenmann dysplasia, Mondini's dysplasia, enlarged vestibular aqueduct and semicircular canal malformations. Maternal factors include infections, drugs during pregnancy, radiation to the mother in first trimester and other factors which include nutritional deficiency, diabetes, toxaemia and thyroid deficiency. Maternal alcoholism is also teratogenic to the developing auditory system. Infections which affect the developing foetus are Toxoplasmosis, Rubella, Cytomegalovirus, Herpes type 1 and 2 and Syphilis. Drugs like Streptomycin, Gentamycin, Tobramycin, Amikacin, Quinine or Chloroquine, when given to the pregnant mother, cross the placental barrier and damage the cochlea. Perinatal causes relate to those during birth or in early neonatal period and include anoxia, prematurity, low birth weight, birth injuries, neonatal jaundice (bilirubin level greater than 20 mg% damages the cochlear nuclei), neonatal meningitis, sepsis, time spent in neonatal ICU and ototoxic drugs. Postnatal causes include viral infections (Measles, Mumps, Varicella, and Influenza), meningitis and encephalitis. Other causes are secretory otitis media, ototoxic drugs, trauma including fracture of temporal bone, middle ear surgery or perilymph leak and noise induced deafness.

2. Material and Methods

Present study included prelingually deafened patients, who attended ENT OPD and underwent cochlear implant in Department of Otorhinolaryngology, SMS Medical College, Jaipur from July 2011 to Dec. 2013. 60 patients (age 2.5 yrs - 11 yrs) underwent cochlear implant in the study period. A detailed history was obtained in reference to prenatal, perinatal and post natal period to find out various risk factors for hearing loss. The etiological diagnosis was obtained by means of an interview carried with the parents and family members. We approached relevant issues such as problems during pregnancy (prenatal factors), problems during delivery and birth of the baby (perinatal factors), problems during postnatal period and hereditary factors associated with the current disease.

3. Results

The study included 60 patients, with male to female ratio of 1.72 and males contributing 63.4% and females were 36.6%. The most common cause of deafness in our study was acquired (56.66%), which predominantly included perinatal risk factors (64.70%), followed by prenatal risk factors (41.17%). The second common cause was hereditary (26.66%), followed by unknown (16.66%) (**Table 1**, **Table 2** and **Figure 1**).

Considering the 14 cases which presented with prenatal risk factors, it was observed that Infection and ototoxic drug history was the most common prenatal risk factor. There were two patients who had congenital rubella syndrome (**Table 3** and **Figure 2**).

Considering the perinatal factors, it was observed that low birth weight, birth asphyxia and prematurity were the important risk factors (**Table 4**). Infection with history of ototoxic drugs, and hyperbilirubenemia requiring phototherapy in neonatal period were the predominant postnatal factors, contributing 80% (**Table 5** and **Figure 3**). 5% of our patients had Waardenburg's syndrome. The distribution of hearing loss in the syndromic verses nonsyndromic group is statistically highly significant (**Table 6**). 13 patients had family history of deaf-mutism, out

Table 1. Etiological factors.

n = 60

Etiological factors for deafness	No. of patients	Percentage
Unknown	10	16.66
Acquired	34	56.66
Hereditary: familial (13) syndromic (3)	16	26.66
Total	60	100

Table 2. Acquired causes of deafness.

n = 34

Causes of hearing loss	No. of patients	Percentage
Prenatal	6	17.64
Perinatal	10	29.41
Postnatal	4	11.76
Prenatal + perinatal	6	17.64
Perinatal + postnatal	4	11.76
Prenatal + perinatal + postnatal	2	5.88
Infant factor	2	5.88
Total	34	100

Prenatal: 14 (41.17); Perinatal: 22 (64.70); Postnatal: 10 (29.41); Infant factor: 2 (5.88).

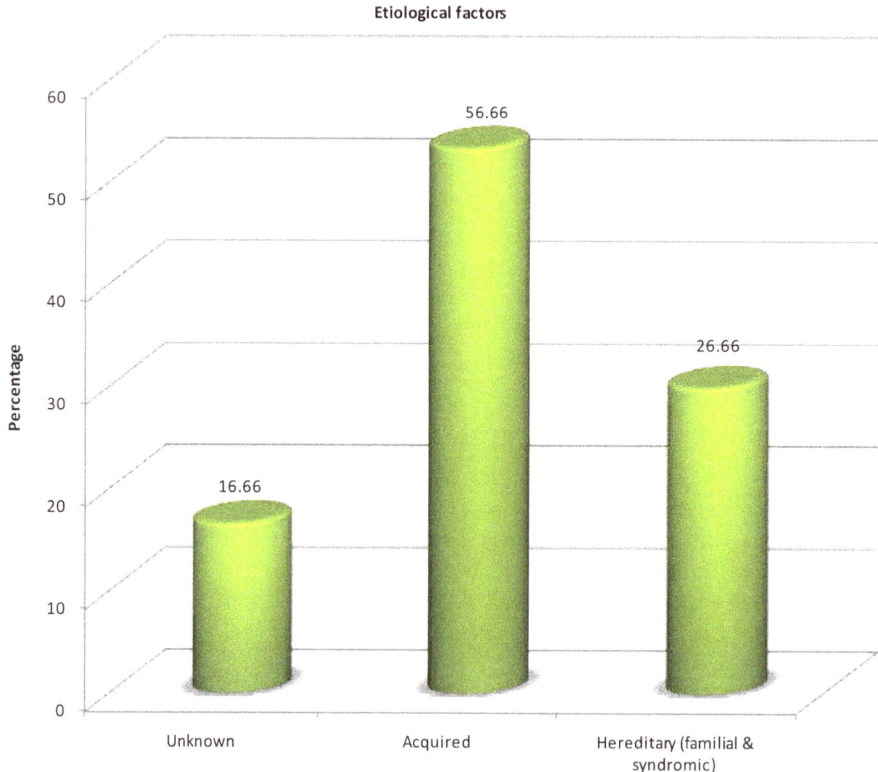

Figure 1. Showing etiological factors.

of them 2 patients had both maternal and sibling factors, these patients were included in sibling group, therefore, out of 13 cases of familial deafness, 69.23% of the patients were in the sibling group (**Table 7**).

4. Discussion

We have performed an institutional study which included prospective review of prelingually deaf children aged 2.5 to 11 years (60 cases), with bilateral severe to profound SNHL who derived minimal to no benefit from conventional amplification *i.e.* using hearing aid and underwent unilateral Cochlear Implant from July 2011 to Dec. 2013. In the present study of 60 patients, male to female ratio was 1.72, with males contributing 63.33% and females were 36.66%, this is in concordance with the gender distribution given by Calhau [1], in which

Table 3. Distribution of prenatal risk factors.

n = 14

Prenatal factors	No. of patients	Percentage
Torch group	2 (rubella)	14.28
Infection and ototoxic drug history (amikacin and tobramycin)	6	42.85
History of repeated abortion	2	14.28
Preeclampsia	2	14.28
History of abortion + preeclampsia	2	14.28
Total No. of patients	14	100

Table 4. Distribution of perinatal risk factors.

n = 22

Perinatal factors	No. of patients	Percentage
Low birth weight	8	36.36
Low birth weight + birth asphyxia	2	9.09
Low birth weight + prematurity	2	9.09
Low birth weight + birth asphyxia + prolonged labour (forceps delivery)	2	9.09
Low birth weight + birth asphyxia + prematurity	4	18.18
Meconium aspiration	2	9.09
Meconium aspiration + low birth + prematurity	2	9.09
Total No. of patients	22	100

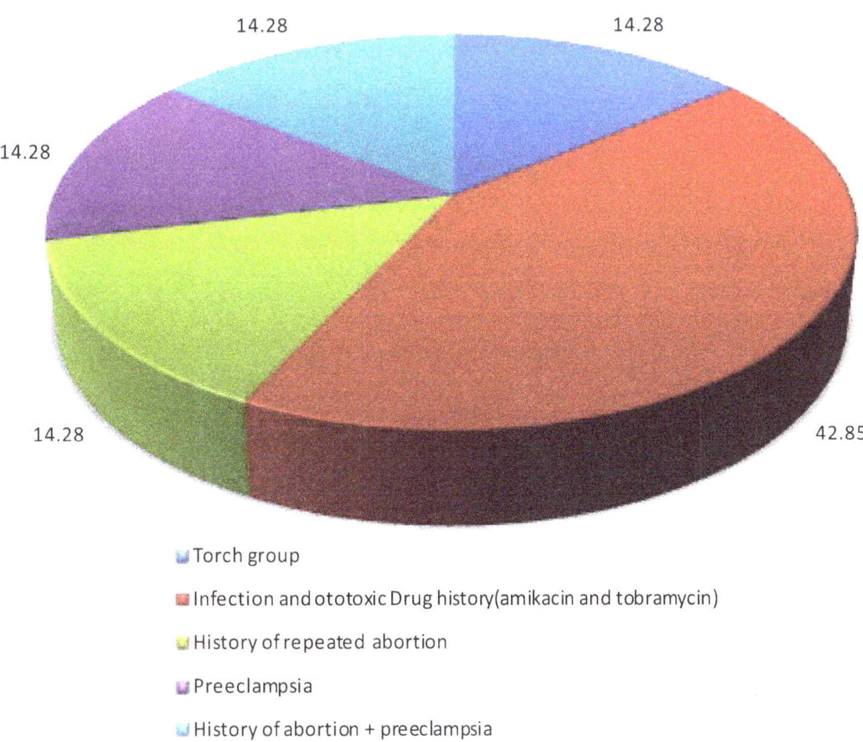

Figure 2. Distribution of prenatal risk factors.

Table 5. Distribution of postnatal risk factors.

n = 10

Postnatal factors	No. of patients	Percentage	
Viral infection	-	-	
Infection and ototoxic drug history	4	40	
Infection with ototoxic drug history and hyperbilirubenemia	2	20	80
Hyperbilirubenemia requiring phototherapy	2	20	
Delayed milestones + ototoxic drug history	2	20	
Total	10	100	

Table 6. Syndromic/nonsyndromic hearing loss.

n = 60

Hearing loss	No. of patients	Percentage	P value (Z test)
Syndromic	3	5	
Nonsyndromic	57	95	0.001 (HS)
Total	60	100	

HS: Highly Significant

Table 7. Familial cases of deafmutism.

n = 13

Familial	No. of patients	Percentage
Paternal	2	15.38
Maternal	2	15.38
Sibling	9	69.23
Total	13	100

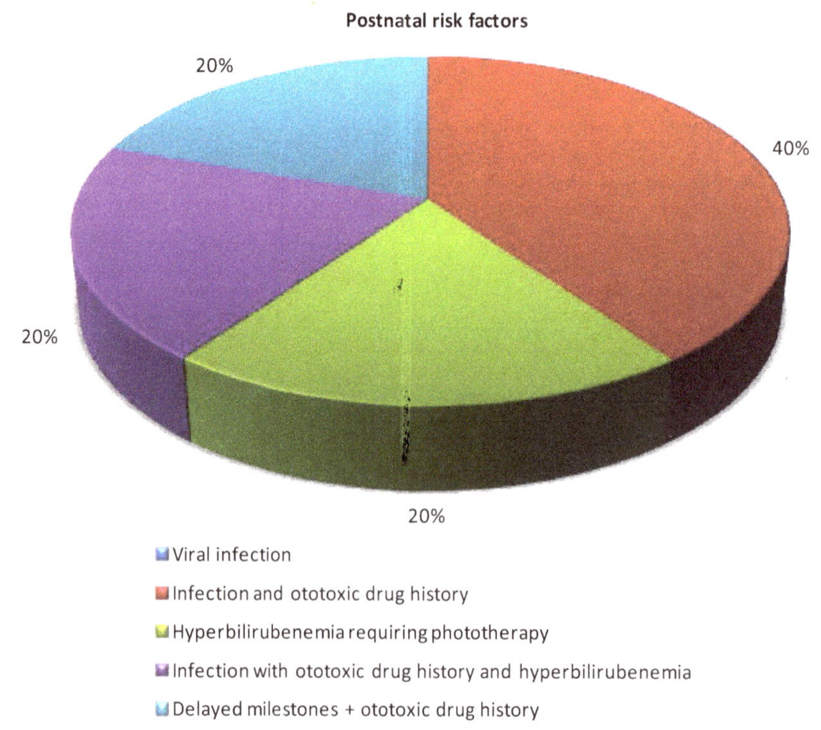

Figure 3. Postnatal risk factors.

male to female ratio was 1.66 with males contributing 62.5% and females were 37.5%; while in a study of 70 cases by Iype [2], male to female ratio was 1.06:1.

There is wide variation across the globe in the incidence and prevalence of childhood hearing loss and its possible etiology. The etiological diagnosis was obtained by means of an interview carried with the parents and family members. We approached relevant issues such as problems during pregnancy (prenatal factors), problems during delivery and birth of the baby (perinatal factors), problems during postnatal period and hereditary factors associated with the current disease.

The most common cause in our study was the acquired (56.66%), corroborating with the prior studies reported by Iype [2], while Taylor [3] reported 41.86% incidence of acquired causes. Studies by Fisch [4], Calhau [1] reported unknown cause as the most common factor. The second most contributing factor was the hereditary cause (26.66%), corroborating with Billings [5], while Calhau [1] reported maternal rubella to be the second most common cause. The third cause is unknown (idiopathic), contributing to 16.66% of the deafness. Fraser [6] in 1960 from U.K reported that in 70% patients, the etiology was congenital and in 30%, it was acquired. Strauss [7] in 1990 from USA reported that the probable cause of congenital deafness in their patients were toxoplasmosis (10% - 15%), rubella (33%) and cytomegalovirus (33% - 48%). He further observed that with introduction of immunization program, the incidence of disease has decreased. As reported by Martin and Davis, the most frequent cause of acquired deafness in childhood was meningitis [8] [9] and according to Dodge [10], 5% to 35% of the patients with bacterial meningitis develop permanent sensorineural hearing loss..

In 34 cases out of 60, an acquired cause for deafness was found. Infant factor in the form of meningitis was found in 2 patients. Prenatal risk factors were identified in 14 cases (41.17%) (**Table 2**), infection and ototoxic drug history was found to be the most common contributing factor (42.85%), next common factors were history of repeated abortion (14.28%) and preeclampsia (14.28%). Serological test results were available for two cases which were positive for rubella infection (**Table 3**).

In 22 cases (64.70%), perinatal risk factors were found, the most common cause was low birth weight followed by birth asphyxia and prematurity (**Table 4**). This is in concordance with the study carried out by Iype [2], in which prenatal risk factors were identified in 45.71%, perinatal factors were found in 71.42%. Birth asphyxia predisposed by prematurity and low birth weight was the most common perinatal risk factor. Majority of their neonatal group had jaundice requiring phototherapy and had delayed motor or personal social development. Bergman [11] found higher incidence of hearing loss in preterm babies than normal because of prolonged hypoxia or acidosis.

In the present study, postnatal risk factors were found in 10 cases (29.41%), infection with history of ototoxic drugs was the most common contributing postnatal risk factors (60%). Ototoxic drugs leading to hearing loss in our study were Gentamycin, Tobramycin and Amikacin, this is in concordance with study by Zahnert [12]. Delayed milestones were found in two patients (**Table 5**). In the study by Iype [2], neonatal risk factors along with antenatal or perinatal risk factors were found in 8 patients. Majority had neonatal jaundice requiring exchange transfusion (6 cases); of these a high proportion had delayed motor or personal social development.

3 patients of the study group had syndromic features with white forelock, dystopia canthorum and heterochromiairidis (Waardenburg's syndrome), contributing to 5% and with the significant P value of 0.001 (**Table 6**). Zeitter [13] reported 3 (4.47%) patients of Waardenburg's syndrome. In a study by Singh [14], syndromic hearing loss were found in 5.4% patients of which, three cases were of Usher syndrome, four Waardenburg's syndrome, two Down syndrome and one patient of Treacher-collin syndrome.

S2-leitlinie, 2011 [15] reported that hearing impairment of genetic cause is due to congenital syndrome in 30% of cases and is nonsyndromic in 70%. Among the nonsyndromic cases, the inheritance pattern is autosomal recessive in 70% - 80%, autosomal dominant in 10% - 25%, and X-linked in 2% - 3%. In our study of 16 cases of hereditary cause 18.75% were of syndromic group.

Nonsyndromic autosomal recessive hearing loss (the most common) is often due to a genetic mutation that impairs the synthesis of transmembrane proteins connexin 26 and 30, which in turn affects the ion transport mechanism in the hair cells and accordingly, connexin 26 and 30 mutations should be sought, whenever hearing impairment of genetic origin is suspected. Genetic hearing impairment is usually severe, being due to sporadic mutation and therefore hard to diagnose [16].

13 patients (21.66%) (**Table 1**) in the study group had familial deafness, including 9 patients with history of deafmutism in sibling, 2 patients with paternal and 2 with maternal history of deafmutism (**Table 7** and **Figure 4**), while study by Singh (2009) [14] reported 10.8% cases of familial deafness.

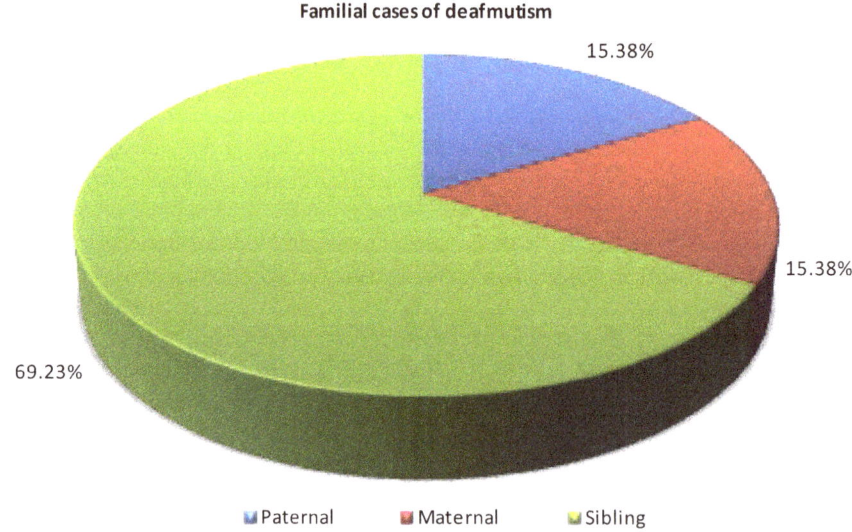

Figure 4. Distribution of familial cases of deafmutism.

5. Summary and Conclusions

The present study included 60 prelingually deafened patients who underwent cochlear implant in Department of Otorhinolaryngology, SMS Medical College, Jaipur. In this study, group perinatal risk factors were (64.7%) most common followed by prenatal (41.17%) and postnatal risk factors.

Infant factors were present in 2 cases (5.88%). Low birth weight along with asphyxia and prematurity was most common perinatal cause. Infection and ototoxic drug history were most common causes in both prenatal and postnatal group. 3 patients (5%) were of syndromic deafness while 13 patients (21.66%) had familial deafness.

References

[1] Ferreira, C.C.M.D., Lima, J.L.R.P., *et al.* (2011) Etiology Profile of the Patients Implanted in the Cochlear Implant Program. *Brazilian Journal of Otorhinolaryngology*, **77**, 13-18.

[2] Mathew, I.E., Sasikumaran, S. and Indira, D.S. (2000) A Clinical Study on Congenital and Neonatal Deafness. *Indian Journal of Otolaryngology and Head and Neck Surgery*, **52**, 242-245.

[3] Taylor, I.G. (1980) The Prevention of Sensorineural Deafness. *Journal of Laryngology and Otology*, **94**, 1327-1343.

[4] Fisch, I.G., Hine, W.D. and Brascer, V.J. (1975) A Study of the Causes of Hearing Loss in a Population of Deaf Children with Special Reference to Genetic Factors. *The Journal of Laryngology and Otology*, **89**, 899-914. http://dx.doi.org/10.1017/S0022215100081184

[5] Billings, K.R. and Kenna, M.A. (1999) Causes of Pediatric Sensorineural Hearing Loss: Yesterday and Today. *Arch Otolaryngol Head Neck Surg.*, **125**, 517-521. http://dx.doi.org/10.1001/archotol.125.5.517

[6] Fraser, G.R., Froggatt, P. and James, T.N. (1964) Congenital Deafness Associated with Electrocardiographic Abnormalities, Fainting Attacks and Sudden Death. *Quart J Med*, **33**, 361-385.

[7] Strauss, M. (1990) Human Cytomegalovirus Labyrinthitis. *American Journal of Otolaryngology*, **11**, 292-329. http://dx.doi.org/10.1016/0196-0709(90)90057-3

[8] Martin, J.A.M. (1982) Aetiological Factors Relating to Childhood Deafness in the European Community. *Audiology*, **21**, 149-158. http://dx.doi.org/10.3109/00206098209072735

[9] Davis, A.C., Wood (1992) The Epidemiology of Childhood Hearing Impairment: Factors Relevant to Planning of Services. *British Journal of Audiology*, **26**, 77-90.

[10] Dodge, P.R., Davis, H., Feigin, R.D., *et al.* (1984) Prospective Evaluation of Hearing Impairment as a Sequela of Acute Bacterial Meningitis. *The New England Journal of Medicine*, **311**, 869-874.

[11] Bergman, L., Hirsch, R.P., Fria, T.J., Shapiro, S.M., Holzman, I. and Painter, M.J. (1985) Cause of Hearing Loss in the High-Risk Premature Infant. *The Journal of Pediatrics*, **106**, 95-101. http://dx.doi.org/10.1016/S0022-3476(85)80476-5

[12] Zanhert, T. (2011) The Differential Diagnosis of Hearing Loss. *Deutsches Arzteblatt International*, **108**, 433-444.

[13] Zeitler, D.M., Anwar, A., *et al.* (2012) Cochlear Implantation in Prelingually Deafened Adolescents. *Archives of Pediatrics and Adolescent Medicine*, **166**, 35-41. http://dx.doi.org/10.1001/archpediatrics.2011.574

[14] Singh, M., Gupta, S.C. and Singla, A. (2009) Assessment of Deafmute Patients: A Study of Ten Years. *Indian Journal of Otolaryngology and Head & Neck Surgery*, **61**, 19-22. http://dx.doi.org/10.1007/s12070-009-0027-3

[15] S2-Leitlinie (2011) Periphere Horstorungen im Kindesalter. AWMF-Register Number 049/010, Stand 02/2005. www.awmf.org/uploads/tx_szleitlinien/049-0101.pdf

[16] Ptok, M. and Ptok, A. (2001) Formen kindlicher Schwerhorigkeit. *Monatsschr Kinderheilkd*, **149**, 870-876.

19

Stylomastoid Foramen Osteoma: Unique Challenges for Appropriate Management

Aisha Larem, Sally Sheta, Abdulsalam Al-Qahtani, Hassan Haidar*

Department of Otolaryngology, Hamad Medical Corporation, Doha, Qatar
Email: *Hahmad2@hamad.qa

Abstract

Osteoma of the temporal bone is a rare and slow-growing benign tumor. It is reported to affect almost all portions of the temporal bone. However, osteoma involving the stylomastoid foramen has never been reported in the literature. We report a case of an osteoma extending from the stylomastoid foramen and occluding the external auditory canal in a young female. Although the osteoma has very close relationship with the facial nerve, it was removed because of the severity of its associated symptomatology; the osteoma was completely removed without any postoperative complications. This report is of interest as it highlights the challenges in the management of osteomas in such localization.

Keywords

Osteoma, Temporal Bone, Stylomastoid Foramen, Facial Nerve

1. Introduction

Osteomas are benign neoplasms formed of mature bone and arising almost exclusively from bone made in membrane, e.g. the skull. In the head and neck region, they are usually found in the front oethmoid area [1] [2]. Temporal bone osteomas are a rare entity [3], and when this occurs, they are most commonly seen in the external auditory canal (canalicular osteomas). Extra canalicular temporal osteomas, such as mastoid osteomas are even more infrequent [4]. Osteomas are usually asymptomatic [5]; in symptomatic cases, typically due to cosmetic deformity, treatment of the osteoma is surgical, but in symptomatic cases involving noble structures, the management can be challenging.

In this report, we present a case of a 43-year-old female patient with a large osteoma extending from the stylomastoid foramen (SMF) and filling the EAC and we discuss the challenges regarding the treatment of this lesion.

*Corresponding author.

2. Case Report

A 43-year-old female, previously healthy, was referred to our center due to a long-standing history of right recurrent otitis externa that become very frequent and invalidating. She reports also progressive right sided hearing loss. There were no accompanying symptoms of vertigo or tinnitus in her medical history.

Otolaryngologic examination revealed a hard, immobile, mildly tender mass with erythematous overlying skin filling the right EAC, occluding view to the tympanic membrane. The left ear was normal. Facial nerve examination was intact bilaterally. No other masses were palpated in the head and neck region. On audiogram, right conductive hearing loss was revealed.

A temporal bone CT scan indicated a well demarcated, dense, sclerotic mass of approximately 2.3 × 2 cm of the right mastoid process filling the EAC and extending inferiorly to the SMF, the mass was very near but not involving the mastoid segment of the fallopian canal. The middle and inner ear were normal. The radiologic appearance was suggestive of osteoma (**Figure 1**).

Because of the severity of her symptoms, especially severe and refractory otitis externa, the patient was asking for definitive treatment. An extensive discussion was done with her on the risk of facial nerve injury because of the critical localization of the lesion. The patient accepted the risk and signed a medical consent of high risk of postoperative facial palsy.

The resection of tumor was performed using posterior transmastoid approach (**Figure 2**). A facial monitor was used due to the close proximity of the facial nerve. After a cortical mastoidectomy, the mastoid segment of the facial nerve was identified and followed down till the SMF. The osteoma was identified in the anteroinferior part of the mastoid process about 1mm lateral to the fallopian canal; the posterior and inferior walls of the EAC were replaced by the tumor which was filling the lateral part of the EAC and extending inferiorly on the vaginal process till the base of styloid process. A gradual drilling around the tumor was performed, taking care of the proximity of the facial nerve, till the mass was complete excised en bloc. Reconstruction of the EAC was done using tragal cartilage and fascia that was covered by the remaining skin. The canal was dressed with gauze with antibiotic and corticoid unguent for 2 weeks (**Figure 2**).

The postoperative period was smooth, facial nerve function was intact. Three weeks later, the EAC dressing was removed; the canal was patent and wide and completely epithelized. Histopathology result confirmed the diagnosis of osteoma (**Figure 3**).

In subsequent follow-up in the 18 ensuing months, patient remained asymptomatic and relieved from the cosmetic, inflammatory and auditory symptoms.

3. Discussion

Temporal bone osteomas are very rare benign osteogenic tumors. When they occur, they are seen most commonly in the EAC. Here they arise from the site lateral to the isthmus of the EAC, with its base being located at

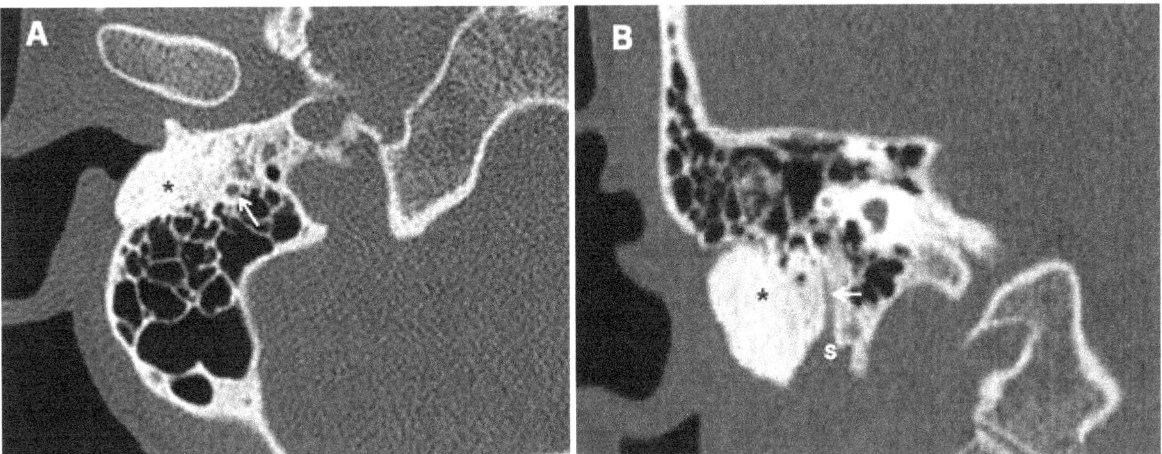

Figure 1. Right Temporal bone CT scan, Axial cut A and saggital cut B showing a hyperdense bony mass (*) occluding the ear canal extending posteriorly into the mastoid in close relationship with the facial nerve(white arrow) and inferiorly to the stylomastoid foramen (S).

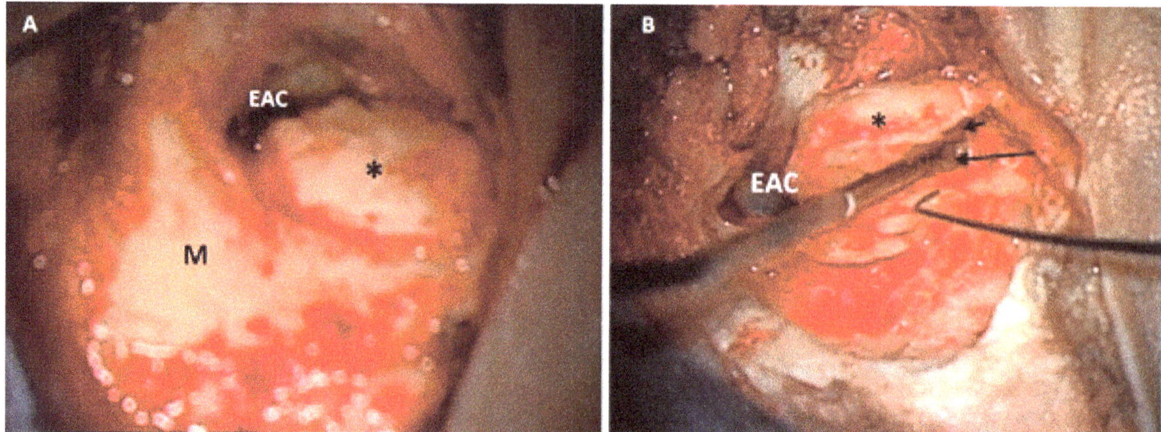

Figure 2. Operative view of posterior approach of right ear. A: a big osteoma (*) filling the ear canal (EAC) and extending to the mastoid cortex (M) and extending inferiorly. B: after cortical mastoidectomy, the mastoid facial nerve is identified till its emergence from the stylomastoid foramen (long arrow); osteoma (*) ;styloid process (short arrow).

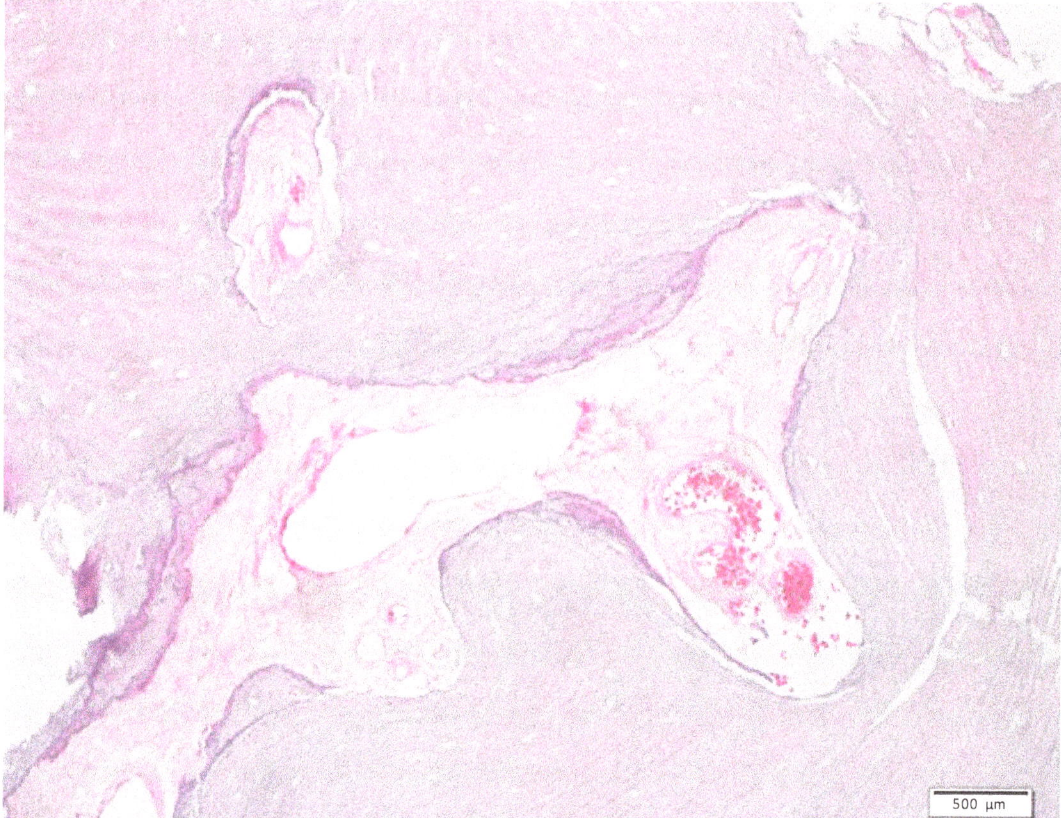

Figure 3. Histopathological assessment of the bony tumor excised. Sections show dense, mature, predominantly lamellar bone. Interosseous space is mostly composed of scant fibrovascular tissue.

the tympanosquamous or tympanomastoid suture lines adjacent to the bony-cartilaginous junction in most cases. An osteoma originates from the preosseous connective tissue in these suture lines as they have a thicker subcutaneous layer and a richer blood supply than the other parts of the bony canal. Canalicular osteomas are usually localized to the external auditory canal; however, canalicular osteomas extending to the stylomastoid foramen have never been reported in literature.

Although an osteoma of the EAC grows slowly and remains stable for many years, symptoms such as conductive hearing impairment or recurrent infection can arise if the osteoma grows to a point of canal obstruction. Hearing loss occurs due to retention of epithelial residues and wax, rather than mechanical obstruction of the conductive passage by the tumor. A secondary cholesteatoma can ensue [6].

Diagnosis is usually confirmed by CT scanwhere osteomas appear as a well circumscribed mass with soft tissue density, egg-shell like density or bone density.

When it comes to histopathological assessment, osteomas are formed of mature bone. Three histological patterns are identified. The compact/ ivoryosteoma consists of dense bone lacking Haversian systems. The cancellous/spongioform osteoma often resembles "normal" bone with central trabeculae containing bone marrow. The mixed osteoma shows both the compact and cancellous variety.

The main treatment for an EAC osteoma is a surgical excision. The size and location of the osteoma as well as the severity of symptoms determine the treatment. Patients with a small osteoma and little or no symptoms may be treated in a conservative manner. Surgical excision is recommended if a growing osteoma results in occlusion of the canal and the patient complains of recurrent infection and/or conductive hearing impairment. When the osteoma is located at the lateral portion of the isthmus and is a peduncular type, it can be easily removed by an osteotome or drilling through the transmeatal approach. When an osteoma is located medial to the isthmus, is huge, or has a broad base, it is safe to remove it through the postauricular approach [7]-[11]. However, for cases with a large posterior wall defect the canal wall down mastoidectomy or canal wall up mastoidectomy with posterior wall reconstruction can be used [12] [13].

It is reported that in cases of osteomas extending into the fallopian canal, complete excision is not indicated since there is risk of damage to the facial nerve [14]. However, it is reported also that partial surgical excision by drilling on the tumor tissue may result in recurrence of tumor that may grow medially to encroach on vital structures making potential future revision excision challenging [14]. The definitive treatment of osteoma remains of complete resection by drilling around the osteoma and avoiding damage to vital structures [15].

In this case, the patient had a huge osteoma occluding almost the entire EAC and an extensive extension posteriorly and inferiorly in a close relationship with the mastoid segment of the fallopian canal till the SMF. Therefore, a canal wall up mastoidectomy and identification of the mastoid segment of the facial nerve from the second genu till the SMF was done first before resection of the osteoma; the inferior and posterior wall of the auditory canal was reconstructed using cartilage.

Prognostically, there are very rare situations where osteomas have recurred post excision, all of which were in long bones and there are no reported cases of recurrence in the head and neck region.

4. Conclusion

In conclusion, osteomas are rare osteogenic tumors that frequently pose no issues for the patient. Symptomatic osteomas in accessible regions can be successfully removed with few complications. Where these tumours involve key structures, as in our case was the facial nerve, surgical management should be planned to complete excise the tumor to avoid recurrence whilst preserving the chief structures.

Disclosure of Interest

There is no conflict of interest to disclose.

Informed Consent

Written informed consent was obtained from the patient who participated in this study.

References

[1] Probst, L.E., Shankar, L. and Fox, R. (1991) Osteoma of the Mastoid Bone. *The Journal of Otolaryngology*, **20**, 228-230.

[2] Burton, D.M. and Gonzalez, C. (1991) Mastoid Osteomas. *Ear, Nose & Throat Journal*, **70**, 161-162.

[3] Unal, O.F., Tosun, F., Yetişer, S. and Dündar, A. (2000) Osteoma of the Middle Ear. *International Journal of Pediatric Otorhinolaryngology*, **52**, 193-195. http://dx.doi.org/10.1016/S0165-5876(00)00286-X

[4] Das, A.K. and Kashyap, R.C. (2005) Osteoma of the Mastoid Bone—A Case Report. *Medical Journal Armed Forces India*, **61**, 86-87.

[5] Güngör, A., Cincik, H., Poyrazoglu, E., Saglam, O. and Candan, H. (2004) Mastoid Osteomas: Report of Two Cases. *Otology & Neurotology*, **25**, 95-97. http://dx.doi.org/10.1097/00129492-200403000-00002

[6] Fenton, J.E., Turner, J. and Fagan, P.A. (1996) A Histopathologic Review of Temporal Bone Exostoses and Osteomata. *The Laryngoscope*, **106**, 624-628. http://dx.doi.org/10.1097/00005537-199605000-00020

[7] Graham, M.D. (1979) Osteomas and Exostoses of the External Auditory Canal. A Clinical, Histopathologic and Scanning Electron Microscopic Study. *Annals of Otology, Rhinology & Laryngology*, **88**, 566-572. http://dx.doi.org/10.1177/000348947908800422

[8] Tran, L.P., Grundfast, K.M. and Selesnick, S.H. (1996) Benign Lesions of the External Auditory Canal. *Otolaryngologic Clinics of North America*, **29**, 807-825.

[9] Fisher, E.W. and McManus, T.C. (1994) Surgery for External Auditory Canal Exostoses and Osteomata. *The Journal of Laryngology & Otology*, **108**, 106-110. http://dx.doi.org/10.1017/S0022215100126027

[10] Sheehy, J.L. (1982) Diffuse Exostoses and Osteomata of the External Auditory Canal: A Report of 100 Operations. *Otolaryngology Head and Neck Surgery*, **90**, 337-342.

[11] Yamamoto, E., Iwanaga, M. and Sato, K. (1986) Osteoma with Cholesteatoma in the External Auditory Canal. *Practica Oto-Rhino-Laryngologica*, **79**, 575-578. http://dx.doi.org/10.5631/jibirin.79.575

[12] Orita, Y., Nishizaki, K., Fukushima, K., Akagi, H., Ogawa, T., Masuda, Y., Fukazawa, M. and Mori, Y. (1998) Osteoma with Cholesteatoma in the External Auditory Canal. *International Journal of Pediatric Otorhinolaryngology*, **43**, 289-293. http://dx.doi.org/10.1016/S0165-5876(98)00022-6

[13] Vrabec, J.T. and Chaljub, G. (2000) External Canal Cholesteatoma. *The American Journal of Otology*, **21**, 608-614.

[14] Mustafa, A. (2012) Osteoma of Mastoid Process Obstructing External Auditory Canal: A Case Report. *Health*, **4**, 222-224. http://dx.doi.org/10.4236/health.2012.44034

[15] Viswanatha, B. (2011) Characteristics of Osteoma of the Temporal Bone in Young Adolescents. *Ear, Nose & Throat Journal*, **90**, 72-79.

20

An Unusually Large Foreign Body in Oesophagus in a 2-Year-Old Male Child

Ajinkya Kelkar[1*], Kalpesh Patil[2]

[1]Department of Otolaryngology and Head and Neck Surgery, Yashwantrao Chavan Hospital, Pune, Maharashtra, India
[2]Department of Paediatric Surgery, Yashwantrao Chavan Hospital, Pune, Maharashtra, India
Email: [*]drajinkyakelkar@gmail.com

Abstract

A large variety of foreign bodies are swallowed by children, but the majority of those pass through the gastrointestinal tract without any adverse effects. The highest incidence of swallowed foreign bodies occurs in children between 6 months and 3 years. We reported to you an unusually large foreign body ingested by a 2-year-old male patient who underwent a rigid oesophagoscopy but the foreign body had to be removed by open surgical technique. It is advisable to have a multidisciplinary approach while dealing with such cases.

Keywords

Foreign Body, Screw, Oesophagoscopy, Gastrostomy

1. Introduction

Foreign bodies in the oesophagus are common in young children and the older age groups. The increased incidence of swallowed foreign bodies in children could be due to their natural propensity to gain knowledge by putting things in their mouth and inadequate control of deglutination as well as tendency to cry, cough or play during eating. Accidental ingestion is common in children due to their habit of putting things in the mouth. The most frequently swallowed foreign bodies in children include coins, safety pins, and toy parts. The peak age in children is between six months and three years.

Older age groups, particularly denture wearers who have less oral sensation, are more susceptible to foreign body ingestion. Fish bone, mutton bone and poorly chewed food are the common foreign bodies.

Since the muscular activity of the upper portion of the oesophagus is weak as compared with pharyngeal

[*]Corresponding author.

musculature, foreign bodies are propelled in the hypopharynx and are more likely to lodge in the cricopharynx. The next most common site is just above the gastro-oesophageal junction.

Failure in identification and management of such foreign bodies results in complications like erosion, perforation, retropharyngeal abscess and pulmonary complications.

The objective of this case report is to have a multidisciplinary approach to foreign body removal so as to prevent the subsequent complications.

2. Anatomy and Pathophysiology

Oesophagus is a vertical muscular tube that extends from the hypopharynx to the stomach. It measures 23 to 25 cm in length in adult [1]. It begins at the lower border of cricoid cartilage at the level of sixth cervical vertebra. It terminates at the cardiac orifice of the stomach at the level of eleventh thoracic vertebra. Normally the lumen of the oesophagus is collapsed in a flattened or stellate pattern. The diameter is reduced at four points: the cricopharynx, crossing of aorta, crossing of left main bronchus and the diaphragm. The average distance from the upper incisor teeth is 16 cm, 23 cm, 27 cm and 38 - 40 cm respectively.

3. Clinical Presentation and Diagnosis

Up to 35% of paediatric patients with oesophageal foreign bodies are asymptomatic. Therefore the history surrounding the foreign body ingestion is extremely important. When and how it occurred, as well as description of the object and subsequent symptoms can give the surgeon, avaluable information. If available, a duplicate of the object can be helpful in choosing the most appropriate instruments for oesophagoscopy and foreign body removal.

Symptoms of foreign body vary with its position and make up. Upper oesophageal foreign bodies produce dysphagia and suprasternal pain on swallowing. With more distal foreign bodies, presentation is vague and orientation and level may not be describable. Rough objects may cause mucosal injury while passing into the stomach and can cause pain which subsides in about 24 hours. Persistent pain suggests that the foreign body has remained lodged. Large objects can obstruct the oesophagus causing salivation and regurgitation of any swallowed liquid including saliva. They may also compress the trachea due to their bulk causing dyspnea.

Disc batteries may lodge in the oesophagus and react with the mucosa resulting in oesophageal burn, perforation and mediastinitis. Such foreign bodies must be removed as soon as possible to reduce the possibility of caustic leak.

Any suspicion of foreign body, its presence must be proved or disproved. Radiologic studies are necessary. Radio-opaque foreign bodies can be visualized in most instances with postero-anterior and lateral neck films from the skull base to thoracic inlet. Non radiopaque objects may also be found, such as increase in the distance between the cervical vertebra and the trachea or air in the cervical oesophagus. Very small radiodense foreign bodies can be visualized on Computed Tomography (CT).

4. Case Report

A 2-year-old male child presented to our casualty with history of ingestion of a metallic screw 4 hours prior. Patient's relative gave history of inability to swallow any liquid or solid food since then. There was no evidence of any respiratory distress.

On examination, air entry was equal in bilateral lung fields. Patient underwent plain roentgenogram in antero-posterior view suggestive of radiodense long metallic foreign body extending from cervical to upper thoracic regionon the left side of trachea, most likely to be in the oesophagus. There was no evidence of pneumomediastinum and soft tissue emphysema (**Figure 1** and **Figure 2**).

After taking a written informed consent for the procedure, patient underwent an emergency oesophagoscopy. Rigid oesophagoscope was passed and the foreign body could be visualized just below the level of cricopharynx. We attempted removal of the foreign body with forceps but could not grasp the head of the screw due to lack of space surrounding the foreign body. An attempt was made passing a dormia basket beyond the head of the screw but the screw was so large that it could not be removed endoscopically. The screw was then pushed distally towards the stomach. C-arm fluoroscopy was used intra operative to confirm the position of the foreign body and decision was taken to remove it by performing a gastrostomy (**Figure 3**).

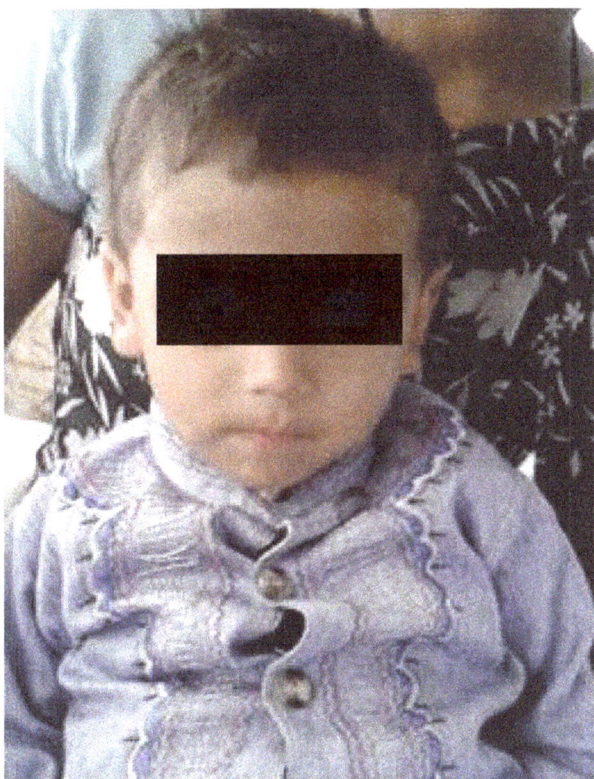

Figure 1. Clinical photograph of the patient.

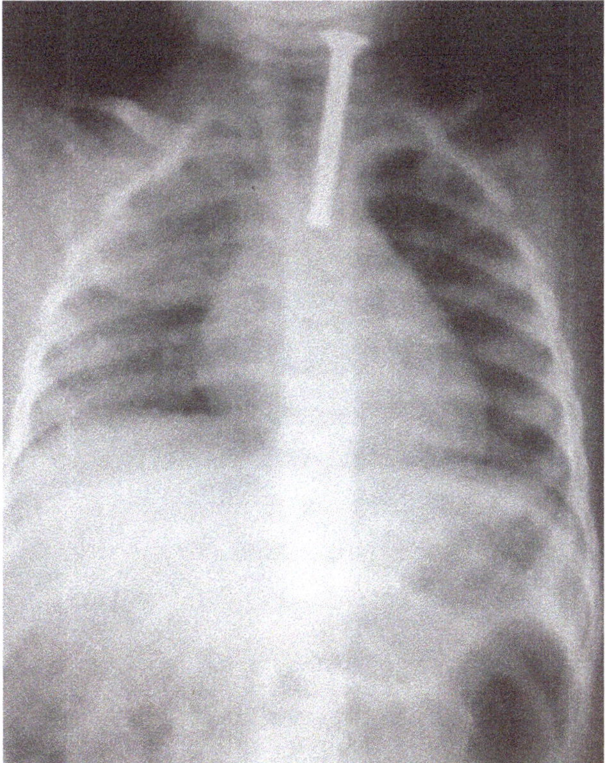

Figure 2. Plain roentgenogram in antero-posterior view in supine position.

The case was handed over to our paediatric surgeon who performed a standard anterior gastrostomy through a left upper abdomen transverse incision. The screw could be palpated at the level of oesophago-gastric junction where the head of the screw remained engaged. By using Babcock's forceps 4.5 cm by 1 cm screw was finally retrieved. Gastrostomy was closed with 3 - 0 vicryl suture and abdominal incision closed in layers. Drain was inserted in the abdominal cavity. Patient was kept nil by mouth for 5 days and started on total parenteral nutrition. Drain was removed on fifth postoperative day after starting with clear oral feeds on the fourth post-operative day. Patient was discharged on seventh post-operative day (**Figure 4** and **Figure 5**).

5. Discussion

A large variety of foreign bodies are swallowed by children, but the majority of those pass through the gastrointestinal tract without any adverse effect [2]. The highest incidence of swallowed foreign bodies occurs in children between 6 months and 3 years [3] [4]. Although 80% to 90% of swallowed foreign bodies will pass spontaneously, there is a definite predilection for swallowed foreign bodies to get impacted at the level of cricopharynx and just below it or at the oesophago-gastric junction.

Foreign bodies less than 2.5 cm in diameter and/or <5 cm in length usually pass through whole gut. The level at which progress is impeded are pylorus, duodenum, duodenojejunoflexure. However any foreign body which is large or sharp may be impacted [5]. In our case, the foreign body was too large to negotiate through the constrictions of the gastro-intestinal tract and there were high chances of impaction and subsequent complications.

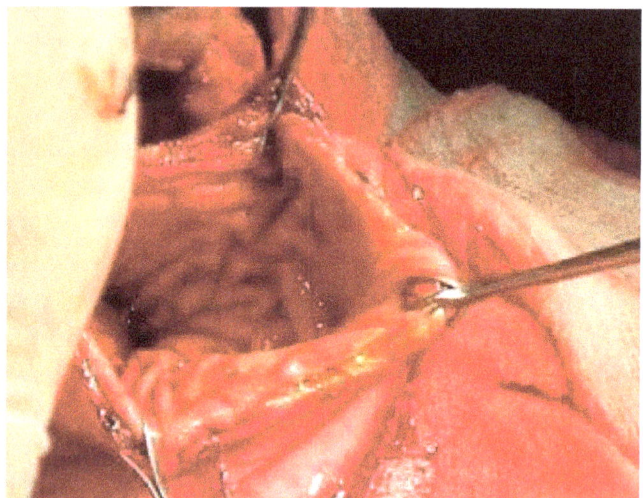

Figure 3. Anterior standard gastrostomy.

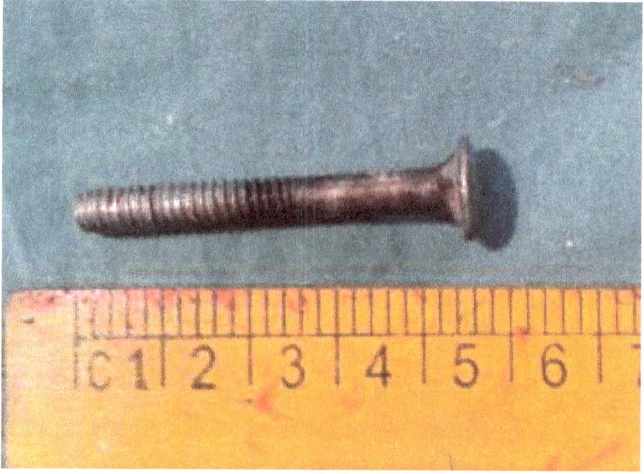

Figure 4. Foreign body (Screw) retrieved length 4.5 cm.

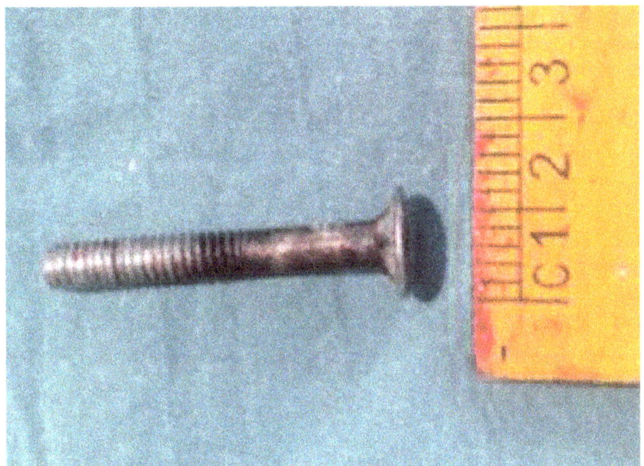

Figure 5. Foreign body (Screw) retrieved breadth 1 cm.

Sharp foreign bodies like fish bone, chicken bone, sharp metallic wire, can be impacted anywhere from base of tongue to lower end of oesophagus. If they are not removed at the earliest, can cause complications such as a retropharyngeal abscess, ulcerative esophagitis, esophago-respiratory fistula, stricture formation, impaction and recurrent pneumonitis. Sharp foreign body can also be removed safely by endoscopic technique in most cases avoiding open surgical methods [6].

But in some cases, locating a sharp foreign body in pharynx or oesophagus is difficult. This may be due to light reflecting from the foreign body or major part of foreign body being hidden in the wall with only a small projection in the lumen. In such cases the C-arm fluoroscopy has to be utilized.

Sharp end of the foreign body has to be taken in the lumen of the endoscope to avoid complications. Partial dentures with sharp hooks, metallic springs, and screws are the most difficult and dangerous object to remove from oesophagus [7]. One can cause laceration and perforation during removal of such objects. Due to the high risk of complication, we took the decision of pushing the foreign body distally towards the stomach and retrieved it with open surgical technique.

6. Conclusion

Early diagnosis and immediate removal of foreign body are key to avoid any complications. Although 80% to 90% of the foreign bodies pass smoothly through the gastrointestinal tract, the nature of foreign body has to be determined. In case of a discbattery, it should be removed surgically if it remains in any one position for more than 24 hours. Sharp and large foreign bodies such as a screw have to be removed to prevent any further complications. It is advisable to have a team approach while dealing with such sharp and impacted foreign bodies.

Disclosure

None of the authors was given an honorarium, grant or other form of payment to produce this paper. We declare no potential conflict of interests, real or perceived.

References

[1] Schild, J.A. and Snow, Jr., J.B. (1996) Esophagology. In: Ballenger, J.J., Ed., *Otorhinolaryngology Head and Neck Surgery*, 15th Edition, Williams and Wilkins, USA, 1221-1235.

[2] Webb, W.A. (1988) Management of Foreign Bodies of the Upper Gastrointestinal Tract. *Gastroenterology*, **94**, 204-216.

[3] Nandi, P. and Ong, G.B. (1988) Foreign Body in the Esophagus: Review of 2394 Cases. *British Journal of Surgery*, **65**, 5-9. http://dx.doi.org/10.1002/bjs.1800650103

[4] Al-Salem, A.H., Qaisarrudin, S., Murugan, A., Hammad, H.A. and Talwalker, V. (1995) Swallowed Foreign Bodies in Children: Aspects of Management. *Annals of Saudi Medicine*, **15**, 419-421.

[5] Tibbling, L. and Stenquist, M. (1991) Foreign Bodies in the Esophagus. A Study of Causative Factors. *Dysphagia*, **6**, 224-227. http://dx.doi.org/10.1007/BF02493532

[6] Sawant, P., Nanivadekar, S.A., Dave, U.R., Kanakia, R.R., Satarkar, R.P., Bhatia, R.S., *et al.* (1994) Endoscopic Removal of Impacted Foreign Bodies. *The Indian Journal of Pediatrics*, **61**, 197-199. http://dx.doi.org/10.1007/BF02843619

[7] Holinger, L.D. (1990) Management of Sharp and Penetrating Foreign Bodies of the Upper Aerodigestive Tract. *Annals of Otology, Rhinology & Laryngology*, **99**, 684-688. http://dx.doi.org/10.1177/000348949009900902

21

Risk Factors of Otitis Media with Effusion in Children

Essam A. Abo el-Magd[1], Yousseria Elsayed Yousef[2], Osama M. El-Asheerr[3], Karema M. Sobhy[4]

[1]Departments of Otorhinolaryngology, Faculty of Medicine, Aswan University, Aswan, Egypt
[2]Pediatric Nursing, Faculty of Nursing, Sohag University, Sohag, Egypt
[3]Pediatrics, Faculty of Medicine, Assiut University, Assiut, Egypt
[4]Public Health, Faculty of Medicine, Aswan University, Aswan, Egypt
Email: esamali801@yahoo.com

Abstract

The aim of this study is to detect the risk factors associated with otitis media with effusion (OME) among children with age ranged from 6 months to 2 years. Materials and Methods: it is a cross-sectional study 500 children were selected from Assiut University Hospital clinics through multi-staged randomized sampling. Parents of these children were interviewed with a structured questionnaire. Clinical examination, including otoscopic examination and tympanometry was performed for each child. Results: There was no statistical significant relationship between OME and gender, age, mother job. There is statistical significant relationship between OME and breast feeding, using pacifier, mother education, sibling of children and exposure to passive smoking. Conclusion: There are multiple risk factors associated with OME in children between 6 months to 2 years of age.

Keywords

Otitis Media with Effusion, Risk Factors

1. Introduction

Otitis media with effusion (OME) is a middle ear disease characterized by presence of serous or mucoid effusion in the middle ear without any signs of acute infection1. This problem occurred because of Eustachian tube dysfunction as well as other problems in the middle ear ventilation. Twenty to fifty percent of children aged 3 - 10 years' experience otitis media with effusion at least once in this period [1] [2].

Vague presentations of otitis media in early stages and coincidence of the disease with the time of learning and speaking of the child cause many problems such as stuttering, delay of speaking, indifference of children at school, and educational problems [3]. Various risk factors are implicated, such as sex, race, premature delivery, passive smoking, allergy, asthma, family size, bottle feeding, socioeconomic status, cleft palate adenoid hypertrophy, which have been studied and are still controversial [4]-[7].

Passive smoking can increase the adherence of bacteria to the respiratory epithelium, depress local immune function and decrease mucociliary action, and thus may be a risk factor for the development of OM [8] [9].

2. Materials and Methods

In this cross-sectional study 500 children whose age ranged from 6 months to 2 years were selected from Aswan University Hospital Clinics through multi-stage randomized sampling in the period between June 2013 and December 2014 after approval from Aswan Faculty of Medicine ethics committee. Informed consent was obtained from the parents who agreed to be interviewed and have their children examined.

Children were considered to have OME in case of:

- Lack of cerumen in their ears
- Intact tympanic membrane
- Type B tympanogram

Retraction of tympanic membrane/or disappearance of cone of light/or presence of air-fluid level in examination.

There were healthy children matched to the case group as the control subjects. They collected information on smoking behavior of parents and other household members. Mothers were asked: "if father's child was smoke?" if he still smoking?" and "Did he/she smoke inside the house, outside only or both?" If the baby's father was part of the family unit, we asked the same questions about the baby's mother.

Lastly, we asked the mother or guardian whether anybody else smoked inside the house. An answer of "yes" to any of these questions was taken to indicate ETS exposure. Information was also collected about feeding practices, parent's education and employment, family history of allergy or atopy, and number, age, and childcare or school attendance of other children in the household. The number of adults and children living in the house as well as the number of rooms in the house were documented to obtain a measure of crowding (number of people/room). Research assistants performed further routine follow-up on study participants at ages 6 - 8 weeks, and 4, 6, 12, 18 and 24 months, when they again enquired about feeding practices and whether the study participant was attending childcare.

At these follow-up visits, we also asked the child's mother or guardian whether they smoked, and whether anybody smoked inside the house. However, as preliminary analysis indicated little change from responses at first interview and, in view of potential bias towards children remaining in the study, analyses were based on the first interview.

We scheduled three routine clinical examinations by an ear, nose and throat (ENT) specialist: before the age of 6 months, at 6 - 11 months and at 12 - 24 months. A clinical diagnosis was established by otoscopy, pneumatic otoscopy and tympanometry at 6 months, 12 months and at 24, and was based on national clinical guideline and approved by the local Ethics committee.

Statistical Analysis

The collected data were computerized and analyzed by using the proper statistical programs such as "SPSS" ver. 16". Data expressed as mean, SD and number, percentage. Using t test to determine significant for numeric variable Using Chi. square to determine significant for non-parametric variable. The difference was considered statistically significant when P-value $\leq 0.05\%$.

3. Result

A total of 250 children were examined. The examined group compared with 250 children of control group. Mean age of cases was 18.16 ± 11.9 months while it was 19.55 ± 9.10 months for controls. 61.6% of cases and 66% of controls were females, with no significant difference between cases and controls ($P > 0.05$). 94% of cases and 92% of controls were Urban with no significant difference ($P > 0.05$). On the other hand, for the higher percentage 28% of cases and 58% of controls, their mothers completed university education with significant statistical difference between them P = 0.000. For more than half, 68.8% of cases and 74.8% of controls, their mothers worked with no statistical significant difference between them (P > 0.05). There was a high significant difference between cases 45.6% versus 34% of controls had family history of second sibling of children P = 0.00. The majority 92.4 % of cases versus 83.6% of controls the number of children per room were 1 - 2 child with high statistical significant difference between them P = 0.02 (**Table 1**). There was a highly statistically significant relationship between OME and breast feeding, use of pacifier, father smoke, exposure to smoke (**Table 2**) (**Figure 1**).

Table 1. Sociodemographic characteristics among study participants and their controls at Assuit University Hospital, 2014.

Variable	Cases (No. 250)		Control (No. 250)		Significant Tests
	No.	%	No.	%	
1-Age "months"					
Mean ± SD	18.16 ± 11.19		19.55 ± 9.10		T-test = 2.54 P = 0.128 n.s
2-Sex:					
Male	96	38.4	85	34.0	x^2 = 1.048 P = 0.176
Female	154	61.6	165	66.0	
3-Residence:					
Rural	15	6.0	20	8.0	x^2 = 0.768 P = 0.242
Urban	235	94.0	230	92.0	
4-Level of education of mother					
Illiterate	29	11.6	21	8.4	**x^2 = 51.965 P = 0.000**
Read and write	38	15.2	22	8.8	
Primary education	58	23.2	20	8.0	
Secondary education	55	22.0	42	16.8	
University	70	28.0	145	58.0	
5-Mother Job					
Work	172	68.8	187	74.8	**x^2 = 2.222**
House wife	78	31.2	63	25.2	**P = 0.082**
6-Sibling of children					
First	58	23.2	63	25.2	x^2 = 32.139 P = 0.000
Second	114	45.6	85	34.0	
Third	39	15.6	61	24.4	
Fourth	20	8.0	40	16.0	
Fifth	19	7.6	1	0.4	
7-No. of room					
1 - 2 rooms	231	92.4	209	83.6	x^2 = 9.167
3 - 4 rooms	19	7.6	41	16.4	P = 0.002

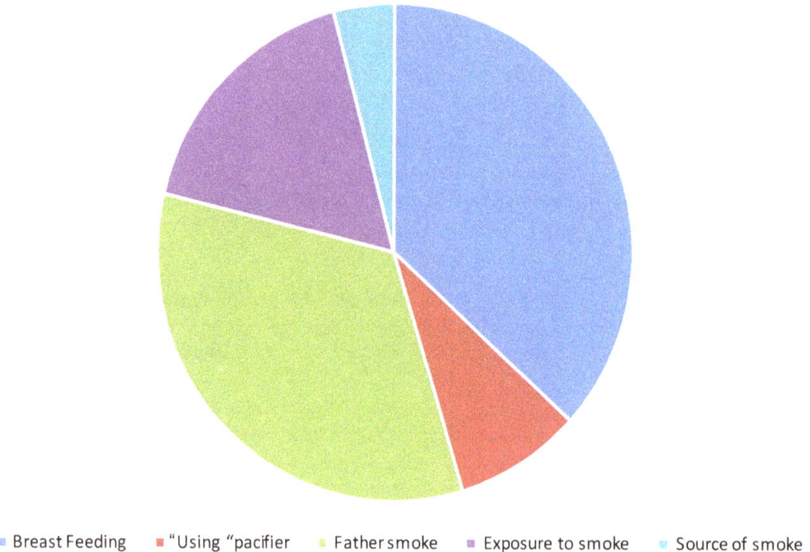

Figure 1. Pie chart for percentage analysis of risk factors among study participants attending Assuit University hospital, 2012.

Table 2. Risk factors among study participants and their controls at Assuit University Hospital, 2014.

Variable	Cases (No. 250)		Control (No. 250)		Significant Tests
	No.	%	No.	%	
1-Breast Feeding:					
Yes	168	67.2	212	84.8	$x^2 = 21.228$ P = 0.000
No	82	32.8	38	15.2	
2-Using "pacifier":					
Yes	39	15.6	21	8.4	$x^2 = 6.136$ P = 0.009
No	211	84.4	229	91.6	
3-Father smoke:					
Yes	153	61.2	106	42.4	$x^2 = 17.695$ P = 0.000
No	97	38.8	144	57.6	
4-Exposure to smoke:					
Yes	78	31.2	42	16.8	$x^2 = 14.211$
No	172	68.8	208	83.2	P = 0.000
5-Source of smoke:					
Yes	19	7.6	1	0.4	$x^2 = 16.875$ P = 0.000
No	231	92.4	249	99.6	

4. Discussion

In the literature, the range of prevalence of OME is wide as the population studied, the countries, environmental factors and climatic factors were different [10]. In our study we did not find any significant difference in the incidence of OME between male and female. Other studies showed higher incidence in male [11]-[13], owing to higher incidence of infectious disease in male. In the same with our results Gultekin *et al.* [14] and Sassen *et al.* [15] showed that higher number of siblings in family increases the risk of OME. Various studies done in the past support the protective role of breast feeding and development of OME [12] [13] [16] [17] but other studies did not establish a significant relationship between the two [14] [15] [18] [19]. Various studies with different designs relating to middle ear disease among young children have a point of consistence in suggesting a modest increase in the risk associated with parental smoking [1] [2] [17].

Hinton *et al.* demonstrated that parental smoking is an influential factor in OME among the children. They require more ventilation tube insertion for OME treatment, comparing with other patients with the same age [20].

This indicates the resistance of OME to suitable therapeutic modalities. Green *et al.* showed the increased risk of OME in case of parental smoking especially with maternal smoking during pregnancy [21].

Moreover, Etzel *et al.* have presented cigarette smoking as an effective factor in extension of the disease period and increasing the frequency of the disease attacks at shorter intervals [22]. Their results are similar to our findings on parental smoking, since both studies indicate increased risk of OME among children with smoker parents. Furthermore, a direct relation exists between pack-years cigarette smoking of parents and the prevalence of the disease. Blackley and Blackley [7], and few others [15] [16] [23] [24] deny any relationship between passive smoking and development of OME. Other studies demonstrated the relationship between the two [24] [25].

Finally, we believe that passive smoking is a preventable cause of otitis media with effusion in children. This seeks further parental attention. The limitations of our study are small number of patients and short period of follow up.

References

[1] Strachan, D.P. and Cook, D.G. (1998) Health Effect of Passive Smoking. *Thorax*, **53**, 50-56. http://dx.doi.org/10.1136/thx.53.1.50

[2] Hinton, A.E. and Buckiey, G. (1988) Parental Smoking and Middle Ear Effusion in Children. *The Journal of Laryngology & Otology*, **102**, 992-996. http://dx.doi.org/10.1017/S0022215100107091

[3] Abbas, S., Ali, S. and Mohsen, V. (2002) Parental Smoking and Risk of Otitis Media with Effusion among Children. *Tanfos*, **1**, 25-28.

[4] Alho, O.-P., Oja, H., Koivu, M. and Sorri, M. (1995) Risk Factors for OME in Infancy. *Archives of Otolaryngology—Head Neck Surgery*, **121**, 839-843. http://dx.doi.org/10.1001/archotol.1995.01890080011002

[5] Aydogan, B., Kirgolu, M. and Yilmaz, M. (2004) The Role of Food Allergy in OME. *Otolaryngology—Head and Neck Surgery*, **130**, 747-750. http://dx.doi.org/10.1016/j.otohns.2004.02.003

[6] Bernstein, J.M. (1992) The Role of IgE Mediated Hypersensitivity in Development of OME. *Otolaryngologic Clinics of North America*, **25**, 197-211.

[7] Blakley, B.W. and Blakley, J. (1995) Smoking and Middle Ear Disease: Are they Related? A Review Article. *Otolaryngology—Head and Neck Surgery*, **112**, 441-446. http://dx.doi.org/10.1016/S0194-5998(95)70281-4

[8] Kum-Nji, P., Meloy, L. and Herrod, H.G. (2006) Envirpmental Tobacco Smoke Exposure: Prevelance and Mechanisms of Causation of Infections in Children. *Pediatrics*, **117**, 1745-1754. http://dx.doi.org/10.1542/peds.2005-1886

[9] Arcavi, L. and Benowitz, N.L. (2004) Cigaret Smoking and Infection. *Archives of Internal Medicine*, **164**, 2206-2216. http://dx.doi.org/10.1001/archinte.164.20.2206

[10] Okur, E., Yildirim, I., Kilic M.A. and Guzelsoy, S. (2004) Prevelance of Otitis Media with Effusion among Primary School Children in Turkey. *International Journal of Pediatric Otolaryngology*, **68**, 557-562. http://dx.doi.org/10.1016/j.ijporl.2003.12.014

[11] Casselbrant, M.L., Brostof, L.M. and Cantekin, E.L. (1985) Otitis Media with Effusion in Preschool Children. *The Laryngoscope*, **95**, 428-436. http://dx.doi.org/10.1288/00005537-198504000-00011

[12] Paradise, J.L, Rockette, H.E. and Calborn, D.K. (1997) Otitis Media in 2253 Infants, Prevelance and Risk Factors. *Pediatrics*, **99**, 318-333. http://dx.doi.org/10.1542/peds.99.3.318

[13] Teele, D., Klein, J. and Rosner, B. (1989) Epidemiology of Otitis Media in Children in Greater Boston: Prospective Study. *The Journal of Infectious Diseases*, **160**, 83-94. http://dx.doi.org/10.1093/infdis/160.1.83

[14] Gultekin, E., Yener, M. and Ozdemir, I. (2010) Prevelance and Risk Factors for Persistent Otitis Media with Effusion in Primary School Children in Turkey. *Auris Nasus Larynx*, **37**, 145-149. http://dx.doi.org/10.1016/j.anl.2009.05.002

[15] Sassen, M., Brand, R. and Grote, J. (1997) Risk Factors for Otitis Media with Effusion in Children 0 to 2 Years of Age. *American Journal of Otolaryngology*, **18**, 324-330. http://dx.doi.org/10.1016/S0196-0709(97)90027-2

[16] Saim, A., Saim, L. and Saim, S. (1997) Prevelance of OME Amongost Pre-School Children in Malasia. *International*

Journal of Pediatric Otorhinolaryngology, **41**, 21-28. http://dx.doi.org/10.1016/S0165-5876(97)00049-9

[17] Rowe-Jones, J.M. and Brockbank, M.J. (1992) Parental Smoking and Persistant OME in Children. *International Journal of Pediatric Otorhinolaryngology*, **24**, 19-24. http://dx.doi.org/10.1016/0165-5876(92)90062-T

[18] Schaefer, O. (1971) Otitis Media and Bottle Feeding. An Epidemiological Study of Infant Feeding Habits and Incedance of Recurrent Middle Ear Diseases in Canadian Escemos. *The Canadian Journal of Public Health*, **62**, 478-489.

[19] Haresten, G., Kalmo, O. and Kornfalt, R. (1989) Recurrent Acute Otitis Media. *Acta Oto-laryngologica*, **107**, 111-119. http://dx.doi.org/10.3109/00016488909127487

[20] Hinton, A.E. (1989) Surgery for Otitis Media with Effusion in Children and Its Relationship to Parental Smoking. *The Journal of Laryngology Otology*, **103**, 556-561. http://dx.doi.org/10.1017/S0022215100109326

[21] Green, R.E. and Cooper, N.K. (1991) Passive Smoking and Middle Ear Effusion in Children. *Journal of the Royal Army Medical Corps*, **137**, 31-33. http://dx.doi.org/10.1136/jramc-137-01-07

[22] Etzel, R.A., Pattishall, E.N. and Haley, N.J. (1992) Passive Smoking and Middle Ear Effusion among Children in Day Care. *Pediatrics*, **90**, 228-232.

[23] Rowe, J. and Brockbank, M. (1992) Parental Smoking and Persistent Otitis Media with Effusion in Children. *International Journal of Pediatric Otorhinolaryngology*, **24**, 19-24.

[24] Iversen, M., Birch, L. and Lundqvist, G. (1985) Middle Ear Effusion in Children and the Indoor Environment: An Epidemiological Study. *Archives of Environmental Health*, **40**, 74-79. http://dx.doi.org/10.1080/00039896.1985.10545893

[25] Uhari, M., Mantysaari, K. and Niemela, M. (1996) A Meta-Analysis Review of the Risk Factors for Acute Otitis Media. *Clinical Infectious Diseases*, **22**, 1079-1083. http://dx.doi.org/10.1093/clinids/22.6.1079

22

New Approach in the Management of Adult Epiglottic Abscess—A Case Report

Ramesh Babu Kalyanasundaram*, Ganesh Kumar Balasubramanian, Ramanathan Thirunavukkarasu, Prabhakharan Saroja Durairaju

Department of ENT and Head & Neck surgery, Thanjavur Medical College, Thanjavur, India
Email: *k.rameshbabu.ent@gmail.com, drganeshkumarb@gmail.com

Abstract

Background: Epiglottic abscess in an otherwise healthy adult is seen as a rare sequelae of acute epiglottitis. It is a life threatening condition which requires emergency management, which if not done early, may result in fatality. Respiratory infections, exposure to environmental chemical or trauma which may lead to inflammation and infection of the structures around the throat which may lead on to epiglottitis, and an epiglottis abscess very rarely. In our case, patient was immediately managed by doing an emergency tracheostomy followed by incision and drainage in the OPD (outpatient department). This emphasizes on need for emergency airway management by doing a tracheostomy there by facilitating incision and drainage in a case of epiglottic abscess as a daycare procedure. **Aim:** The primary aim of this clinical record is to emphasize the need for immediate airway management in epiglottic abscess there by facilitating incision and drainage as an OPD (out-patient department) Procedure. **Case Presentation:** A 45-year-old man presented to the OPD (outpatient department) with complaints of dysphagia, odynophagia, muffled voice, noisy breathing for the previous 7 hours. On clinical examination pt was in stridor & respiratory distress. Since the pt was in stridor, it was immediately shifted to the OT (operation theatre), and an emergency tracheostomy was done and the airway was secured, following which a video laryngoscopic examination was done in the OPD, which revealed oedematous enlarged epiglottis with pus pointing obscuring the laryngeal inlet. Abscess was incised and drained, and pus was sent for culture & sensitivity. Pt was treated with I. V (intravenous) antibiotics as per culture reports and subsequent video laryngoscopic examination revealed near normal epiglottis with an adequate laryngeal inlet. **Conclusion:** Patients with epiglottic abscess are at increased risk of airway compromise, hence in such patients airway should be immediately secured by doing an emergency tracheostomy. This case shows the benefits of an emergency tracheostomy for doing incision and drainage for epiglottic abscess as an OPD procedure.

*Corresponding author.

Keywords

Epiglottic Abscess, Epiglottitis, Tracheostomy, Incision and Drainage

1. Introduction

Epiglottic abscess is a rare complication of acute epiglottitis. Epiglottitis is an acute inflammation of the supraglottic region of the larynx involving epiglottis, arytenoids, vallecula and aryepiglottic folds. The development of epiglottic abscess from epiglottitis secondary to radiotherapy has previously been described in literature. Epiglottic abscess incidence among patient with acute epiglottitis is around 4%. It is due to respiratory infections, exposure to environmental chemicals and trauma. Previously, the incidence was reportedly more common in children. But recently the incidence of epiglottic abscess is found to be more common in adults. The incidence in adults is 1 case per 100,000 per year. Incidence is more common in males than in females with a ratio of 3:1. We present a case report of a 45-year-old male with epiglottic abscess, managed with emergency tracheostomy followed by endoscopic assisted incision and drainage of the abscess as an OPD (out-patient department) procedure.

2. Case Report

A 45-year-old male presented to the OPD (out-patient department) with complaints of dysphagia, odynophagia, muffled voice, noisy breathing for the previous 7 hours. On clinical examination, patient was in stridor, tachycardia. O_2 saturation was 90%. X-Ray STNL (soft tissue neck lateral view) revealed edema of the epiglottis (thumb sign) (**Figure 1**) with airway obstruction.

Since the patient was in stridor, after doing basic investigations, patient was shifted to the OT (operation theatre) and an emergency tracheostomy was done and the airway was secured.

Post tracheostomy (**Figure 2**), In the OPD a video laryngoscopic examination using a 30 degree/4 mm Hopkins rod was done and it revealed an edematous, enlarged yellowish red appearing epiglottis with pus pointing (**Figure 3**) on the lingual surface, obscuring the laryngeal inlet.

Abscess was incised and about 10 - 15 ml of frank pus was drained (**Figure 4**) and the purulent material was sent for culture and antibiotic sensitivity.

In the post operative period, patient was stable and was managed with I.V (intravenous) third generation cephalosporins and I.V metronidazole.Culture report showed *Klebsiella pneumonia* growth, sensitive to ciprofloxacin, co-trimoxazole and ceftriaxone. Four days later, repeat video laryngoscopy was done which revealed a decrease in the edema of the epiglottis, enabling the visualisation of the laryngeal inlet which was found to be adequate. Three days later, another repeat video laryngoscopy revealed a near normal epiglottis (**Figure 5**) with a healthy slough covering. Decannulation was done on the 10th POD (**Figure 6**) and the patient was discharged on the 14th day (**Figure 7**).

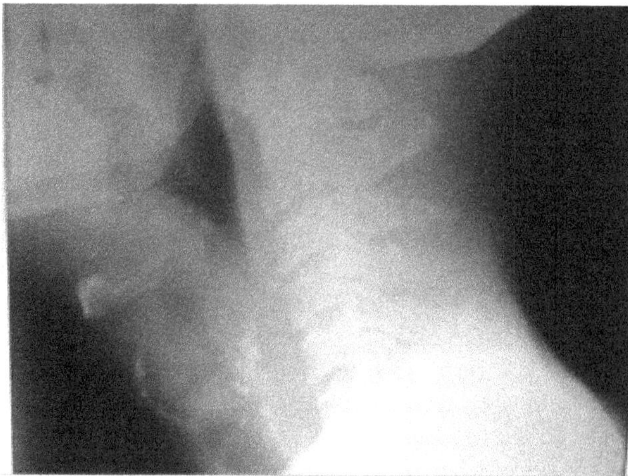

Figure 1. X-Ray STNL showing edema of the epiglottis (thumb sign).

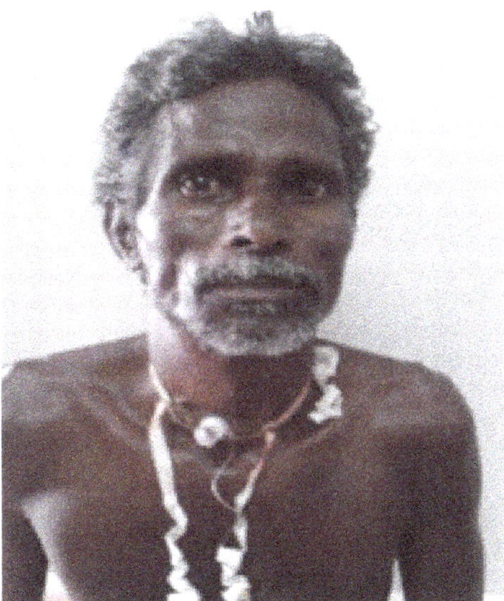

Figure 2. Post tracheostomy.

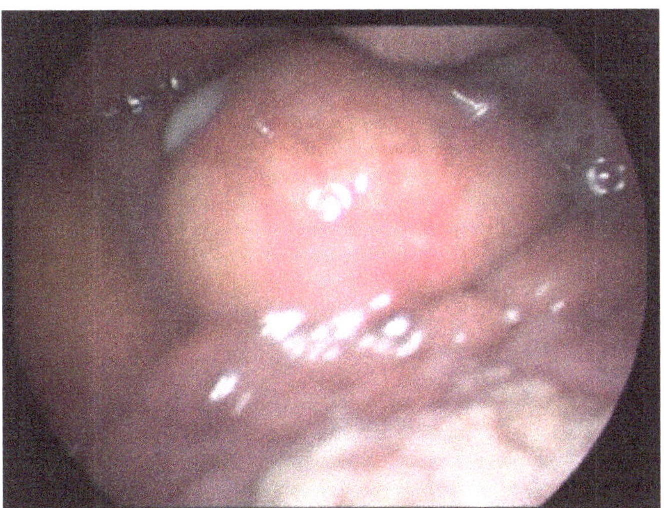

Figure 3. Edematous epiglottis with puspointing.

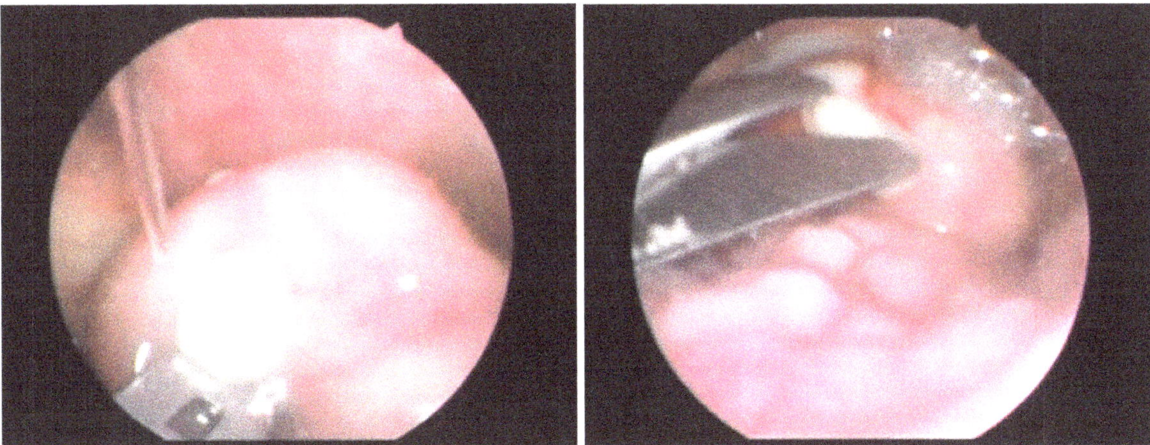

Figure 4. Incision and drainage.

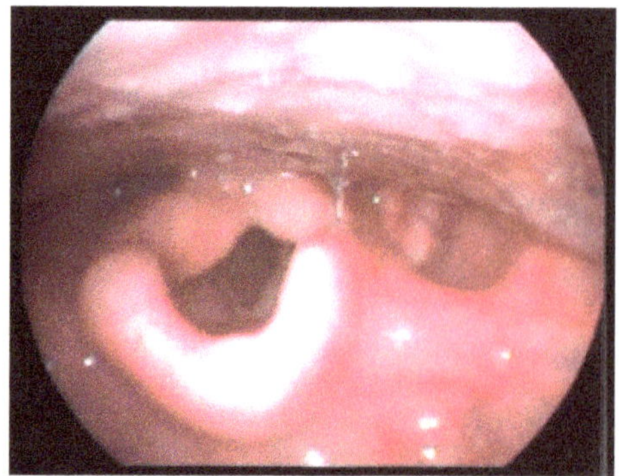

Figure 5. Post operative day 7—near normal epiglottis.

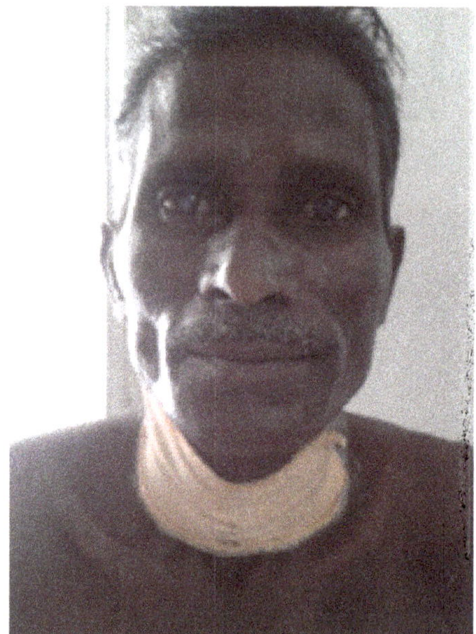

Figure 6. Post operative day-10.

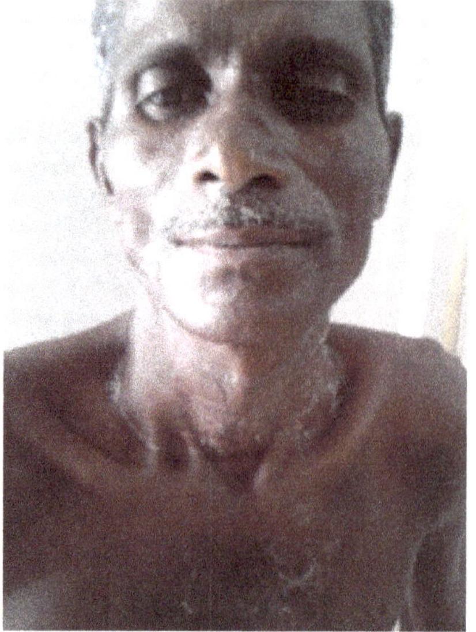

Figure 7. Post operative day-14.

3. Discussion

Epiglottic abscess is a sequelae of acute epiglottitis, precisely known as supraglottitis. Supraglottitis is the acute inflammation involving the epiglottitis, arytenoids, vallecula and the aryepiglottic fold. The development of epiglottic abscess from epiglottitis secondary to radiotherapy has previously been described in the literature [1]. Epiglottic abscess incidence among patient with acute epiglottitis is around 4%. It is due to respiratory infections [2], exposure to environmental chemicals and trauma. The rising incidence of adult epiglottic abcess has risen between 1986 and 2000. This seems unrelated to Haemophilus influenzae Type B, but related to miscellaneous bacteria [3]. Clinical features include sore throat, respiratory difficulty, dyphagia, change in voice. Fatal air way obstruction can occur without warning, indicating a need for early need for early protection of airway in adults as well in children. Incidence was more common in children previously, but recently there has been a steady increase in incidence in the adults [4]. The decrease in incidence in the pediatric age is probably due to the introduction of the H. influenza B vaccine in children [4]. Incidence is more common in males than in females with a ratio of 3:1, the average age group being 45 years [5]. Physical findings are epiglottic asymmetry, a yellow colored epiglottis, prominent median glossoepiglottic furrow and taut appearing epiglottic mucosa [5]. The organisms causing epiglottc abscess were due to streptococcus hemolyticus which was found in pure culture in most of the cases.other organisms isolated were Hemophilus influenza, Escherichia coli, Pseudomonas aeruginosa, Micrococcus catarrhalis, Staphylococcus aureus, *klebsiella pneumoniae* and pneumococci [6]. Risk factors include adult age at onset, diabetes mellitus, presence of foreign body, immune compromised state [6].

A diagnosis of epiglottic abscess should be considered in a patient with sore throat, epiglottitis, dyspnea, stridor. CT and MRI may reveal thickening of the epiglottis, obliteration of the pre-epiglottic fat and thickening of the subcutaneous tissue and muscles [7]. Lateral neck radiographs and CT imaging may be helpful but a prompt and accurate diagnosis can be established with flexible fibreoptic Nasopharyngo laryngoscope. The lingual surface is the most commonly involved site [7]. Differential diagnosis includes abscess of deep neck space, peritonsillar abscess, lingual tonsillitis, laryngitis, ingested foreign body.

The principles of treatment for patients with epiglottic abscess are immediate airway management, direct laryngoscopy with incision and drainage of the abscess and intravenous administration of broad spectrum antibiotics.

4. Outcome and Follow Up

By doing an emergency tracheostomy followed by incision and drainage the patient was managed promptly. Patient has been on follow up for the past two months in the OPD and subsequent video laryngoscopic examinations revealed a normal epiglottis with an adequate laryngeal inlet.

5. Conclusions

- Patients with epiglottic abscess are at increased risk of airway compromise, hence in such patients airway should be immediately secured by doing an emergency tracheostomy.
- Any undue manipulation would lead to or precipitate glottic spasm.
- In previously managed epiglottic abscesses, incision and drainage were done in the OT under general anesthesia, but we did this procedure in the OPD under local anesthesia.
- This case shows the benefits of an emergency tracheostomy for doing incision and drainage for epiglottic abscess as an OPD procedure.

References

[1] Harvey, M., Quagliotto, G. and Milne, N. (2012) Fatal Epiglottic Abscess after Radiotherapy for Laryngeal Carcinoma. *American Journal of Forensic Medicine & Pathology*, **33**, 297-299. http://dx.doi.org/10.1097/PAF.0b013e318221be6a

[2] Ellenbogen Ram, N.C., Raim, J. and Lytton, L. (1955) Abscess of the Epiglottis-Problem in Differential Diagnosis. *JAMA*, **159**, 1289-1290. http://dx.doi.org/10.1001/jama.1955.02960300035009a

[3] Berger, G., Landau, T., Berger, S., Finkelstein, Y., Bernheim, J. and Ophir, D. (2003) The Rising Incidence of Adult Acute Epiglottitis and Epiglottic Abscess. *American Journal of Otolaryngology*, **24**, 374-383.

[4] Mayo-Smith, M.F., Spinale, J.W., Donskey, C.J., Yukawa, M., Li, R.H. and Sciffman, F.J. (1995) Aute Epiglottitis. *The New England Journal of Medicine*, **108**, 1640-1647.

[5] Vaileadis, I., Kapetanakis, S., Vaileiadis, D., Petousis, A. and Karatzas, T. (2013) Epiglottic Abscess Causing Airway Obstruction in an Adult. *Journal of the College of Physicians and Surgeons Pakistan*, **23**, 673-675.

[6] Deepalakshmi, T., Devan, P.P. and Prasad, M. (2014) An Unusual Case of Acute Epiglottic Abscess. *Iranian Journal of Otorhinolaryngology*, **26**, 56.

[7] Al-Qudah, M., Shetty, S., Alomari, M. and Alqdah, M. (2010) Acute Adult Supraglottitis: Current Management and Treatment. *Southern Medical Journal*, **103**, 800-804.

23

Carotid Artery Prolapse and Myringocarotidopexy in Osteogenesis Imperfecta

Hassanin Abdulkarim[1*], Hassan Haidar[1], Maryam Abdulraheem[1], Ahmad Abualsoud[1], Ahmed Elsotouhy[2], A. Salam Alqahtani[1]

[1]Department of Otorhinolaryngology, Head & Neck Surgery, Hamad Medical Corporation, Doha, Qatar
[2]Department of Radiology, Hamad Medical Corporation, Doha, Qatar
Email: [*]hassanainh2@hotmail.com

Abstract

Osteogenesis Imperfecta is a rare genetic disorder of connective tissue that is caused by an error in collagen formation. The disease is characterized by abnormal bone fragility, osteopenia, blue discoloration of the sclerae and hearing loss. Chronic non-suppurative otitis media is frequent in Osteogenesis Imperfecta patients and usually attributed to Eustachian tube dysfunction due to cranial molding and deformities. In some cases of severe Osteogenesis Imperfecta, the fragile bone of the petrous carotid canal can be broken down by the pulsations of the carotid artery, this may result in prolapse of the carotid artery into the protympanum with resultant Eustachian tube obstruction and tympanic membrane retraction with adhesion to prolapsed carotid artery, a condition called myringocarotidopexy.

Keywords

Eustachian Tube, Carotid Artery, Osteogenesis Imperfecta, Chronic Otitis Media, Myringocarotidopexy, Hearing Loss

1. Introduction

Osteogenesis Imperfecta (OI) is a rare genetic disorder of connective tissue that is caused by an error in collagen formation. The disease is characterized by abnormal bone fragility, osteopenia, blue discoloration of the sclerae and hearing loss.

[*]Corresponding author.

Hearing loss is a common problem in patients with OI and it affects 30% - 60% of patients [1]-[5]. The majority of OI patients usually develop a conductive hearing loss in the second to forth decade of life which gradually progress to mixed hearing loss [6]-[8].

Conductive hearing loss (CHL) in OI is often attributed to otosclerosis-like stapes fixation, ossicular discontinuity and chronic otitis media [2].

Chronic non-suppurative otitis media (COM) is frequent in young OI patients and usually attributed to eustachian tube (ET) dysfunction cranial molding and deformities [9].

In this report we present a 45-year-old lady with bilateral COM bilateral eustachian tube dysfunction caused by prolapsed Internal Carotid Arteries (ICA) with resultant adhesive otitis media and myringocarotidopexy.

2. Case Report

A 45-year-old Qatari female patient who is a known case of osteogenesis imperfecta, presented to the clinic complaining of reduced hearing in the right ear for long time, not associated with any other symptoms.

Examination of the ear revealed adhesive tympanic membrane with retrotympanic pinkish opacity in the right ear and retracted tympanic membrane in the left.

Pure tone audiogram showed bilateral moderate to severe mixed hearing loss. Impedance tympanometry showed bilateral flat (type B). Fiberoptic nasopharyngeal examination was done to rule out nasopharyngeal mass and was normal.

Temporal bone CT scan was ordered to discover the nature of the retrotympanic opacity. After that, CT angiogram was done and showed ET obstruction by a prolapsed ICA in the middle ear which confirmed our presumption of prolapsed ICA in the middle ear (**Figure 1**).

Patient was referred to the audiologist for hearing aid.

3. Discussion

Most of the ICA in the middle ear reported cases described as an aberrant ICA in the middle ear. Aberrant ICA is a variant of the ICA that passes through the middle ear. In this case we are presenting for the first time a bilateral prolapsed ICA in the middle ear. Presence of the carotid artery in the neck "CT angiogram" confirmed that the carotid artery in the middle ear is a prolapsed not aberrant carotid artery (**Figure 2**).

Patients with OI disease characterized by having brittle bones for that, the chance of getting spontaneous bone fractures is very high. Histopathologic studies of 8 temporal bones from 5 patients of OI, showed evidence of both deficient and abnormal ossification was found in the bony walls of middle ear and ossicles. Microfractures were found in the otic capsule and in the ossicles [9]. Depending on that, we assume that these microfractures can also happen in the ICA canal.

Computerized tomography (CT) of the temporal bone in an OI patient demonstrated otic capsule demineralization that appeared to progress as hearing diminished. Band-like areas of lucency were seen surrounding the cochlea, semicircular canals, the distal internal auditory canal, and oval window in an individual with hearing loss of mixed origin.

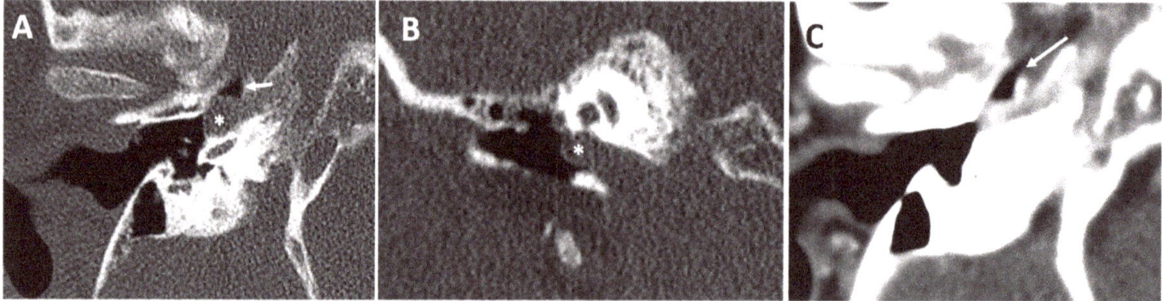

Figure 1. Right temporal bone Ct scan in axial (A), coronal (B), and after IV contrast in axial cut (C) showing dehiscence of the carotid canal and prolapse of the first genu of the petrous carotid artery (*) into the middle ear and encroaching upon the hypo-tympanic and protympanic spaces and occluding the bony part of Eustachian tube (arrow). IV contrast injection confirms the prolapse of the carotid into the Eustachian tube. Note the diffuse decrease in the bone density of the skull base bones in this patient with Osteogenesis Imperfecta.

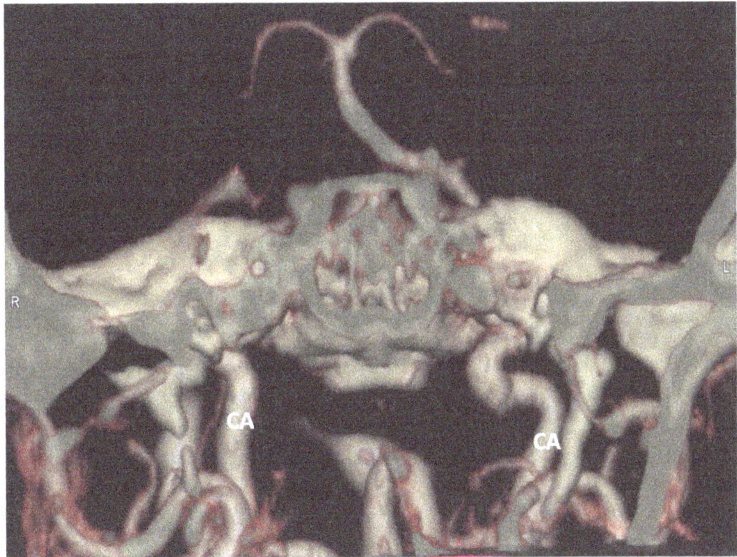

Figure 2. Colored 3D reconstruction of angio CT scan of skull base confirm the presence of both internal carotid arteries in the neck (CA).

Similarly, magnetic resonance imaging (MRI) examination of the otic capsule in type I OI demonstrated demineralized pericochlear lesions with soft tissue signal intensity and contrast enhancement

Postgadolinium T1-weighted MR imaging have shown symmetrical, band-like, homogeneously enhancing pericochlear areas, corresponding to the demineralization on CT, similar to retrofenestral or cochlear otosclerosis. High-resolution T2-weighted imaging may show irregularities in the outline of the labyrinthine and focal narrowing at the proximal basal turn of the cochlea, reflecting spongiotic foci.

The ICA wall itself is weak and thin due to collagen formation defect. Also the bony wall which separating the ICA canal and ET is naturally very thin. The thin wall canal, brittle bone and pulsation of the ICA all can contribute to the fracture of the canal and prolapse of the ICA.

This is the first report to show ICA prolapse as a cause of bilateral ET dysfunction, we suggest for patients with OI presented with AOM to do CT scan before myringotomy or ventilation tube insertion to avoid life threating/disastrous complications especially in those with craniofacial deformities or abnormalities.

The case at hand has already been approved by our institution's medical research and ethics committee at the research center with the reference number of (#14332/14), the patient consent was taken for the publication of the case report and the figures and Authors and co-authors don't have any conflict of interest or financial interest to disclose.

4. Disclosure

The case at hand has already been approved by our institution's medical research and ethics committee at the research center with the reference number of (#14332/14), the patient consent was taken for the publication of the case report and the figures and Authors and co-authors don't have any conflict of interest or financial interest to disclose. None of the authors was given an honorarium, grant or other form of payment to produce this paper. We declare no potential conflict of interests, real or perceived.

5. Conclusion

Computed tomography will guide us in identifying the cause of hearing loss in patients with osteogenesis imperfecta, also it plays a crucial role in avoiding a disastrous intervention like insertion of ventilation tube in such cases or craniofacial deformities. The role of temporal CT scan is major to rule out a nasopharyngeal mass in adult patients with a unilateral retracted tympanic membrane.

References

[1] Carey, M.C., Fitzgerald, O. and McKiernan, E. (1968) Osteogenesis Imperfecta in Twenty Three Members of a Kin-

dred with Heritable Features Contributed by a Non-Specific Skeletal Disorder. *Quarterly Journal of Medicine*, **37**, 437-449.

[2] Stoller, F.M. (1962) The Ear in Osteogenesis Imperfecta. *Laryngoscope*, **72**, 855-869. http://dx.doi.org/10.1288/00005537-196207000-00002

[3] Carruth, J.A., Lutman, M.E. and Stephens, S.D. (1978) An Audiological Investigation of Osteogenesis Imperfecta. *The Journal of Laryngology & Otology*, **92**, 853-860. http://dx.doi.org/10.1017/S0022215100086229

[4] Cox, J.R. and Simmons, C.L. (1982) Osteogenesis Imperfecta and Associated Hearing Loss in Five Kindreds. *Southern Medical Journal*, **75**, 1222-1226. http://dx.doi.org/10.1097/00007611-198210000-00016

[5] Quisling, R.W., Moore, G.R., Jahrsdoerfer, R.A. and Cantrell, R.W. (1979) Osteogenesis Imperfecta: A Study of 160 Family Members. *Archives of Otolaryngology*, **105**, 207-211. http://dx.doi.org/10.1001/archotol.1979.00790160041011

[6] Kuurila, K., Kaitila, I., Johansson, R. and Grenman, R. (2002) Hearing Loss in Finnish Adults with Osteogenesis Imperfecta: A Nationwide Survey. *Annals of Otology, Rhinology & Laryngology*, **111**, 939-946. http://dx.doi.org/10.1177/000348940211101014

[7] Pedersen, U. (1984) Hearing Loss in Patients with Osteogenesis Imperfecta. A Clinical and Audiological Study of 201 Patients. *Scandinavian Audiology*, **13**, 67-74. http://dx.doi.org/10.3109/01050398409043042

[8] Stewart, E.J. and O'Reilly, B.F. (1989) A Clinical and Audiological Investigation of Osteogenesis Imperfecta. *Clinical Otolaryngology & Allied Sciences*, **14**, 509-514. http://dx.doi.org/10.1111/j.1365-2273.1989.tb00414.x

[9] Berger, G., Hawke, M., Johnson, A. and Proops, D. (1985) Histopathology of the Temporal Bone in Osteogenesis Imperfecta Congenita: A Report of 5 Cases. *Laryngoscope*, **95**, 193-199. http://dx.doi.org/10.1288/00005537-198502000-00014

24

Acquired Hemophilia A Simulating Retropharyngeal Abscess: Importance of Differential Diagnosis of Neck Masses before Surgery

Isabel López-Sánchez[1], José-Ramón Alba-García[1], Cristina Vázquez-Romero[1], Miguel Armengot-Carceller[2*]

[1]ENT Department, General and University Hospital, Valencia, Spain
[2]Rhinology Unit, ENT Department, General and University Hospital.Valencia University, Valencia, Spain
Email: isa.lopez.85@gmail.com, joseramon43@hotmail.com, crisvazquez50@hotmail.com, [*]miguel.armengot@uv.es

Abstract

The coexistence of acquired hemophilia A with a secondary retropharyngeal hematoma is an extremely unusual condition with important clinical implications. The purpose of this paper is to present a case involving a patient whose first clinical manifestation, namely dysphagia, along with specific clinical examination and imaging findings, led to an incorrect initial diagnosis of a retropharyngeal abscess. However, performance of a more thorough clinical examination led to the correct diagnosis of a hematoma secondary to acquired hemophilia A. This allowed surgery to be avoided in a patient at a high risk of bleeding. Conclusions: Acute neck masses require meticulous differential diagnosis assessing the possible presence of various causative systemic diseases before the most appropriate therapy can be determined.

Keywords

Dysphagia, Cervical Inflammation, Coagulopathy, Hematoma, APTT, Parapharyngeal Spaces

1. Introduction

The acute or subacute development of a neck mass usually indicates an infectious or congenital problem. When

[*]Corresponding author.

acute evolution, poor mass demarcation, and dysphagia develop simultaneously in a patient with a neck mass, the first clinical diagnosis considered is a cervical abscess. One of the less common causes of such a mass is a retropharyngeal hematoma, which is a rare clinical entity [1]. Acquired hemophilia A is an uncommon autoimmune disorder characterized by the presence of autoantibodies to circulating factor VIII [2]. The coexistence of acquired hemophilia A with a secondary retropharyngeal hematoma is an extremely unusual condition with important clinical implications. A literature search of PubMed revealed only one such published case; however, the clinical manifestation involved airway obstruction [3].

The purpose of this paper is to present a case involving a patient whose first clinical manifestation, namely dysphagia, along with specific clinical examination and imaging findings, led to an incorrect initial diagnosis of a retropharyngeal abscess. However, the atypical evolution of the patient's clinical condition and the subsequent performance of a more thorough clinical examination led to the correct diagnosis of a hematoma secondary to acquired hemophilia A. This allowed surgery to be avoided in a patient at a high risk of bleeding.

2. Case Report

A 45-year-old woman with no medical history presented to the emergency department with a 48-h history of dysphagia and malaise without other symptoms. Clinical examination revealed thickened lateral and posterior pharyngeal walls extending to the larynx. MRI revealed an extensive inflammatory cervical retropharyngeal abscess extending to the parapharyngeal spaces and upper mediastinum without objectified images of an abscess (**Figure 1**).

Laboratory examination revealed no signs of infection. The only laboratory abnormalities were a high activated partial thromboplastin time (APTT) (64.2 s; reference range, 24 - 36 s) and a low hemoglobin level of 8.3 g/dL. However, these findings were not considered to be significant at that point in time. Considering these data, the patient was diagnosed with a retropharyngeal abscess with extension to the parapharyngeal spaces. She was hospitalized for intravenous antibiotic treatment and monitoring.

At 48 h after admission, the patient had developed bruises on her cervical and upper thoracic skin as well as in the posterior pharyngeal wall (**Figure 2**). Such clinical findings were associated with the previously recognized laboratory abnormality (the prolonged APTT). The Department of Hematology initiated clinical investigation of a possible coagulopathy. The patient had a significantly low level of coagulation factor VIII (4.5%; reference

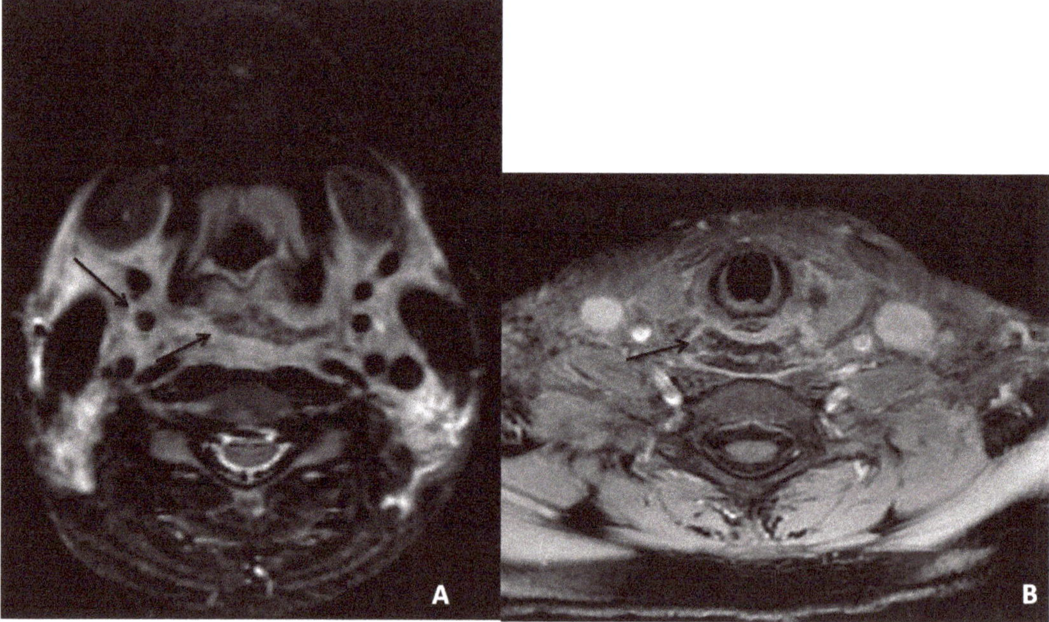

Figure 1. Magnetic resonance imaging: A space-occupying lesion exhibiting diffuse and extensive signal alterations was present in the parapharyngeal, retropharyngeal (A, arrows), and periesophageal spaces (B, arrow). The lesion caused enlargement of the prevertebral space, which extended to all fat cervical planes. These findings were suggestive of an extensive inflammatory cervical abscess extending to the upper mediastinum.

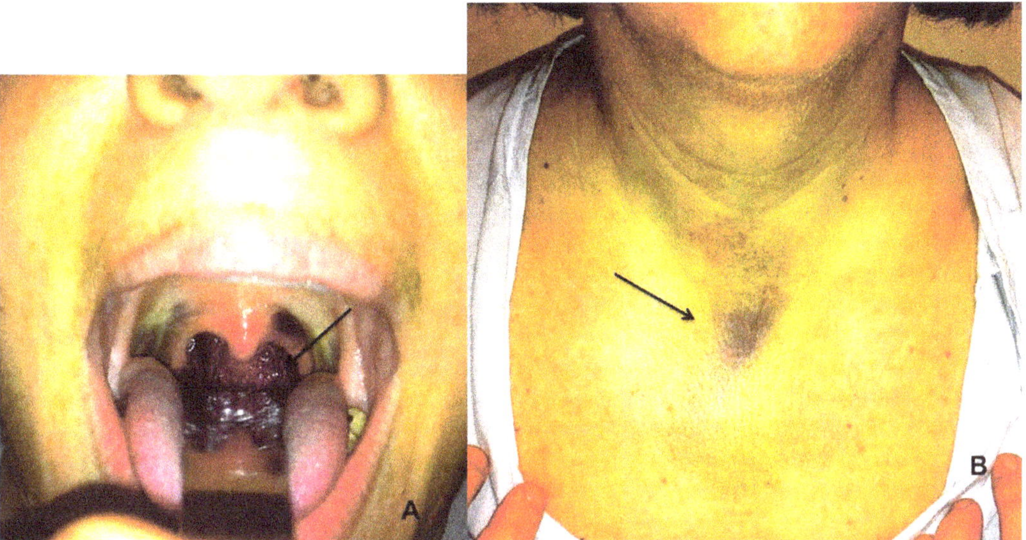

Figure 2. Clinical examination 48 h after admission. Bruises on the cervical and upper thoracic skin (A, arrow) and in the posterior pharyngeal wall (B, arrow) were suggestive of subcutaneous and submucosal hematomas.

range, 70% - 150%). Immunologically, the Bethesda test was positive for inhibitors of coagulation factor VIII (1.5 IU Bethesda).

The patient was diagnosed with acquired hemophilia A, and "factor eight inhibitor bypassing activity" (FEIBA) was administered for 24 h. Adjunctive treatment was commenced (corticosteroids and cyclophosphamide). The hemoglobin level increased, and the factor VIII concentration rose to 25%. The patient's clinical symptoms rapidly diminished. A CT scan taken at 48 h after diagnosis showed a significant reduction in the size of the retropharyngeal hematoma.

After 3 months of monitoring, the APTT and hemoglobin level had normalized, and the factor VIII inhibitory factors had disappeared. She remains clinically asymptomatic at the time of writing.

3. Discussion

Diagnosis of acquired hemophilia A is established by the presence of low levels of coagulation factor VIII together with inhibitors of this factor, as determined by the Bethesda test. Our patient met both criteria. In these patients there may be a prolonged activated partial thromboplastin time [4]. Acquired hemophilia A is a serious disease with a mortality rate of up to 9%, mainly because of the development of severe digestive tract and pulmonary hemorrhage (2.5).

Acquired hemophilia A is rare, with an estimated incidence of 1.5 cases per million people per year [5]. The typical manifestation of the disease is development of multiple small foci of spontaneous subcutaneous bleeding [6]. However, manifestation as dysphagia secondary to a retropharyngeal and parapharyngeal hematoma is rare [7].

This case is notable because, initially, our clinical suspicion was a retropharyngeal and parapharyngeal abscess possibly requiring surgical treatment. If an otolaryngologist had decided to perform surgical drainage of the mass based on this initial diagnosis, serious harm to the patient may have resulted from uncontrollable bleeding.

Acute neck masses require meticulous differential diagnosis assessing the possible presence of various causative systemic diseases before the most appropriate therapy can be determined. If the clinical course is not typical and the patient's general condition is not serious, we can delay the surgery a few hours after establishing a medical treatment. During this time we must review all the diagnostic tests carried out to reach a more accurate diagnosis.

Conflict of Interests

The authors declare no conflict of interest.

References

[1] Kubota, H., Endo, H., Noma, M., *et al.* (2013) Airway Obstruction by a Retropharyngeal Hematoma Secondary to Thoracic Aortic Aneurysm Rupture. *Journal of Cardiothoracic Surgery*, **8**, 232. http://dx.doi.org/10.1186/1749-8090-8-232

[2] Franchini, M., Gandini, G., Di Paolantonio, T. and Mariani, G. (2005) Acquired Hemophilia A: A Concise Review. *American Journal of Hematology*, **80**, 55-63. http://dx.doi.org/10.1002/ajh.20390

[3] Harper, M., Oblensky, L., Roberts, P. and Mercer, M. (2007) A Case of Acute Upper and Lower Airway Obstruction Due to Retropharyngeal Haemorrhage Secondary to Acquired Haemophilia A. *Anaesthesia*, **6**, 627-630. http://dx.doi.org/10.1111/j.1365-2044.2007.05053.x

[4] Freeman, A. (2015) Acquired Haemophilia A Presenting at a District General Hospital. *BMJ Case Reports*, 17 Feb. 2015, pii: bcr2014208001.

[5] Collins, P.W., Hirsch, S., Baglin, T.P., *et al.* (2007) Acquired Hemophilia A in the United Kingdom: A 2-Year National Surveillance Study by the United Kingdom Haemophilia Centre Doctors' Organisation. *Blood*, **109**, 1870-1877. http://dx.doi.org/10.1182/blood-2006-06-029850

[6] Vitry, A., Valois, A., Weinborm, M., *et al.* (2014) Acquired Haemophilia A: Two Cases. *Annales de Dermatologie et de Vénéréologie*, **141**, 441-445.

[7] Mulliez, S.M., Vantilborgh, A. and Devreese, K.M. (2014) Acquired Hemophilia: A Case Report and Review of the Literature. *International Journal of Laboratory Hematology*, **36**, 398-407. http://dx.doi.org/10.1111/ijlh.12210

25

Locally Advanced Anaplastic Thyroid Carcinoma with Long-Term Survival of More Than 7 Years after Combined Surgery Including Tracheal Resection and Radiotherapy: Case Report

Weizhong Ernest Fu[1*], Ming Yann Lim[1], Khoon Leong Chuah[2], Li-Chung Mark Khoo[1]

[1]Department of Otolaryngology, Tan Tock Seng Hospital, Singapore City, Singapore
[2]Department of Pathology, Tan Tock Seng Hospital, Singapore City, Singapore
Email: [*]ernest.fu@gmail.com

Abstract

Background: Anaplastic thyroid carcinoma (ATC) is one of the most aggressive human malignancies with a mean survival time of 6 months regardless of treatment. Aim: To present a case of locally advanced anaplastic thyroid carcinoma with long-term survival. A 10-year literature review of locally advanced ATC with long-term survival (more than 2 years) is also presented. Case presentation: We present a case of locally advanced anaplastic thyroid carcinoma (ATC) with tracheal invasion in a 67-year-old elderly Chinese man who was treated with radical surgery encompassing total thyroidectomy, neck dissection and tracheal resection followed by adjuvant radiotherapy. Long-term disease-free survival is more than 7 years to date. Conclusion: The prognosis of ATC remains poor as it is characterized by aggressive and extensive disease at presentation, the inability in most patients to perform radical enough surgery in order to achieve clear margins, high morbidity of complete extirpation and limited response to radiotherapy or chemotherapy. However, if complete surgical resection is possible, patients should be treated aggressively with a combination of surgery and adjuvant radiotherapy.

Keywords

Anaplastic, Thyroid, Survival, Trachea

[*]Corresponding author.

1. Introduction

Anaplastic thyroid carcinoma (ATC) accounts for about 2% of all thyroid carcinomas and is one of the most aggressive human malignancies [1]-[4]. In most series, mean survival time from diagnosis is 6 months regardless of treatment [5]-[13]. Peak incidence is usually more than 60 years of age and it occurs more commonly in females than males. Patients usually present with symptoms of extensive local invasion such as pain, dysphagia, hoarseness, respiratory distress and a rapidly enlarging neck mass.

In this paper, we present a case of locally advanced ATC with trachea invasion in an elderly male that was treated with radical surgery and adjuvant radiotherapy with long-term disease-free survival of more than 7 years. A 10-year literature review of locally advanced ATC with long-term survival (more than 2 years) is also presented.

2. Case report

A 67-year-old Chinese man first presented to us with a left sided neck mass of 2 months' duration associated with hoarseness and compressive symptoms since 1 month.

He was a smoker and had a history of bilateral pulmonary silicosis, having previously worked in a granite quarry for more than 25 years. He has no family history of thyroid disease or previous exposure to irradiation.

On examination, there was a hard 4 cm left thyroid mass that was fixed to the larynx and trachea. There were no palpable cervical nodes. Nasoendoscopy examination revealed left vocal cord paresis in the adducted position. Computed tomography (CT) revealed a left thyroid lesion with possible tracheal invasion (**Figure 1**). The left vocal fold was adducted. There were no evidence of metastatic cervical lymphadenopathy and systemic examination was negative for distant metastasis. Fine-needle aspiration cytology (FNAC) showed features of a high-grade malignant tumour with necrosis favouring an anaplastic carcinoma of the thyroid. Thyroid function tests were normal.

He underwent elective total thyroidectomy, bilateral level 6 neck dissection, and tracheal resection with primary end-to-end anastomosis. There was frank tracheal invasion with gross tumour seen intra-luminally. Frozen section analysis showed a malignant high-grade neoplasm. The post-operative period was uneventful and he was discharged after 12 days.

Final histology showed anaplastic carcinoma of the isthmus and left hemithyroid measuring 5 × 3.7 × 2.5 cm.

On microscopic examination, it was a high-grade neoplasm composed of epithelioid and spindle cells with marked anisonucleosis. Necrosis and mitotic activity including tripolar mitotic figures were present (**Figure 2**). The tumour had infiltrated posteriorly into the adjacent trachea reaching the connective tissue below the epithelial lining of the trachea and was 2 mm from the closest tracheal margin. No follicular or papillary component

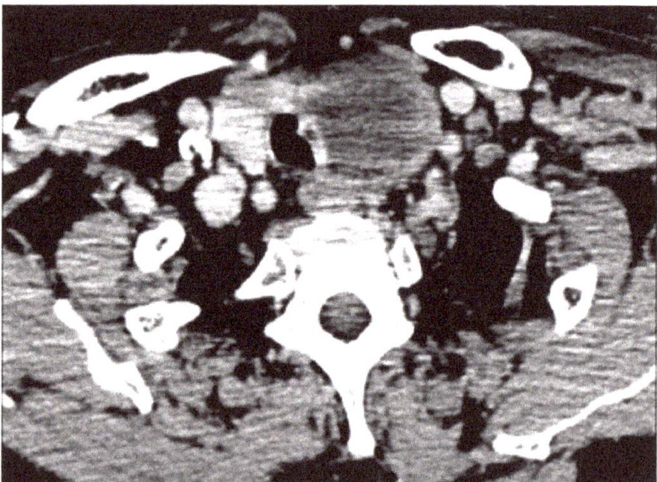

Figure 1. Hypodense left thyroid lesion 4.0 × 3.9 cm causing displacement of the trachea to the right with invasion of left lateral wall of the trachea with a polypoidal enhancing mass of tissue seen protruding into the tracheal lumen.

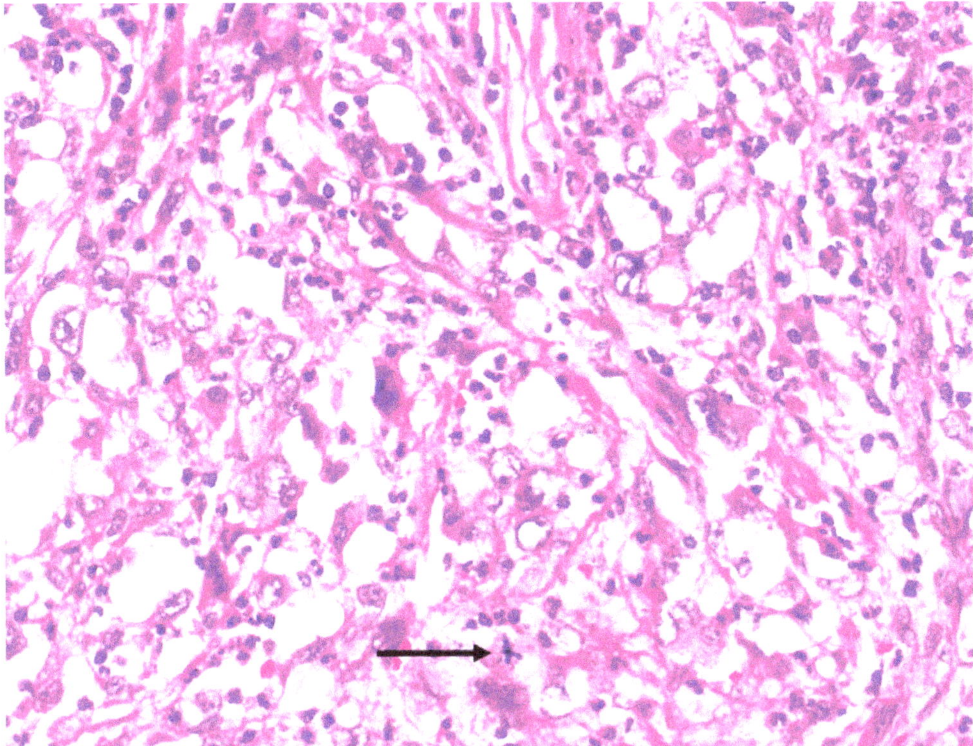

Figure 2. High-powered view of thyroid neoplasm disclosing a proliferation of epithelioid and spindle cells with nuclear pleomorphism amidst a fibrotic background. Note the presence of a tripolar mitotic figure (arrow). (Haematoxylin and eosin stain).

was noted despite extensive sampling. On immunohistochemistry, the tumour was positive for cytokeratin AE 1/3 but not CD31. A total of 11 level 6 lymph nodes were negative for tumour.

He subsequently underwent adjuvant intensity-modulated radiation therapy (IMRT) of 66 Gy over 33 fractions. He has since been on regular follow-up and to date has been disease-free for more than 7 years. Post-treatment CT scans has showed no evidence of local recurrence or distant metastasis. He is on thyroxine replacement.

3. Discussion

ATC is one of the most lethal human cancers and to date, the management remains challenging and controversial. Based on the American Thyroid Guidelines on ATC published in 2012 [14], in patients with extra-thyroidal invasion, an en bloc resection should be considered if grossly negative margins (R1 resection) could be achieved.

There have been many studies looking at various prognostic factors affecting survival. Kebebew *et al.* [5] studied a cohort of 516 patients with ATC wherein multivariate analysis showed that although most patients with ATC had an extremely poor prognosis, patients less than 60 years old with intra-thyroidal tumours survived longer. Surgical resection with external beam radiotherapy was associated with lower cause-specific mortality.

Other studies have variably shown that younger age, tumour size less than 6 cm, localized disease, female gender, and tumour resectability are independent predictors of lower cause-specific mortality [8] [15]-[17]. In particular, complete surgical resection appears to be an important determinant of survival. Haigh *et al.* [18] reported that the primary factor associated with survival was potential curative surgery. In their study, neither tumour size nor age had influenced survival. Kobayashi *et al.* [19] also observed that complete tumour resection achieved better prognosis and that age did not significantly impact survival.

In contrast to the above findings, Sugitani *et al.* [9] performed a retrospective analysis of 44 patients with ATC and devised a novel prognostic index (PI) based on four prognostic factors to select patients for aggressive multimodal treatment. The features were the presence of acute symptoms, large tumour size (>5 cm), distant metastasis, and leukocytosis (white blood cell count >10,000/mm^3), but notably did not include complete surgical resection. The presence of acute symptoms and large tumour size probably reflect rapid disease progression. Smaller tumour size may correlate with resectability. Patients with distant metastasis inevitably do poorly and the presence of leukocytosis likely represent the late stage of specific subtypes of ATC secreting granulocyte colony-stimulating factor (G-CSF) or related cytokines. The PI is calculated by totaling the number of unfavourable prognostic factors a given patient possessed: 0 to 4. The study showed that patients whose PI was ≤s1 had a 62% survival rate at 6 months. No patients whose PI was ≥3 survived more than 6 months and all patients whose PI was 4 died within 3 months. The authors also noted that the mean PI of the patients treated by multimodal therapy was 0.6 (either 0 or 1), whereas the PI of those who were not was 2.3, and hence proposed that multimodal treatment be advocated for PI of ≤1 while aggressive treatment is avoided when PI is ≥3.

Orita *et al.* [20] recently published the prospective application of this PI in the treatment strategy of 74 patients with ATC. 6-month survival rates for PI ≤1 and PI ≥3 were 72% and 12%, respectively. Both groups (P1 ≤1 and ≥3) demonstrated significantly better disease-specific survival as compared to the previous study above. Within each group, the survival rates did not differ between stages. The authors thus concluded that the PI is valid for anticipating prognosis and aiding timely decisions on treatment policy for ATC.

In the present case, long-term survival with no evidence of disease after 7 years is unusual, especially considering the presence of tracheal invasion. However, based on the above PI, he has a PI of 1 for tumour size, which indicated that he would have benefitted from the multimodal treatment he received.

In the past, there has been anecdotal evidence of cases of ATC with long-term survival. Since the mid-1980s, a group of poorly differentiated thyroid cancers (PDTC) has been recognized and considered to be tumours of biological aggressiveness intermediate between the more indolent well-differentiated thyroid carcinomas and ATC [21]. Historically, the distinction between poorly differentiated thyroid cancer (PDTC) and ATC has always been difficult. In our patient, there was no question that the tumour was an ATC.

We carried out a literature review of all ATC cases with survival greater than 2 years. Prior to review, we identified several features thought to influence survival as discussed above, namely age, tumour size, extent of tumour spread, adequacy of surgical resection, histopathology and neoadjuvant/adjuvant therapy. We restricted our review to papers published after January 1990. Exclusion criteria included papers not published in peer-reviewed journals as well as any case series in which the prognostic factors for the longest surviving cases were not specified. Medical subject headings and main keywords used were: "undifferentiated", "anaplastic" and "thyroid", with variants of the main keywords also applied.

The initial review yielded a total of 37 articles, 10 case reports and 21 case series. 13 case series were further excluded due to insufficient data. We further excluded 3 case reports and 1 case series with only intra-thyroidal ATC tumours (T4a) for ease of comparison. A total of 7 case reports and 7 case series remained for our review.

A total of 22 cases of locally advanced ATC (T4b) with long-term survival of more than 2 years were compiled from the remaining 14 articles (**Table 1**). The length of survival varied from more than 2 to 12 years. The age at diagnosis ranged from 26 to 85 years. 4 cases [22]-[24] were diagnosed with ATC incidentally after surgery for presumed benign thyroid disease. Of cases that were known, most did not present with acute symptoms, usually that of a rapidly enlarging neck mass. Only 3 cases [22] [25]-[26] had evidence of tracheal invasion while 1 case [27] had tumour extending to the cervical esophagus.

All cases received multi-modality treatment with most cases being treated with radical surgery followed by either concurrent chemoradiation or radiotherapy or radioactive iodine ablation. Only 3 cases [27]-[29] received neoadjuvant chemoradiation followed by surgery. The extent of thyroidectomy performed also differed and ranged from lobectomy to total thyroidectomy. All patients with clinically or radiologically positive cervical lymph nodes underwent neck dissections. Surgical resection included debulking surgery, macroscopically complete resections and microscopically complete resections. In general, most studies concluded that although the prognosis of most patients with ATC continues to be poor, complete resection combined with adjuvant chemotherapy and radiotherapy resulted in better survival.

There have been 3 cases with comparable survival in the literature with survival of more than 9, 10 and 12 years [23] [24]. All cases were characterized by having just an incidental focus of ATC within an otherwise well-differentiated thyroid carcinoma with limited extra-thyroidal spread. Our case however, was different as our patient presented with a gross ATC tumour with tracheal invasion and we were fortunate that the disease was still surgically resectable.

A widely cited staging system by Shin *et al.* [30] for papillary thyroid cancer is based on the depth of tracheal

Table 1. Cases of locally advanced (T4b) ATC with long-term survival of >2 years.

S N	Journal	Age/ Gender	Presentation	Extent of surgery	Positive margins	Neoadjuvant/ Adjuvant Therapy	Tumour size (cm)	Formal Histopathology	Presence of extrathyroidal spread & location	TMN Stage	Length of survival
1	Kanaseki *et al.* [25]	52/F	Enlarging anterior neck mass with vocal cord palsy	TT with tracheal wall resection Interval upper mediastinal LN dissection	No	Adjuvant CTX followed by CRT	9.0 × 6.5 × 3.0	ATC with tracheal invasion Positive superior mediastinal LN	Yes Tracheal wall and mediastinal LN	Stage IVB T4bN1bM0	>2 years
2	Shinohara *et al.* [27]	53/F	Anterior neck pain with left thyroid nodule	Total pharyngo–laryngo–esophagectomy with bilateral neck and upper mediastinum LN dissection	No	Neoadjuvant CTX followed by RT Tumour regrowth on MRI after RT, proceeded with surgery	4.1	Tumour replaced by granulation tissue and necrosis, no cancer cells (ATC on initial fine-needle aspiration cytology)	Yes Cervical esophagus	Stage IVB T4bN0MO	>2 years
3	Kurukahvecioglu *et al.* [22]	35/F	Rapidly growing right thyroid nodule initially Tracheal mass 9 months later Suspicious right neck nodes on PET-CT 5 months later	Right lobectomy Interval radical excision of tracheal mass and left lobectomy Interval right radical ND	No	Adjuvant CTX and RT after 2nd surgery	2.1 × 1.5	Right thyroid nodule: benign Tracheal mass: ATC, 3 LN positive Right ND: negative	Yes Trachea and strap muscles	Stage IVB T4bN1aM0	>3 years after second surgery
4	Noguchi *et al.* [28]	51/M	Rapidly growing right thyroid nodule with mild tenderness	Right lobectomy with right levels 2 - 4 and level 6 ND with intraoperative RT	No	Oral valproic acid daily Neoadjuvant CRT Adjuvant CTX	3 × 4.1 × 3.5	Tumour surrounded by fibrous tissue divided by thin ring of PTC; encapsulating fibrous tissue contained remnants of ATC LN: 4 out of 26 positive	Yes Strap muscles	Stage IVB T4bN1M0	>2 years
5	Olthof *et al.* [31]	76/F	Enlarging anterior neck mass	TT with left modified radical neck dissection (levels 2-6)	Yes	Adjuvant radioactive iodine therapy I131 Adjuvant RT	7 × 6 × 4	Hürthle cell carcinoma dedifferentiated to ATC with differentiation along rhabdomyoblastic cell lines Level 2 LN positive	Yes Regional cervical LN	Stage IVB T4aN1aM0	>3 years
6	Liu *et al.* [23]	68/M	Anterior neck mass with compressive symptoms and dyspnoea	TT with removal of enlarged LNs	No	Adjuvant RT	5 × 3 × 4	ATC LN negative	Yes Strap muscles	Stage IVB T4bN0M0	>10 years
7	Pichardo-Lowden *et al.* [26]	26/F	Rapidly growing anterior neck mass with odynophagia and voice change	TT and left modified radical ND	No	Adjuvant CRT	5 × 4	Undifferentiated carcinoma LN negative	Yes Tracheal wall, strap and sternocleidomastoid muscles, encasing left internal jugular vein and adhering to common carotid artery	Stage IVB T4bN0M0	>2 years
8	Akaishi *et al.* [24]	48/F	Not known	Now known but completely resected	No	No	<5	Incidental small focus of ATC	Yes Not known	Stage IVB	>12 years 7 months
9	Akaishi *et al.* [24]	68/F	Not kwown	Not known but debulking done	Not known	Adjuvant RT and CTX	<5	Incidental small focus of ATC	Yes Not known	Stage IVB	9 years
10	Akaishi *et al.* [24]	66/F	Not known	Not known but completely resected	No	Adjuvant RT and CTX	>5	ATC	Yes Not known	Stage IVB	>3 years
11	Kihara *et al.* [32]	82	Immobile thyroid mass	Subtotal thyroidectomy	Not known	Adjuvant CRT	4.9	ATC	Yes Surrounding muscle	Stage IVB T4bN0M0	6 years 4 months

Continued

12 Kim *et al.* [33]	57/F	Not known	TT	Not known	Adjuvant RT and CTX	5	ATC	Yes Not known	Stage IVB	4 years 4 months
13 Kim *et al.* [33]	55/F	Not known	TT	Not known	Adjuvant RT	4	ATC	Yes Not known	Stage IVB	>3 years 5 months
14 Siironen *et al.* [34]	85/F	Not known	Thyroid lobectomy	Not known	Adjuvant RT	Not known	ATC	Yes Recurrent laryngeal nerve	Stage IVB T4bN0M0	>6 years 6 months
15 Siironen *et al.* [34]	62/M	Not known	Radical surgery including TT	Not known	Adjuvant CRT	Not known	ATC	Yes Not known	Stage IVB T4bN0M0	5 years 4 months
16 De Crevoisier *et al.* [29]	75/M	Not known	Macroscopically complete resection	Not known	Adjuvant CRT	Not known	ATC concomitant with PTC or FTC	Yes Not known	Stage IVB T4bN1M0	6 years 6 months
17 De Crevoisier *et al.* [29]	72/F	Not known	Incomplete resection	No	Adjuvant CRT	Not known	ATC concomitant with PTC or FTC	Yes Not known	Stage IVB T4bN0M0	>4 years
18 De Crevoisier *et al.* [29]	52/F	Not known	Macroscopically complete resection	Not known	Neoadjuvant CRT	Not known	ATC	Yes Regional cervical LN	Stage IVB T4bN1M0	2 years 3 months
19 De Crevoisier *et al.* [29]	75/F	Not known	Macroscopically complete resection	Not known	Adjuvant CRT	Not known	ATC	Yes Regional cervical LN	Stage IVB T4bN1M0	2 years 1 month
20 De Crevoisier *et al.* [29]	58/M	Not known	Incomplete resection	No	Adjuvant CRT	Not known	ATC concomitant with PTC or FTC	Yes Regional cervical LN	Stage IVB T4bN1M0	2 years 1 month
21 Ito *et al.* [35]	77/F	Not known	TT and ND	Yes	Adjuvant CRT	Not known	ATC	Yes Local spread and regional cervical LN	Stage IVB T4bN1M0	>4 years 6 months
22 Rodriguez *et al.* [36]	58/M	Not known	Total thyroidectomy and multiple LN dissections (5)	Not known	Adjuvant CTX	Not known	ATC with associated PTC	Yes Local spread and regional cervical LN	Stage IVB T4bN1M0	>5 years 10 months

ATC: anaplastic thyroid carcinoma, CRT: concurrent chemoradiation, CTX: chemotherapy, FTC: follicular thyroid carcinoma, LN: lymph node, MRI: magnetic resonance imaging, ND: neck dissection, PTC: papillary thyroid carcinoma, RT: radiotherapy, TT: total thyroidectomy

invasion. Stage I disease abuts the external perichondrium of the trachea but without cartilaginous erosion. Stage II disease invades into the cartilage or causes cartilage destruction. Stage III disease extends into the lamina propria of the tracheal mucosa. Stage IV disease is full-thickness invasion through the tracheal mucosa. There is no similar staging system for ATC but based on the above, the degree of tracheal invasion for the present case would be classified as Stage 3. Based on the histological examination, the tumour was about 2 mm from the closest tracheal resection margin with tumour seen beneath the epithelium of the trachea. The involved tracheal segment was completely resected and primary anastomosis was performed.

Our case represents an anecdotal case wherein it is possible to achieve cure with clear surgical margins. Although there is general reluctance to attempt surgical resection in anaplastic carcinoma due to uniformly poor prognosis, our case concurs with the American Thyroid Guidelines on ATC [14] in which patients with ATC and extra-thyroidal invasion should have en bloc resection if grossly negative margins can be achieved. In our opinion, being able to achieve clear negative margins is the single most important prognostic factor for patients with ATC.

4. Conclusion

The prognosis of ATC remains poor as it is characterized by aggressive and extensive disease at presentation, the inability in most patients to perform radical enough surgery in order to achieve clear margins, high morbidity of complete extirpation and limited response to radiotherapy or chemotherapy. However, if complete surgical resection is possible, patients should be treated aggressively with a combination of surgery and adjuvant radiotherapy.

References

[1] Pasieka, J.L. (2003) Anaplastic Thyroid Cancer. *Current Opinion in Oncology*, **15**, 78-83. http://dx.doi.org/10.1097/00001622-200301000-00012

[2] Ain, K.B. (1998) Anaplastic Thyroid Carcinoma: Behavior, Biology, and Therapeutic Approaches. *Thyroid*, **8**, 715-726. http://dx.doi.org/10.1089/thy.1998.8.715

[3] Giuffrida, D. and Gharib, H. (2000) Anaplastic Thyroid Carcinoma: Current Diagnosis and Treatment. *Annals of Oncology*, **11**, 1083-1089. http://dx.doi.org/10.1023/A:1008322002520

[4] O'Neill, J.P., O'Neill, B., Condron, C., Walsh, M. and Bouchier-Hayes, D. (2005) Anaplastic (Undifferentiated) Thyroid Cancer: Improved Insight and Therapeutic Strategy into a Highly Aggressive Disease. *Journal of Laryngology & Otology*, **119**, 585-591. http://dx.doi.org/10.1258/0022215054516197

[5] Kebebew, E., Greenspan, F.S., Clark, O.H., Woeber, K.A. and McMillan, A. (2005) Anaplastic Thyroid Carcinoma. Treatment Outcome and Prognostic Factors. *Cancer*, **103**, 1330-1335. http://dx.doi.org/10.1002/cncr.20936

[6] Goutsouliak, V. and Hay, J.H. (2005) Anaplastic Thyroid Cancer in British Columbia 1985-1999: A Population-Based Study. *Clinical Oncology*, **17**, 75-78. http://dx.doi.org/10.1016/j.clon.2004.07.013

[7] Besic, N., Auersperg, M., Us-Krasovec, M., Golouh, R., Frkovic-Grazio, S. and Vodnik, A. (2001) Effect of Primary Treatment on Survival in Anaplastic Thyroid Carcinoma. *European Journal of Surgical Oncology*, **27**, 260-264. http://dx.doi.org/10.1053/ejso.2000.1098

[8] McIver, B., Hay, I.D., Giuffrida, D.F., *et al.* (2001) Anaplastic Thyroid Carcinoma: A 50-Year Experience at a Single Institution. *Surgery*, **130**, 1028-1034. http://dx.doi.org/10.1067/msy.2001.118266

[9] Sugitani, I., Kasai, N., Fujimoto, Y. and Yanagisawa, A. (2001) Prognostic Factors and Therapeutic Strategy for Anaplastic Carcinoma of the Thyroid. *World Journal of Surgery*, **25**, 617-622. http://dx.doi.org/10.1007/s002680020166

[10] Passler, C., Scheuba, C., Prager, G., *et al.* (1999) Anaplastic (Undifferentiated) Thyroid Carcinoma (ATC). A Retrospective Analysis. *Langenbeck's Archives of Surgery*, **384**, 284-293. http://dx.doi.org/10.1007/s004230050205

[11] Nilsson, O., Lindeberg, J., Zedenius, J., Ekman, E., Tennvall, J., Blomgren, H., *et al.* (1998) Anaplastic Giant Cell Carcinoma of the Thyroid Gland: Treatment and Survival over a 25-Year Period. *World Journal of Surgery*, **22**, 725-730. http://dx.doi.org/10.1007/s002689900460

[12] Junor, E.J., Paul, J. and Reed, N.S. (1992) Anaplastic Thyroid Carcinoma: 91 Patients Treated by Surgery and Radiotherapy. *European Journal of Surgical Oncology*, **18**, 83-88.

[13] Demeter, J.G., De Jong, S.A., Lawrence, A.M. and Paloyan, E. (1991) Anaplastic Thyroid Carcinoma: Risk Factors and Outcome. *Surgery*, **110**, 956-961.

[14] Smallridge, R.C., Ain, K.B., Asa, S.L., Bible, K.C., Brierley, J.D., Burman, K.D., *et al.* (2012) American Thyroid Association Anaplastic Thyroid Cancer Guidelines Taskforce. American Thyroid Association Guidelines for Management of Patients with Anaplastic Thyroid Cancer. *Thyroid*, **22**, 1104-1139. http://dx.doi.org/10.1089/thy.2012.0302

[15] Venkatesh, Y.S., Ordonez, N.G., Schultz, P.N., Hickey, R.C., Goepfert, H. and Samaan, N.A. (1990) Anaplastic Carcinoma of the Thyroid: A Clinicopathologic Study of 121 Cases. *Cancer*, **66**, 321-330. http://dx.doi.org/10.1002/1097-0142(19900715)66:2<321::AID-CNCR2820660221>3.0.CO;2-A

[16] Are, C. and Shaha, A.R. (2006) Anaplastic Thyroid Carcinoma: Biology, Pathogenesis, Prognostic Factors, and Treatment Approaches. *Annals of Surgical Oncology*, **13**, 453-464. http://dx.doi.org/10.1245/ASO.2006.05.042

[17] Tan, R.K., Finley III, R.K., Driscoll, D., Bakamjian, V., Hicks Jr., W.L. and Shedd, D.P. (1995) Anaplastic Carcinoma of the Thyroid: A 24-Year Experience. *Head Neck*, **17**, 41-47; Discussion 47-48. http://dx.doi.org/10.1002/hed.2880170109

[18] Haigh, P.I., Ituarte, P.H., Wu, H.S., Treseler, P.A., Posner, M.D., Quivey, J.M., *et al.* (2001) Completely Resected Anaplastic Thyroid Carcinoma Combined with Adjuvant Chemotherapy and Irradiation Is Associated with Prolonged Survival. *Cancer*, **91**, 2335-2342. http://dx.doi.org/10.1002/1097-0142(20010615)91:12<2335::AID-CNCR1266>3.0.CO;2-1

[19] Kobayashi, T., Asakawa, H. and Umeshita, K. (1996) Treatment of 37 Patients with Anaplastic Carcinoma of the Thyroid. *Head Neck*, **18**, 36-41. http://dx.doi.org/10.1002/(SICI)1097-0347(199601/02)18:1<36::AID-HED5>3.0.CO;2-#

[20] Orita, Y., Sugitani, I., Amemiya, T. and Fujimoto, Y. (2011) Prospective Application of Our Novel Prognostic Index in the Treatment of Anaplastic Thyroid Carcinoma. *Surgery*, **150**, 1212-1219. http://dx.doi.org/10.1016/j.surg.2011.09.005

[21] Patel, K.N. and Shaha, A.R. (2006) Poorly Differentiated and Anaplastic Thyroid Cancer. *Cancer Control*, **13**, 119-128.

[22] Kurukahvecioglu, O., Ege, B., Poyraz, A., Tezel, E. and Taneri, F. (2007) Anaplastic Thyroid Carcinoma with Long Term Survival after Combined Treatment: Case Report. *Endocrine Regulations*, **41**, 41-44.

[23] Liu, A.H., Juan, L.Y., Yang, A.H., Chen, H.S. and Lin, H.D. (2006) Anaplastic Thyroid Cancer with Uncommon Long-Term Survival. *Journal of the Chinese Medical Association*, **69**, 489-491. http://dx.doi.org/10.1016/S1726-4901(09)70314-4

[24] Akaishi, J., Sugino, K., Kitagawa, W., Nagahama, M., Kameyama, K., Shimizu, K., *et al.* (2011) Prognostic Factors and Treatment Outcomes of 100 Cases of Anaplastic Thyroid Carcinoma. *Thyroid*, **21**, 1183-1189. http://dx.doi.org/10.1089/thy.2010.0332

[25] Kanaseki, T., Harabuchi, Y., Wakashima, J., Asakura, K., Kataura, A. and Satoh, M. (1999) A Case of Anaplastic Thyroid Carcinoma Surviving Disease Free for over 2 Years. *Auris Nasus Larynx*, **26**, 217-220. http://dx.doi.org/10.1016/S0385-8146(98)00074-1

[26] Pichardo-Lowden, A., Durvesh, S., Douglas, S., Todd, W., Bruno, M. and Goldenberg, D. (2009) Anaplastic Thyroid Carcinoma in a Young Woman: A Rare Case of Survival. *Thyroid*, **19**, 775-779. http://dx.doi.org/10.1089/thy.2009.0025

[27] Shinohara, S., Kikuchi, M., Naito, Y., Fujiwara, K., Hori, S., Tona, Y., *et al.* (2009) Successful Treatment of Locally Advanced Anaplastic Thyroid Carcinoma by Chemotherapy and Hyperfractionated Radiotherapy. *Auris Nasus Larynx*, **36**, 729-732. http://dx.doi.org/10.1016/j.anl.2009.02.001

[28] Noguchi, H., Yamashita, H., Murakami, T., Hirai, K., Noguchi, Y., Maruta, J., *et al.* (2009) Successful Treatment of Anaplastic Thyroid Carcinoma with a Combination of Oral Valproic Acid, Chemotherapy, Radiation and Surgery. *Endocrine Journal*, **56**, 245-249. http://dx.doi.org/10.1507/endocrj.K08E-016

[29] De Crevoisier, R., Baudin, E., Bachelot, A., Leboulleux, S., Travagli, J.-P., Caillou, B. and Schlumberger, M. (2004) Combined Treatment of Anaplastic Thyroid Carcinoma with Surgery, Chemotherapy, and Hyperfractionated Accelerated External Radiotherapy. *International Journal of Radiation Oncology*Biology*Physics*, **60**, 1137-1143. http://dx.doi.org/10.1016/j.ijrobp.2004.05.032

[30] Shin, D.H., Mark, E.J., Suen, H.C. and Grillo, H.C. (1993) Pathologic Staging of Papillary Carcinoma of the Thyroid with Airway Invasion Based on the Anatomic Manner of Extension to the Trachea: A Clinicopathologic Study Based on 22 Patients Who Underwent Thyroidectomy and Airway Resection. *Human Pathology*, **24**, 866-870. http://dx.doi.org/10.1016/0046-8177(93)90136-5

[31] Olthof, M., Persoon, A.C., Plukker, J.T., van der Wal, J.E. and Links, T.P. (2008) Anaplastic Thyroid Carcinoma with Rhabdomyoblastic Differentiation: A Case Report with a Good Clinical Outcome. *Endocrine Pathology*, **19**, 62-65. http://dx.doi.org/10.1007/s12022-008-9017-3

[32] Kihara, M., Miyauchi, A., Yamauchi, A. and Yokomise, H. (2004) Prognostic Factors of Anaplastic Thyroid Carcinoma. *Surgery Today*, **34**, 394-398. http://dx.doi.org/10.1007/s00595-003-2737-6

[33] Kim, T.Y., Kim, K.W., Jung, T.S., Kim, J.M., Kim, S.W., Chung, K.-W., *et al.* (2007) Prognostic Factors for Korean Patients with Anaplastic Thyroid Carcinoma. *Head Neck*, **29**, 765-772. http://dx.doi.org/10.1002/hed.20578

[34] Siironen, P., Hagström, J., Mäenpää, H.O., Louhimo, J., Heikkilä, A., Heiskanen, I., *et al.* (2010) Anaplastic and Poorly Differentiated Thyroid Carcinoma: Therapeutic Strategies and Treatment Outcome of 52 Consecutive Patients. *Oncology*, **79**, 400-408. http://dx.doi.org/10.1159/000322640

[35] Ito, K., Hanamura, T., Murayama, K., Okada, T., Watanabe, T., Harada, M., *et al.* (2012) Multimodality Therapeutic Outcomes in Anaplastic Thyroid Carcinoma: Improved Survival in Subgroups of Patients with Localized Primary Tumours. *Head Neck*, **34**, 230-237. http://dx.doi.org/10.1002/hed.21721

[36] Rodriguez, J.M., Piñero, A., Ortiz, S., Moreno, A., Sola, J., Soria, T., *et al.* (2000) Clinical and Histological Differences in Anaplastic Thyroid Carcinoma. *European Journal of Surgery*, **166**, 34-38.

Nuclear Features in the Diagnosis of Follicular Variant of Papillary Thyroid Carcinoma—The Diagnostic Dilemma

Chaganti Padmavathi Devi[1], Karri Maruthi Devi[1], Madabhushi Venugopal[1], Mulukutla Partha Akarsh[2]

[1]Guntur Medical College, Guntur, India
[2]Siddhartha Medical College, Vijayawada, India
Email: drcpd60@gmail.com, ratnakumardevi@gmail.com, mvgopal@yahoo.com, akarsh316@yahoo.com

Abstract

Aim: Follicular variant of papillary thyroid carcinoma [FVPC] as a diagnostic entity has been beset by many controversies. In this study, we describe the nuclear features essential for the diagnosis and analyze the difficulties that confront pathologists as it is important to avoid pitfalls because appropriate management protocol depends upon on an accurate diagnosis of this variant. Materials and Methods: A total of 30 cases, diagnosed as FVPC over a period of two years in the Department of Pathology, were taken for the study. Haematoxylin and Eosin stained sections were reviewed. The extent and distribution of nuclear features were analyzed. Results: The 30 cases of FVPC were categorized into encapsulated and infiltrative groups basing on the presence or lack of capsule and capsular invasion and vascular invasion. Conclusion: FVPC is diagnosed basing on specific nuclear features and hence histopathology still remains the gold standard for the accurate diagnosis.

Keywords

Nuclear Features, Follicular Variant, Papillary Carcinoma, Encapsulation, Vascular Invasion Capsular Invasion

1. Introduction

Papillary thyroid carcinoma [PTC] is conventionally diagnosed basing on cytological features rather than architectural pattern whereas Follicular carcinoma of thyroid is diagnosed basing on the presence of invasion [1]. Lindsay [2] first described the entity of follicular variant of papillary thyroid carcinoma (FVPC) which was later defined by Chen and Rosai [3]. During the last three decades either infiltrative or encapsulated thyroid tumors with follicular pattern were diagnosed as papillary carcinoma basing on the nuclear features like enlargement, elongation, nuclear clearing, intranuclear grooves, inclusions, micronucleoli and thick nuclear membranes [4] [5]. However, problems cropped up in the diagnosis of completely encapsulated tumors because of variability among pathologists due to the lack of agreement on the minimal diagnostic criteria [4] [6]. Chan proposed criteria for the diagnosis of encapsulated FVPC which include clear nuclei, round to oval nuclei, crowded nuclei, intranuclear grooves, psammoma bodies and secondary features like irregular follicles, thick colloid and multinucleated histiocytes [1]. A scoring system was applied for the diagnosis of PTC by Verhulst *et al.* who observed that follicular patterned PTC was at or below the threshold score [7].

The inter- and intra-observer variability often leads to confusion among clinicians regarding the management of FVPC. To overcome this grey zone, the term "well differentiated thyroid tumor of uncertain malignant potential" was coined by Chernobyl Pathologist group for encapsulated follicular patterned tumor with incomplete or unconvincing features of PTC [8]. Livolsi VA proposed that FVPTC is a heterogeneous group and defined 6 histologic subtypes basing on variation in architectural pattern and distribution of nuclear features [9].

Hung-Yu Chang *et al.* found that, though the clinical behavior of FVPC hovers between that of pure papillary carcinoma and follicular carcinoma, prognosis following aggressive treatment was similar to pure papillary cancer [10]. As such a thorough and diligent scrutiny of sections sampled from representative areas and strict adherence to the specific criteria are imperative for an accurate diagnosis of FVPC which is of paramount importance in planning of an appropriate and personalized treatment protocol.

Aim: This study is undertaken to reclassify FVPC basing on architectural and cytological features and discuss the spectrum of nuclear features in the diagnosis of FVPC and the difficulties encountered in the evaluation of subtypes of FVPC.

2. Material and Methods

In this study the tumors which were diagnosed as FVPC between January, 2011 and December, 2012 were taken. The cases included total thyroidectomy or hemithyroidectomy surgical specimens. Tumor size was measured in the greatest diameter. Surgical margins were also inked. The sections were stained with hematoxylin and eosin.

Exclusion Criteria-Tumors with presence of necrosis and increased mitotic activity of more than 5 per 10 HPF were excluded from the present study. Tumors showing papillary configurations constituting more than 1% of tumor area were excluded from the diagnosis of FVPC [4].

3. Results

A total of 30 cases diagnosed as FVPC reported during the period of two years were selected for the present study. The cases were subdivided in to encapsulated and infiltrative tumors. We classified them as encapsulated if the tumor was completely surrounded by a capsule and infiltrative if there was no capsule or incomplete capsulation with tongues of tumor tissue infiltrates in to non-neoplastic thyroid. Tumors that were grossly encapsulated with no microscopic evidence of capsular and vascular invasion were designated as noninvasive encapsulated FVPC. Tumors that were grossly encapsulated but showing microscopic evidence of capsular or vascular infiltration were classified as invasive encapsulated (**Figure 1**).

In our study twenty seven cases were found to be encapsulated tumors while the remaining three cases showed infiltrative features. Encapsulated tumors were again subdivided in to noninvasive and invasive groups basing on absence or presence of capsular and vascular invasion. Non invasive encapsulated tumors were 21 in number where as the remaining six were identified as invasive encapsulated tumors.

Complete infiltration of entire thickness of tumor capsule is taken as capsular infiltration (**Figure 2**). However tumor nests embedded within the tumor capsule and irregularity of the contour along the inner border of the capsule were not considered as evidence of capsular invasion. Vascular invasion implies invasion of a vessel with in or out side tumor capsule with covering by endothelium or attachment to the vessel wall [3] (**Figure 3**).

In our study women outnumbered men and the commonest age group was 20 to 30 years.

The size of the tumor in our cases is less than 4 cms in 28 cases and more than 4 cms in 2 cases.

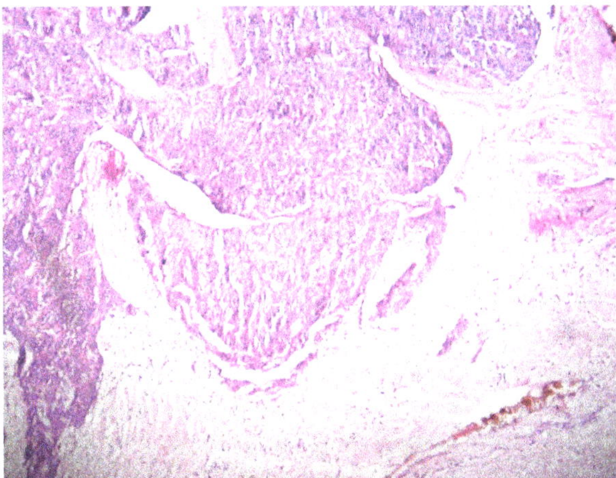

Figure 1. Infiltrative tumor.

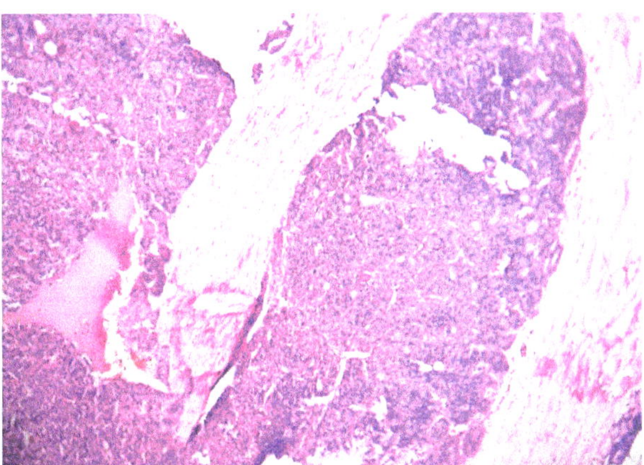

Figure 2. Full thickness capsular infiltration.

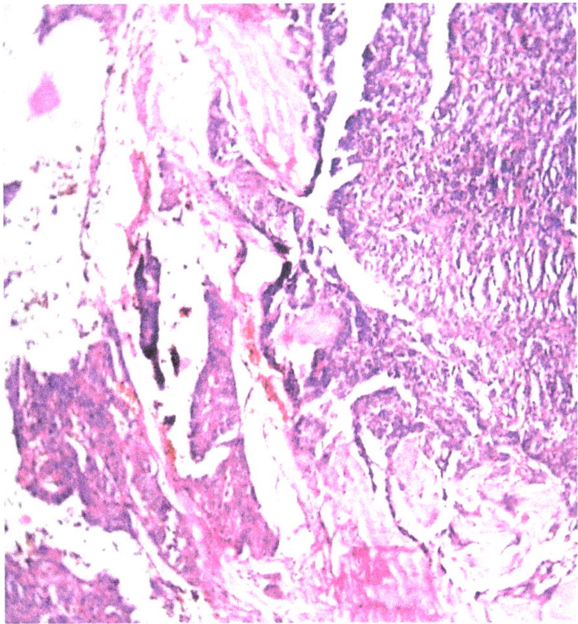

Figure 3. Vascular infiltration—Tumor attached to the wall of the blood vessal.

The nuclear and other morphological features which favored the diagnosis of FVPC in the descending order of frequency in our cases were pale nuclei, crowding of nucleus (**Figure 4**), thick colloid (**Figure 5**), nuclear grooves, round to oval nuclei, psammoma bodies and multicentricity.

4. Discussion

The differential diagnosis of thyroid neoplasms with follicular architecture includes adenomatous hyperplasias, Follicular Adenoma [FA], Follicular Carcinoma [FC] and FVPC. Tumors which were predominantly composed of follicles with nuclear features of PTC were classified under the category of FVPC [11].

In the study of Liu Jeffery, the median age of the patients was 43.1 years and females outnumbered males and constituted 76% of cases [12]. In our study also females outnumbered males and most cases were seen in third decade.

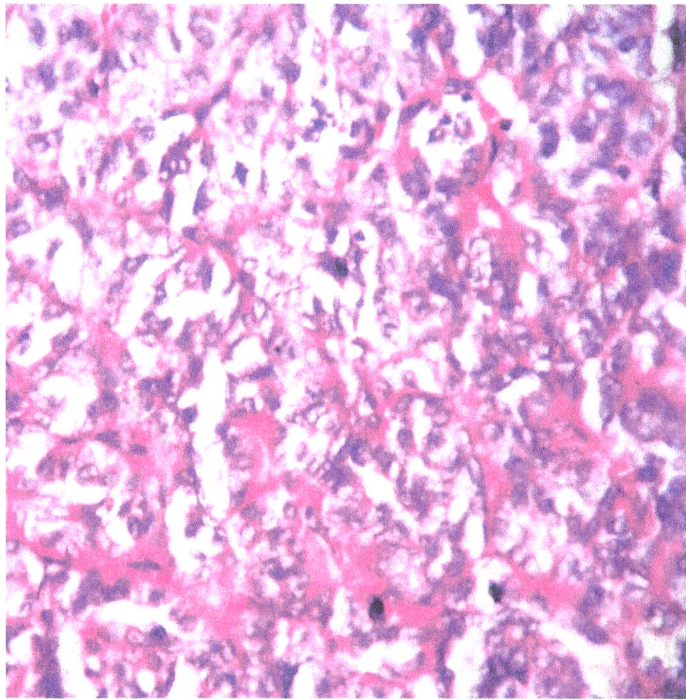

Figure 4. Pale nuclei,oval nuclei and crowding of nuclei.

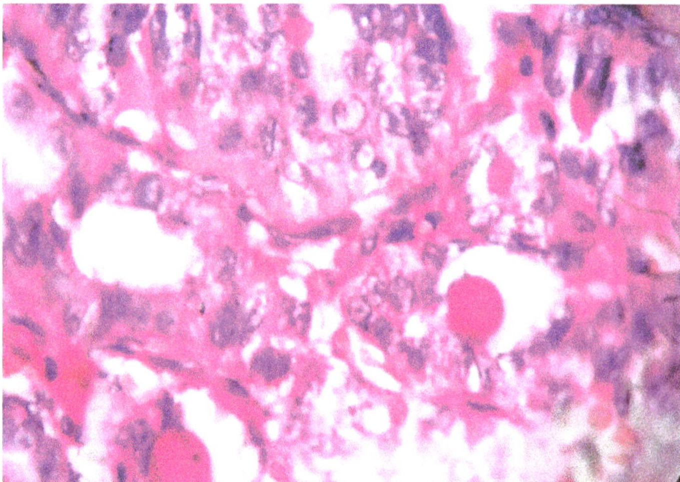

Figure 5. Nuclear grooves and thick colloid.

FVPC clinically, histologically and on molecular basis are divided into two distinct groups. The first group is encapsulated and the second one is non-encapsulated which includes infiltrative and diffuse forms [12]. The infiltrative growth resembles classic PTC in its invasive growth and metastasis to lymph nodes. FVPC has more favorable clinicopathological features in the form of frequent encapsulation, lower rates of lymph node metastases and less frequent extra thyroidal extension [13] [14]. However, some encapsulated FVPC behave like follicular neoplasm and may even metastasize to distant sites [11]. In the studies of Chen and Rosai [3] and Jeffery Liu [12] encapsulated FVPC accounted for more number of tumors than infiltrative type. In our study also encapsulated tumors outnumbered infiltrative tumors. This finding is in concordance with the world literature.

Nuclear features: FVPC can be easily diagnosed when nuclear features of papillary carcinoma are classic and diffuse. However the diagnosis of FVPC becomes very difficult if the nuclear features are not well developed and when they are focally present [4].

Some authors believe that there is an increase in the reporting of FVPC because of lowering of thresholds [4]. Renshaw *et al.* observed that lack of minimum histological definition and reports of rare aggressive clinical behavior resulted in a marked lowering of diagnostic threshold of FVPC and consequent over diagnosis of this entity [15]. Elsheikh TM *et al.* noted that there are no strict guidelines regarding the quantitative criteria to diagnose FVPC including the percentage of tumor showing nuclear features of papillary carcinoma [NFPC], the degree of nuclear pallor, the number of nuclear grooves and optically clear nuclei [4].

According to Livolsi *et al.* strict criteria for specific nuclear features comprising of ovoid nuclei, crowded nuclei, clear nuclei, intranuclear grooves and inclusions should be applied to diagnose FVPC [7]. They also observed that other favorable features included psammoma bodies and secondary features such as elongated irregularly shaped follicles, dark staining colloid, and multinucleated histiocytes in the lumen of the follicles [5]. In the decreasing order of preference the histological features taken in to consideration for the diagnosis of FVPC are cytoplasmic invaginations, abundant nuclear grooves, ground glass nuclei, psammoma bodies, enlarged overlapping nuclei, and irregularly shaped nuclei [5].

In the study of Tarik M. Elsheikh *et al.*, nuclear features in the decreasing order of frequency were nuclear clearing, very fine powdery chromatin, nuclear grooves, nuclear overlapping, nuclear membrane irregularity, and nuclear enlargement [4]. The secondary features comprised chromatin margination, distorted follicular architecture and fibrosis/sclerosis [4]. According to Chan JK the features necessary to make the diagnosis of FVPC include ovoid nuclei rather than round nuclei, crowded nuclei with lack of polarization, nuclei which show pale or clear chromatin pattern with the nuclear clearing not to be confined to the centre, nuclear grooves and psammoma bodies [1]. The additional features that should be taken in to consideration, if the above features were lacking, include abortive papillae, elongated or irregularly shaped follicles, dark staining colloid, presence of rare and multinucleated histiocytes in the lumen of the follicles.

In our study features seen in the decreasing order of frequency were pale nuclei, nuclear grooves, abortive papillae, nuclear pseudo inclusions, nuclear clearing, followed by crowded nucleus, Psammoma bodies and thick colloid. Sclerosis was consistently seen in all invasive cases.

Rosai *et al.* subscribe to the view that ground glass nuclei should be seen in most areas to diagnose a lesion as PTC. Plain vesicular nuclei are seen both in benign and malignant thyroid lesions and hence should not be taken as diagnostic marker for FVPC [16].

In view of the various morphological presentations of FVPC and controversies Virginia A Livolsi proposed that FVPC is a heterogeneous group and classified them into six variants [9].

Type 1: Unencapsulated invasive tumor where the lesion grows in infiltrative pattern [16].

Type 2: Encapsulated invasive tumors with diffuse classical features

Type 3: Encapsulated invasive tumors showing either classical or unconvincing nuclear features which are present in multifocal areas

Type 4: Encapsulated noninvasive tumors with classical and diffuse nuclear features

Type 5: Encapsulated noninvasive tumors with classical or unconvincing nuclear features which are present multifocally.

FVPC—Type 2 to 5: They represent a group of capsulated tumors which are invasive or noninvasive. They present diagnostic difficulty when the nuclear features are present in multiple locations in the same tumor. Cases of noninvasive encapsulated variant of FVPC with multifocal but incomplete nuclear features are the ones which caused diagnostic problems and greatest inter observer variability. In such cases, Lioyd *et al.* and Elsheikh observed that the best developed nuclear features were seen in the rim of tumor closest to the tumor capsule [4] [6].

Livolsi also suggests that encapsulated FVPC may represent a hybrid of papillary carcinoma and follicular adenoma or carcinoma [9].

Type 6: Capsulated lesion of thyroid in which subcentimeter area shows classical nuclear features of PTC, the lesion was designated as papillary microcarcinoma in Follicular Adenoma [11]. In our study we did not come across type 6 cases.

Baloch and Livolsi found that encapsulated FVPC with multifocal nuclear features developed distant metastasis [11]. Rivera *et al.* observed that invasive encapsulated tumors do possess metastatic potential but the sites of secondary deposits vary from the classic papillary cancer. They also found that FVPC without capsular or vascular invasion lacked lymph node deposits and did not recur [17].

Chernobyl Pathologist Group classified neoplasms which showed questionable nuclear features and lack of vascular or capsular invasion as well differentiated tumors of uncertain malignant potential or hybrid tumors [1]. In our study, one noninvasive tumor with unconvincing nuclear features was reported as well differentiated tumor of uncertain malignant potential.

According to Livolsi, even when the nuclear change is multifocal but not diffuse, the entire lesion could be malignant [9]. This possibility is supported by different molecular and immunohistochemical studies [18] [19]. Markers like high molecular weight cytokeratin, cytokeratin 19, HBME1, CD 57, CD 44, and CD 15 are commonly expressed in PTC when compared to non neoplastic lesions of thyroid. But their expression is not sufficient for the diagnosis of FVPC because in classic PTC also they are focally expressed [20]. CD 56 is considered a negative marker for the diagnosis of PTC as it is expressed in 93% of benign lesions and while it is expressed in only 5% of cases of PTC [20].

A Salajegheh *et al.* believe that FVPTC has different molecular changes compared to conventional papillary thyroid carcinoma which lead to phenotypic differences [21]. Adeniran AJ observed that BRAF, RET/PTC, and RAS mutations are associated with distinct microscopic, clinical, and biologic features of thyroid papillary carcinomas and RAS mutations characterize exclusively FVPC and correlate with less prominent nuclear features [22]. Livolsi *et al.*, however, are of the view that the field is still evolving and molecular studies of subtypes of FVPC are required to define these tumors [5].

5. Conclusion

Follicular variant of papillary thyroid carcinoma can present as uncapsulated infiltrative variant or partly capsulated or encapsulated variants. The diagnosis of FVPC is made primarily basing on nuclear features. However nuclear features when incomplete or borderline and multifocal can pose diagnostic difficulty. Immunohistochemical markers, either positive or negative, are not 100% diagnostic of FVPC. Better understanding of molecular basis of FVPC will help in identifying precise markers. As such histopathology still remains the gold standard for the accurate diagnosis of FVPC.

References

[1] Chan, J.K. (2002) Strict Criteria Should Be Applied in the Diagnosis of Encapsulated Follicular Variant of Papillary Carcinoma of Thyroid. *American Journal of Clinical Pathology*, **117**, 16-18. http://dx.doi.org/10.1309/P7QL-16KQ-QLF4-XW0M

[2] Lindsay, S. (1960) Carcinoma of the Thyroid Gland. A clinical and Pathological Study of 239 Patients at the University of California Hospital. Charles C Thomas, Springfield, IL.

[3] Chen, K.T. and Rosai, J. (1977) Follicular Variant of Thyroid Papillary Carcinoma: A Clinicopathological Study of Six Cases. *American Journal of Surgical Pathology*, **1**, 171-175. http://dx.doi.org/10.1097/00000478-197706000-00003

[4] Elsheikh, T.M., Asa, S.L., Chan, J.K., *et al.* (2008) Interobserver and Intraobserver Variation among Experts in the Diagnosis of Thyroid Follicular Lesions with Borderline Nuclear Features of Papillary Carcinoma. *American Journal of Clinical Pathology*, **30**, 736-744. http://dx.doi.org/10.1309/AJCPKP2QUVN4RCCP

[5] Livolsi, V.A. and Baloch, Z.W. (2009) The Many Faces of Follicular Variant of Papillary Thyroid Carcinoma. *Pathology Case Reviews*, **14**, 214-218. http://dx.doi.org/10.1097/PCR.0b013e3181c75e9b

[6] Lioyd, R.V., Erickson, L.A., Casey, M.B., *et al.* (2004) Observer Variation in the Diagnosis of Follicular Variant of Papillary Thyroid Carcinoma. *American Journal of Surgical Pathology*, **28**, 1336-1340. http://dx.doi.org/10.1097/01.pas.0000135519.34847.f6

[7] Verhulst, P., Devos, P., Aubert, S., *et al.* (2008) A Score Based on Microscopic Criteria Proposed for Analysis of Papillary Carcinoma of Thyroid. *Virchows Archiv*, **452**, 233-240. http://dx.doi.org/10.1007/s00428-008-0577-x

[8] Williams, E.D., Abrosimov, A., Bogdanova, T.I., *et al.* (2000) Two Proposals Regarding the Terminology of Thyroid Tumors [Guest Editorial]. *International Journal of Surgical Pathology*, **8**, 181-183. http://dx.doi.org/10.1177/106689690000800304

[9] Livolsi, V.A. and Baloch, Z.W. (2009) The Many Faces of Follicular Variant of Papillary Thyroid Carcinoma. *Pathology Case Reviews*, **14**, 214-218. http://dx.doi.org/10.1097/PCR.0b013e3181c75e9b

[10] Chang, H.-Y., Lin, J.-D., Chou, S.-C., Chao, T.-C. and Hsueh, C. (2006) Clinical Presentations and Outcomes of Surgical Treatment of Follicular Variant of the Papillary Thyroid Carcinomas. *Japanese Journal of Clinical Oncology*, **36**, 688-693. http://dx.doi.org/10.1093/jjco/hyl093

[11] Baloch, Z.W. and Livolsi, V.A. (2002) Follicular-Patterned Lesions of the Thyroid. *American Journal of Clinical Pathology*, **117**, 143-150. http://dx.doi.org/10.1309/8VL9-ECXY-NVMX-2RQF

[12] Liu, J., Singh, B., Tullini, G., Curlson, D.L., *et al.* (2006) Follicular Variant of Papillary Thyroid Carcinoma: A Clinicopathological Study of a Problematic Entity. *Cancer*, **6**, 1255-1264. http://dx.doi.org/10.1002/cncr.22138

[13] Passler, C., Prager, G., Scheuba, G., *et al.* (2003) Follicular Variant of Papillary Thyroid Carcinoma: A Long Term Follow-Up. *Archives of Surgery*, **138**, 1362-1366. http://dx.doi.org/10.1001/archsurg.138.12.1362

[14] Zidan, J., Karen, D., Stein, M., *et al.* (2003) Pure versus Follicular Variant of Papillary Thyroid Carcinoma: Clinical Features, Prognostic Factors, Treatment, and Survival. *Cancer*, **97**, 1181-1185. http://dx.doi.org/10.1002/cncr.11175

[15] Renshaw, A.A. and Gould, E.W. (2002) Why There Is the Tendency to "Overdiagnose" the Follicular Variant of Papillary Thyroid Carcinoma. *American Journal of Clinical Pathology*, **117**, 19-21. http://dx.doi.org/10.1309/CJEU-XLQ7-UPVE-NWFV

[16] Rosai, J., Carcangiu, M.L. and Delellis, R.A. (1992) Follicular Carcinomas, Papillary Carcinomas. In: Rosai, J., Sobin, J. and Sobin, L.H., Eds., *Tumors of Thyroid Gland, Atlas of Tumor Pathology*, Armed Forces Institute of Pathology, Washington DC, 49-121.

[17] Rivera, M., Tuttle, R.M. and Patel, S., *et al.* (2009) Encapsulated Papillary Thyroid Carcinoma: A Clinic-Pathologic Study of 106 Cases with Emphasis on Its Morphologic Subtypes (Histologic Growth Pattern). *Thyroid*, **19**, 119-127. http://dx.doi.org/10.1089/thy.2008.0303

[18] Fusco, A., Chiappetta, G., Hui, P., *et al.* (2002) Assessment of RET/PTC Oncogene Activation and Clonality in Thyroid Nodules with Incomplete Morphological Evidence of Papillary Carcinoma: A Search for the Early Precursors of Papillary Cancer. *American Journal of Pathology*, **160**, 2157-2167. http://dx.doi.org/10.1016/S0002-9440(10)61164-9

[19] Barroeta, J.E., Baloch, Z.W., Lal, P., *et al.* (2006) Diagnostic Value of Differential Expression of CK19, Galectin-3, HMBE-1, ERK, RET, and p16 in Benign and Malignant Follicular Derived Lesions of the Thyroid: An Immunohistochemical Tissue Microarray Analysis. *Endocrine Pathology*, **17**, 225-234. http://dx.doi.org/10.1385/EP:17:3:225

[20] Shahebrahimi, K., Madani, S.H., Fazaeli, A.R., Khazaei, S., *et al.* (2013) Diagnostic Value of CD56 and nm23 Markers in Papillary Thyroid Carcinoma. *Indian Journal of Pathology and Microbiology*, **56**, 2-5. http://dx.doi.org/10.4103/0377-4929.116139

[21] Salajegheh, A., Pectu, E.B., Smith, R.A. and Lam, A.K.Y. (2008) Follicular Variant of Papillary Thyroid Carcinoma: A Diagnostic Challenge for Clinicians and Pathologists. *Postgraduate Medical Journal*, **84**, 78-82. http://dx.doi.org/10.1136/pgmj.2007.064881

[22] Adeniran, A.J., Zhu, Z., Gandhi, M., Steward, D.L., Fidler, J.P., Giordano, T.J., Biddinger, P.W. and Nikiforov, Y.E. (2006) Correlation between Genetic Alterations and Microscopic Features, Clinical Manifestations, and Prognostic Characteristics of Thyroid Papillary Carcinomas. *American Journal of Surgical Pathology*, **30**, 216-222. http://dx.doi.org/10.1097/01.pas.0000176432.73455.1b

27

Post-Stapedectomy Granuloma: A Rare Case Report

Kartik Parelkar, Smita Nagle, Mohan Jagade, Poonam Khairnar, Madhavi Pandare, Rajanala Nataraj, Reshma Hanwate, Bandu Nagrale, Devkumar Rangaraja

Department of ENT, Grant Govt Medical College & Sir J J Group of Hospitals, Mumbai, India
Email: kartikparelkar@ymail.com

Abstract

Reparative granuloma in the oval window region is an uncommon complication of stapes surgery, which usually develops within one to eight weeks after operation and causes a sudden hearing loss and disturbance of balance. It may also cause otalgia. Because of its rarity, no single centre would be able to give conclusive evidence regarding this complication. Hence we would like to report our experience and hope to get a better understanding regarding the stapes surgery induced granulation.

Keywords

Stapes Surgery, Granulation Tissue, Post-Stapedectomy, Otalgia, Otosclerosis

1. Introduction

Since the advent of stapedectomy and its use in the treatment of otosclerosis, a few complications have been reported in the literature. Among them, the granulomatous reaction, described by Harris and Weiss in 1962 [1], is rare. It is an excessive inflammation that forms granulation tissue around the prosthesis and the oval window [2].

The term reparative granuloma is a misnomer [2] as the lesion does not involve granulomatous inflammation and stapes surgery induced granulation tissue is a more appropriate term.

Although the etiology is uncertain, several authors believe that the main cause is a foreign body reaction to the material used in filling the oval window region [3]. Other theories include pyogenic inflammation, autoimmune and allergic reactions or an over exuberant healing process.

The incidence is 0.1% for stapedectomy and 0.07% for stapedectomy cases [3]; it generally manifests after surgery as sensorineural dysacusis and vertigo.

It may be confirmed by exploratory tympanotomy to visualize granulation tissue near the prosthesis and the oval window region in a symptomatic patient [3].

2. Case Report

A 32-year-old female patient, a known case of unilateral otosclerosis who had undergone left stapedectomy at another institute 6 months back presented with complaints of progressive hearing hearing loss, vertigo and otalgia post-surgery.

Patient had the above complaints 1 to 2 weeks after the stapedectomy, the hearing loss was gradually progressive and constant in nature. While the vertigo had partially subsided with anti-vertiginous drugs, the otalgia affected her daily life. The pain was of throbbing type, over the left post-auricular region, radiating over the temporal region and upper neck on the left side. The symptoms were not relieved by medications. She had no associated ear discharge, tinnitus, facial weakness, nausea or visual complaints.

After ruling out orthopaedic and neuromedical causes for her symptoms a thorough ENT examination was conducted.

On otoscopy bilateral tympanic membranes were intact and hazy. Tympanometery was within normal limits and stapedial reflex was absent on the left side.

Pure tone audiogram (PTA) showed severe to moderate mixed hearing loss in the left ear while the right ear hearing sensitivity was within normal limits. (note: patient did not have sensory component before the stapedotomy; her pre-stapedectomy PTA showed left moderate conductive hearing loss).

High resolution computed tomography (HRCT) of temporal bones showed left ear stapes surgery defect with the piston in situ and in proper position. Minimal soft tissue density at the oval window region near the prosthesis and an partially dehiscent fallopian canal were noted.

After meticulous routine blood investigations and pre-anaesthetic check up an exploratory tympanotomy was scheduled. A written informed consent was taken from the patient.

Procedure was performed under local anaesthesia with intravenous sedation, endomeatal incision was made and the tympanomeatal flap was raised to visualize the middle ear cavity. Exposed facial nerve and the piston in situ were noted, piston was gently removed (**Figure 1**). A granuloma/granulation tissue was visualized under the over hanging facial nerve on the oval window area where the prosthesis was seated (**Figure 2**). The granuloma was removed and hemostasis was achieved. Also after removal of the piston necrosed lenticular process of incus was clearly visible (**Figure 3**).

The tympanomeatal flap was reposited and betadine soaked gelfoam was kept in the external auditory canal. The postoperative period was insignificant. Patient was relieved of otalgia and was started on oral steroids in tapering fashion with antibiotics during the post-op period.

3. Discussion

The incidence of reparative granuloma varies from 0.1% for stapedectomy and 0.07% for stapedectomy [3]. However certain studies have estimated the incidence up to 1.3% [4] to 1.8% [5]. Because of such low incidence rates this complication is rare even for a surgeon who frequently does stapes surgery.

Presenting symptoms usually surface one to eight weeks following surgery and most commonly involve vertigo but may include sensorineural hearing loss, progressive mixed hearing loss, sudden hearing loss and tinnitus [3] [6]. Our patient presented with progressive mixed hearing loss, vertigo and otalgia. Otoscopic findings may be inaccurate and variable as in our case but sometimes dull reddish discolouration in the posterosuperior quadrant of the tympanic membrane or granulations extending into the external auditory canal may also be present.

Reparative granuloma causes hearing impairment in 70 to 100 percent of the cases in early post-stapes surgery period. Vertigo may affect 20 - 35 percent of the cases and sometimes tinnitus, otalgia may also be present [7].

The differential diagnosis is made with perilymphatic fistula and stapedectomy long prosthesis. High resolution computed tomography may be used, since this method makes it possible to identify these conditions [8].

A foreign body reaction has been suggested as the hypothesis, although autoimmune reactions, infection and local inflammation have not been discarded [1]. The most common filling materials in stapedectomy that have been associated with granuloma are blood and gelfoam; in stapedectomy, these materials are fat and gelfoam [3].

They are used to fill in the oval window and to decrease the risk of a perilymphatic fistula. An animal experimental model showed that gelfoam placed in the open oval window niche caused injury to the basilar membrane on histology [9].

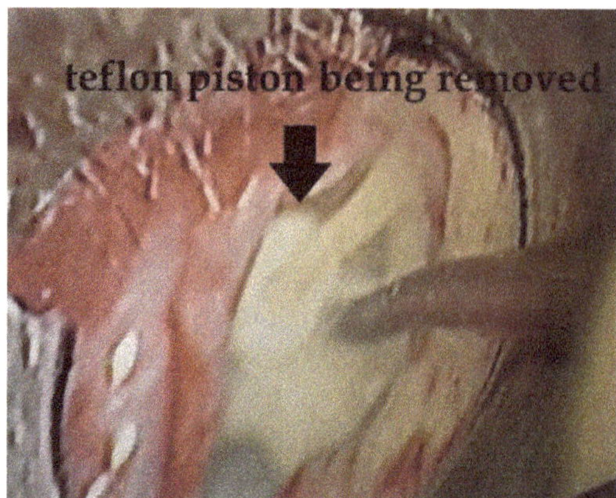

Figure 1. Piston removal.

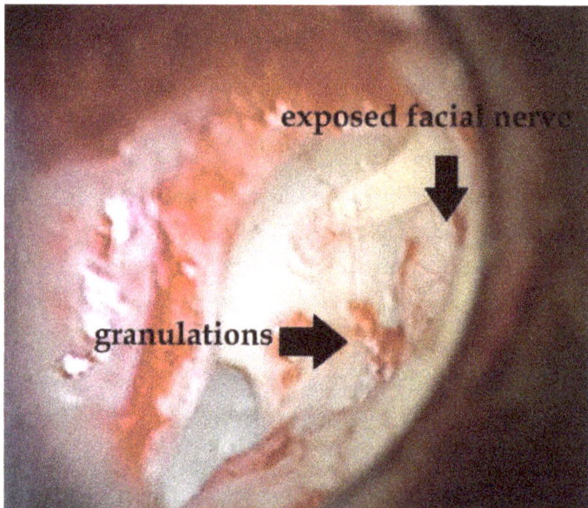

Figure 2. Granuloma.

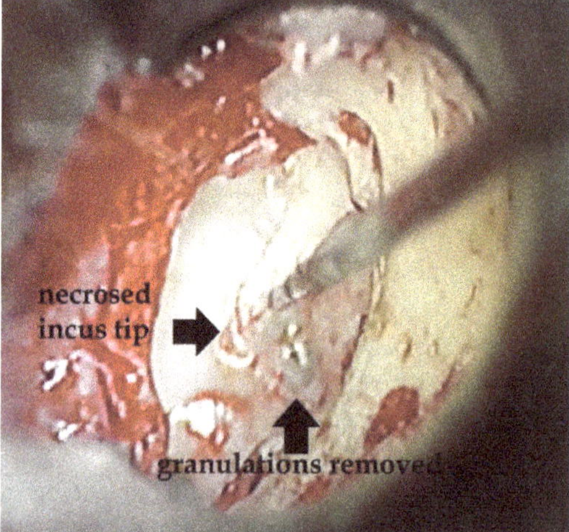

Figure 3. After removal.

Accidental foreign bodies including cotton wool fibers, linen fibers from drapes, glove powder (talc or starch) [10] and fractured Teflon fragments have been considered to stimulate foreign body granuloma. However, Kaufman *et al.* [6] and Buntner *et al.* [5] found these materials to be non-contributory.

Though in our case granulations weren't sent for investigation, if frank granulations are present, a bacterial culture along with histopathological reporting is advisable.

In our case we presume that the friction between teflon piston and the nerve sheath of the exposed facial nerve could have induced the granulation tissue formation.

There is disagreement regarding the mode of management of reparative granuloma. While Kaufman *et al.* [6] advocate immediate surgical exploration and removal of granulation with replacement of prosthesis. Seicshnaydre *et al.* [3] mentioned the use of high-dose steroids and antibiotics followed by delayed surgery. Hough and Dyer [11] considered surgery to be contra-indicated in such patients.

According to Fenton *et al.* [2] immediate exploration and meticulous removal of granulations followed by delayed ossiculoplasty if there is residual hearing is the appropriate line of management.

As in our case the lenticular process of incus was necrosed with minimal anterior displacement and the facial nerve was exposed, we decided to avoid putting a new piston during this surgery.

Since our patient has a normally functioning opposite ear, if she prefers, we plan to give her a hearing aid trial before going ahead with revision stapes surgery.

Even though there are no published papers specifically on the treatment of granulomas, several authors, based on their experience, have obtained better results by combining corticosteroids and early revision with removal of the granuloma and placement of a new prosthesis [3] [4].

4. Conclusion

Though rare is the post-stapedectomy/stapedectomy, granulations/reparative granuloma is an important cause of sensorineural hearing loss in operated cases of otosclerosis. Unfortunately, there aren't predictive patterns for its occurrence. We should be ready to deal with this situation if it arises in spite of its rarity.

References

[1] Harris, I. and Weiss, L. (1962) Granulomatous Complications of the Oval Window Fat Grafts. *The Laryngoscope*, **72**, 870-885. http://dx.doi.org/10.1288/00005537-196207000-00003

[2] Fenton, J.E., Turner, J., Shirazi, A. and Fagan, P.A. (1996) Post-Stapedectomy Reparative Granuloma: A Misnomer. *The Journal of Laryngology & Otology*, **110**, 185-188. http://dx.doi.org/10.1017/S0022215100133134

[3] Seicshnaydre, M.A., Sismanis, A. and Hughes, G.B. (1994) Update of Reparative Granuloma: Survey of the American Otological Society and the American Neurotology Society. *American Journal of Otology*, **15**, 155-160.

[4] Tange, R.A., Schimanski, G., van Lange, J.W., Grolman, W. and Zuur, L.C. (2002) Reparative Granuloma Seen in Cases of Gold Piston Implantation after Stapes Surgery for Otosclerosis. *Auris Nasus Larynx*, **29**, 7-10. http://dx.doi.org/10.1016/S0385-8146(01)00106-7

[5] Burtner, D. and Goodman, M.L. (1974) Etiological Factors in Post-Stapedectomy Granulomas. *Archives of Otolaryngology*, **100**, 171-173. http://dx.doi.org/10.1001/archotol.1974.00780040179003

[6] Kaufman, R.S. and Schuknecht, H.F. (1967) Reparative Granuloma Following Stapedectomy: A Clinical Entity. *Annals of Otology, Rhinology & Laryngology*, **76**, 1008-1017. http://dx.doi.org/10.1177/000348946707600511

[7] Scott-Brown (2008) Otosclerosis. In: *Michael Gleeson Scott-Brown's Otorhinolaryngology, Head and Neck Surgery*, 7th Edition, Hodder Arnold, London, 3477.

[8] Mann, W.J., Amedee, R.G., Fuerst, G. and Tabb, H.G. (1996) Hearing Loss as a Complication of Stapes Surgery. *Otolaryngology—Head and Neck Surgery*, **115**, 324-328. http://dx.doi.org/10.1016/S0194-5998(96)70046-3

[9] Bellucci, R.J. and Wolff, D. (1960) Tissue Reaction Following Reconstruction of the Oval Window in Experimental Animals. *Annals of Otology, Rhinology & Laryngology*, **69**, 517-539. http://dx.doi.org/10.1177/000348946006900217

[10] Dawes, J.D.K., Cameron, D.S., Curry, A.R. and Rannie, I. (1973) Poststapedectomy Granuloma of the Oval Window. *The Journal of Laryngology & Otology*, **87**, 365-378. http://dx.doi.org/10.1017/S002221510007701X

[11] Hough, J.V.D. and Dyer, R.K. (1993) Stapedectomy, Causes of Failure and Revision Surgery in Otosclerosis. *Otolaryngologic Clinics of North America*, **26**, 453-470.

28

Squamous Cell Carcinoma of the External Ear in a Child

Waheed Rahman, Rashid Sheikh*, Hassen Mohammed, Zeynel Abidin Dogan

Department of Otorhinolaryngology and Head & Neck Surgery, Hamad Medical Corporation, Doha, Qatar
Email: *rsheikh@hamad.qa

Abstract

Tumors involving the head and neck are uncommon in children. Furthermore, those which involve the external ear are extremely rare. In the external ear itself, the most commonly encountered malignancy is Squamous Cell Carcinoma, both in the adult and pediatric age groups. We encountered one such case of a 14 years old male with a recurring skin lesion involving the right external ear. In this report, we wish to highlight and address the difficulty in recognizing and managing such an unwonted pathology as Squamous Cell Carcinoma in the pediatric age group.

Keywords

Squamous Cell Carcinoma, External Ear, External Auditory Canal

1. Introduction

Squamous cell carcinoma (SCC) is a common malignancy arising from malignant proliferation of the keratinocytes of the epidermis. It is primarily a disease of older adults, occurring most frequently in patients older than age 45 years. Epidemiological studies over the last 20 years have shown a steady rise in the incidence of these cancers in younger adults [1].

Many reports had been published on the cause(s), risk factors, progression and prognosis of SCC in young adults since this disease was previously recognized as a distinct clinical entity, but they were inconsistent. Younger patients often do not present with the conventional risk factors of alcohol and/or tobacco exposure. This leads to a suspicion that other potential agents, such as genetic factors, infections, and behavioral factors may be involved [2]-[4].

Furthermore, if SCC involves the head and neck region, in particular the external ear, it can be potentially lethal. Therefore, managing such a case requires an early and aggressive interventionist approach. In this report,

*Corresponding author.

we focus on the presentation, diagnosis, existing literature and the tailored management of such a rare pathology in a 14 years old male.

2. The Case

A 14 year old male presented with an isolated, rapidly recurring, painless, raised, hyperpigmented and ulcerated lesion which was approximately 2 cm × 2 cm in size on his right tragus involving the preauricular skin and the external auditory canal (EAC) (**Figure 1**). It was increasing in size over the preceding 3 months. The patient underwent excision of a lesion in the same location 6 months before presenting to our Otolaryngology service. He had also undergone 5 prior excisions of similar lesions in the same location. The child's parents had lost the records of most of the histopathology results. The available results of 3 out of 6 presumed excisional biopsies were: pyogenic granuloma, atypical dysplasia and basal cell carcinoma.

Informed verbal and written consents were taken from the parents. Radiological imaging ensued (**Figure 2**). It was decided to proceed with excisional biopsy of the lesion under general anesthesia. Subsequent histopathology result showed moderately differentiated SCC that involved the tragus, preauricular skin and external auditory canal. The tumor was invading the cartilagenous part of the right EAC encroaching upon the parotid capsule without gross invasion. Medially the tumor extended to the skin of the bony EAC without gross erosion of the bone.

A detailed discussion in the multidisciplinary tumor board meeting occurred prior to initiating definitive management. High risk features in this case included recurrence, location and cartilage invasion. Eventually, with a therapeutic and curative intent, subtotal right external ear canal excision with reconstruction along with right supraomohyoid neck dissection and right total parotidectomy was done with tumor free margins on frozen section and final histopathology.

Microscopic examination of the sections revealed the tumor to be residual invasive carcinoma with squamous differentiation. Scar and changes consistent with previous biopsy site were noted. It was unifocal with 1.0 cm in greatest dimension with no adjacent squamous dysplasia or carcinoma in-situ. Histologic grade was poorly differentiated. It was adjacent to the parotid gland with invasion of the capsule and surrounding soft tissue while bone and cartilage was spared. Margins were free of the tumor. While tumor necrosis was focally present, there was no lymphovascular or perineural invasion. The tumor consisted of sheets, islands and trabeculae of abnormal squamous cells showing pleomorphism, nucleomegaly and frequent mitotic figures (**Figure 3**). The cells showed cytoplasmic keratinization and focal squamous pearls (**Figure 4**). The tumor infiltrated the subepithelial stroma where it extended to the cartilaginous plate. Immuohistochemical staining showed positive staining with CK5/6, CK14, AE1/AE3, p63 and EMA (antibodies that support squamous nature for the tumor) (**Figure 5** & **Figure 6**). The tumor cells were negative with CK7, CK20, HPV, and EBV. Ki-67 index > 50%. Insitu hybridization was performed using special antibody against EBV (EBER antibody). There was no staining with the antibody. Appropriate positive and negative controls were working. The pathologic stage (pTNM) was verified to be was pT1, N0.

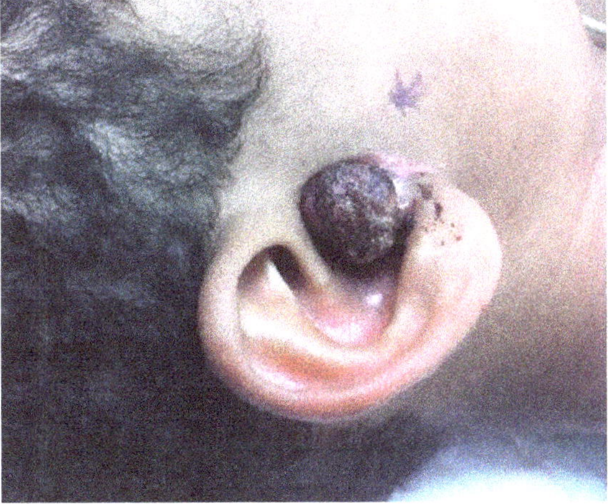

Figure 1. Appearance of the lesion at presentation.

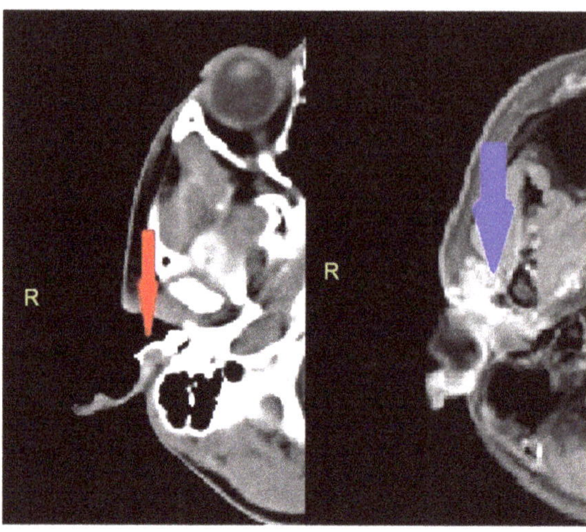

Figure 2. Imaging of the right side of the head. CT Scan showing the lesion invading the external ear canal (red arrow) and MRI showing the same lesion (blue arrow).

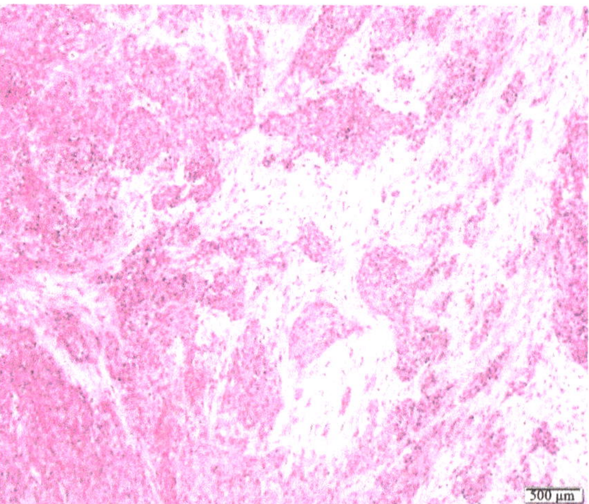

Figure 3. Sections show islands and sheets of tumor cells invading the stroma (H & E ×100).

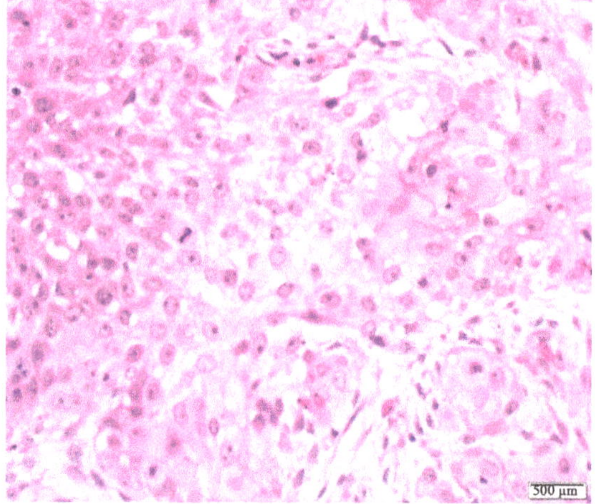

Figure 4. High power view showing the atypical squamous cells with cytoplasmic keratinization (right side of slide) (H & E ×400).

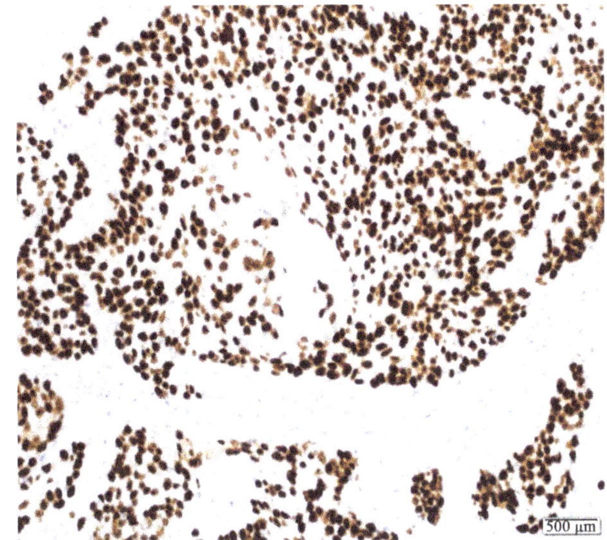

Figure 5. Diffuse nuclear staining with p63 antibody (immuoperoxidase ×200).

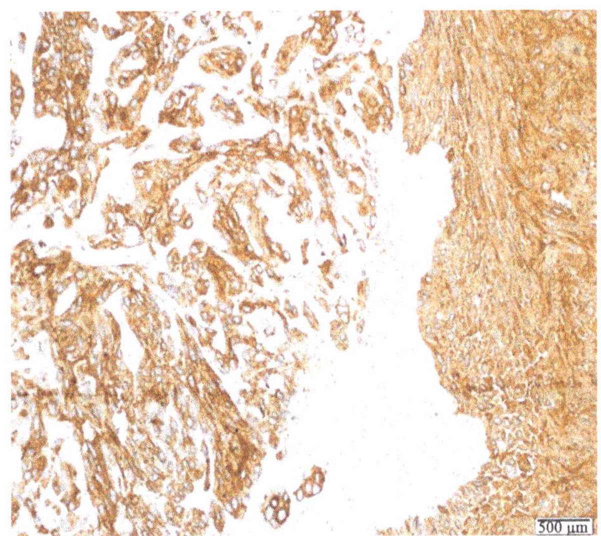

Figure 6. Diffuse membranous and cytoplasmic staining with CK14 antibody ×200.

To date and a year on from the definitive surgery, the child has had no signs of local or distant recurrence of the tumor and the surgical wound has healed well. Two of the patient's six monthly followup radiology surveillance imaging reports suggested no evidence of local or distant recurrence.

3. Discussion

SCC of the head and neck region is unusual in young patients and extremely rare in the pediatric age group, the upper limit of which varies in different centers let alone countries and regions [5]. SCC of the head and neck is a disease of middle age and beyond usually in patients who are exposed to its primary risk factors which are smoking and alcohol consumption. A portion of patients who are younger, however, develop SCC of the head and neck without the use of tobacco or alcohol and it is this population in which the etiology of their cancer comes into question. Debate regarding the tumor nature in this group of patients and its effects on progression and survival is open-ended [6]. Like most cancers, there isn't a single etiology and it has been determined that multiple factors may be involved.

EAC carcinomas, let alone SCC as in this case, are frequently misdiagnosed. A retrospective study to review misdiagnosed cases and analyze the factors involved was done by Zhang T. *et al.* [7]. Eighteen of 44 EAC carcinoma cases seen were misdiagnosed: Six as otitis media, five as otitis externa and two as EAC cholesteatomas. Other misdiagnoses were stenosis of the EAC, ear neuralgia, furuncle of the EAC, benign neoplasm of the EAC and pre-auricular fistula. Our case stands unique as the clinical presentation was of a recurring lesion despite excisional biopsies and at the same time histopathology results differed repeatedly. No particular reason, apart from the age of the patient, was outlined to explain this. It leads us to believe that the pathologists were not cautious in making the diagnosis as the microscopic description did not provide any clue as to why the diagnosis was missed.

Young patients with SCC reported in literature are isolated cases and their management is difficult because there is no large study to support treatment decision for every child [5]. A CT scan and/or MRI of the head and neck is recommended to note bony erosion and/or soft tissue involvement of a suspected tumor of the EAC. A low threshold of suspicion for possible underlying malignancy should exist for otitis media or externa cases, especially those with bloody ear discharge and/or otalgia, which do not respond to routine anti-bacterials. A prompt biopsy should be conducted to obtain a histopathological diagnosis [7] [8].

Upto 75 cases of SCC of the external ear were reviewed to determine patterns of occurrence and treatment failure in a series by Shockley *et al.* Forty patients had adequate follow-up for determination of cancer control rates. Local control was successful with initial treatment in 85% of the cases. The incidence of lymph node metastases was 10%, whereas distant metastasis occurred in only one patient (2.5%) [9]. It has been observed that young patients with SCC of the head and neck have an analogous prognosis to older patients. However, a higher regional recurrence in young patients has been noted in recent times which has prompted surgeons to utilize prophylactic neck dissection to halt the unusual rise in recurrence [6]. Adding to that, Federspil *et al.* showed that tumor excision with wide margins (5 - 10 mm) as first-line treatment is recommended. He also noted that neck dissection with parotidectomy is indicated when suspicious lymph nodes are detected, the tumor diameter is >4 cm, cartilaginous invasion is present, and vertical tumor thickness is >5 mm [10].

Keeping in view existing knowledge of the management of such a case, it is pertinent and worthwhile to mention that the management of SCC of the skin differs from SCC of the external auditory canal. In this case, repeated surgical intervention had obscured the path of progression of the disease, whether it was from the skin to the external ear canal or vis versa. We approached the case as an EAC SCC which propelled us to take a more aggressive approach. Another dilemma which we encountered was whether to give the patient adjuvant radiotherapy or not. Thus far, after following the patient for over 12 months, there are no signs of recurrence and the patient has not received radiotherapy. We can also safely assume that if the margins of the excised tumor are clear, then such cases may not merit use of radiotherapy and can be considered tumor free or in remission.

4. Conclusion

This case has been reported to sensitize the reader, the histopathologist and the otorhinolaryngologist and head & neck surgeon that the possibility of Squamous Cell Carcinoma should be high on their differential list even in the pediatric age group. Misdiagnosis may lead both the patient and doctor off track with regards to the best course of management of the disease especially in cases where intervention is indicated. Tools of diagnosis and staging including imaging and histopathology should be utilized effectively prior to commencing on the management of such a disease. In order to prevent recurrence, a more radical and aggressive approach should be taken which has been seen to cause remission of the disease without utilizing adjuvant radiotherapy.

Disclosure

The case at hand has already been approved by our institution's medical research and ethics committee at the research center with the reference number of MRC0575/2015. The patient's father's consent was taken for the publication of the case report and the figures. None of the authors was given an honorarium, grant or other form of payment to produce this paper. We have no conflict of interest or financial interest, real or perceived, to disclose.

References

[1] Chaturvedi, A.K., Engels, E.A., Anderson, W.F. and Gillison, M.L. (2008) Incidence Trends for Human Papillomavirus-Related and -Unrelated Oral Squamous Cell Carcinomas in the United States. *Journal of Clinical Oncology*, **26**, 612-619. http://dx.doi.org/10.1200/JCO.2007.14.1713

[2] Myers, J.N., Elkins, T., Roberts, D. and Byers, R.M. (2000) Squamous Cell Carcinoma of the Tongue in Young Adults: Increasing Incidence and Factors that Predict Treatment Outcomes. *Otolaryngology—Head and Neck Surgery*, **122**, 44-51. http://dx.doi.org/10.1016/S0194-5998(00)70142-2

[3] Sturgis, E.M. and Cinciripini, P.M. (2007) Trends in Head and Neck Cancer Incidence in Relation to Smoking Prevalence. *Cancer*, **110**, 1429-1435. http://dx.doi.org/10.1002/cncr.22963

[4] Byers, R.M. (1975) Squamous Cell Carcinoma of the Oral Tongue in Patients Less than Thirty Years of Age. *The American Journal of Surgery*, **130**, 475-478. http://dx.doi.org/10.1016/0002-9610(75)90487-0

[5] de Carvalho, M.B., de Andrade Sobrinho, J., Rapoport, A., *et al.* (1998) Head and Neck Squamous Cell Carcinoma in Childhood. *Medical and Pediatric Oncology*, **31**, 96-99. http://dx.doi.org/10.1002/(SICI)1096-911X(199808)31:2<96::AID-MPO9>3.0.CO;2-U

[6] Goldstein, D.P. and Irish, J.C. (2005) Head and Neck Squamous Cell Carcinoma in the Young Patient. *Current Opinion in Otolaryngology & Head and Neck Surgery*, **13**, 207-211. http://dx.doi.org/10.1097/01.moo.0000170529.04759.4c

[7] Zhang, T., Dai, C. and Wang, Z. (2013) The Misdiagnosis of External Auditory Canal Carcinoma. *European Archives of Oto-Rhino-Laryngology*, **270**, 1607-1613. http://dx.doi.org/10.1007/s00405-012-2159-4

[8] Hosokawa, S., Mizuta, K., Takahashi, G., *et al.* (2012) Surgical Approach for Treatment of Carcinoma of the Anterior Wall of the External Auditory Canal. *Otology & Neurotology*, **33**, 450-454. http://dx.doi.org/10.1097/MAO.0b013e318245ccbf

[9] Shockley, W.W. and Stucker Jr., F.J. (1987) Squamous Cell Carcinoma of the External Ear: A Review of 75 Cases. *Otolaryngology—Head and Neck Surgery*, **97**, 308-312.

[10] Federspil, P.A., Pauli, U.C. and Federspil, P. (2001) Squamous Epithelial Carcinomas of the External Ear. *HNO*, **49**, 283-288. http://dx.doi.org/10.1007/s001060050747

29

A Case of Maxillary Sinus Cholesteatoma Originating from the Retromaxillary Sinus Wall

Jun Myung Lee, Nam Gyu Ryu, Ick Soo Choi

Department of Otorhinolaryngology-Head and Neck Surgery, Inje University College of Medicine, Ilsanpaik Hospital, Goyang, Korea
Email: leochoics@gmail.com

Abstract

Cholesteatomas are often observed in the middle ear or mastoid cavity. However, cholesteatomas in areas other than the middle ear or mastoid are extremely rare and thus are not often reported in the literature. We recently treated an 18-year-old female patient with an incidentally detected maxillary sinus mass. A paranasal sinus computed tomography examination revealed a cystic lesion in the left maxillary sinus infiltrating the posterolateral walls of the left maxillary sinus. An endoscopic operation was performed for definitive diagnosis. Histopathological examination of the mass confirmed the diagnosis of cholesteatoma. Despite the rarity of paranasal cholesteatoma in comparison with cholesteatomas in the tympanum, a few cases involving the frontal sinus have been reported. However, retromaxillary cholesteatoma is even less common than sinus cholesteatoma and is reported rarely. To our knowledge, this is the first reported case of a maxillary cholesteatoma originating from the retromaxillary area. For this reason, we present this case along with a literature review.

Keywords

Cholesteatoma, Paranasal Sinus, Retromaxillary Sinus, Paranasal Sinus Computed Tomography

1. Introduction

A cholesteatoma is a mass formed by keratin layers within a hyper-keratinized squamous epithelium that partially or entirely replaces the normal mucous membrane [1]. These masses are commonly formed in the middle ear or mastoid cavity. However, there are reports of cholesteatomas originating outside the middle ear or mastoid cavity. Cholesteatomas in the maxillary sinus are rare and those in the retromaxillary sinus are extremely rare [2]. A few hypotheses have tried to explain the likely causes of nasal sinus cholesteatomas, but a clear cause has not been identified yet [2] [3].

Symptoms of nasal sinus cholesteatoma depend on the location and can include rhinorrhea, nasal obstruction, facial edema, tenderness on palpation, exophthalmos, and oculomotor dysfunction [2] [4]. This case report describes the histopathological characteristics of a cholesteatoma in the retromaxillary space that is incidentally detected by brain computed tomography (CT). A mass in the retromaxillary space, which grew while pushing the maxillary sinus outward, was removed. We report the findings in this case and provide a literature review.

2. Case

An 18-year-old woman presented to the hospital with persistent dizziness and underwent a brain CT examination. The CT images incidentally showed a mass in the left maxillary sinus, which appeared as a radiopaque lesion containing relatively homogeneous soft tissues inside the left maxillary sinus. The patient was referred to the department of otorhinolaryngology for further evaluation, and her dizziness was found to be secondary to orthostatic hypotension. She denied experiencing headache, facial pain, nasal obstruction, and toothache. She also reported no other medical history or familial disorders.

Endoscopic examination revealed hypertrophy of both inferior turbinates, deviation of the nasal septum, and absence of nasal polyps. The blood test did not show any abnormal findings. For detailed characterization of nasal sinus mass, a paranasal sinus (PNS) CT examination was performed. The PNS CT images showed a cystic lesion in the left maxillary sinus (MS) infiltrating into the posterolateral walls of the left MS. The mass showed contrast enhancement in the outer edges, with radiopaque soft tissue shading partially inside. There was no maxillary sinus expansion except for a bony defect on the posterolateral wall of the left MS (**Figure 1**).

To make a definitive diagnosis, an endoscopic operation was performed. After widening the natural ostium, we explored the lesion endoscopically. In the left MS, a fibrous, homogeneous membrane was observed, appearing thin and solid like an eggshell. The posterolateral bony wall of the left MS was protruding into the sinus, forming a part of the cystic wall. The cystic mass pushed into the sinus from its posterior portion and contained a cavity filled with a keratin-like material. The mass was removed and the findings of the histologic review were consistent with cholesteatoma (**Figure 2**).

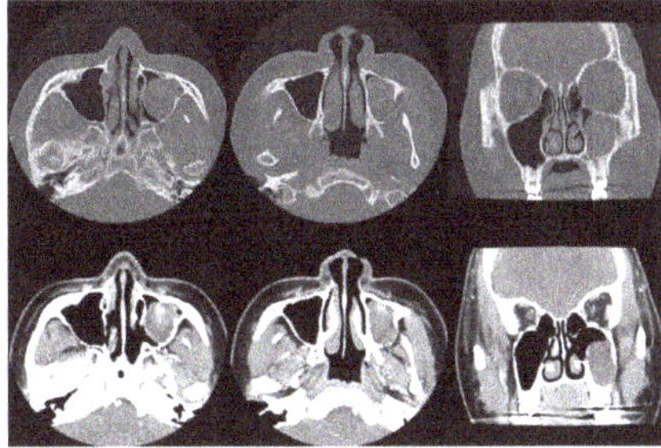

Figure 1. Cystic lesion invading posterior and lateral left maxillary wall.

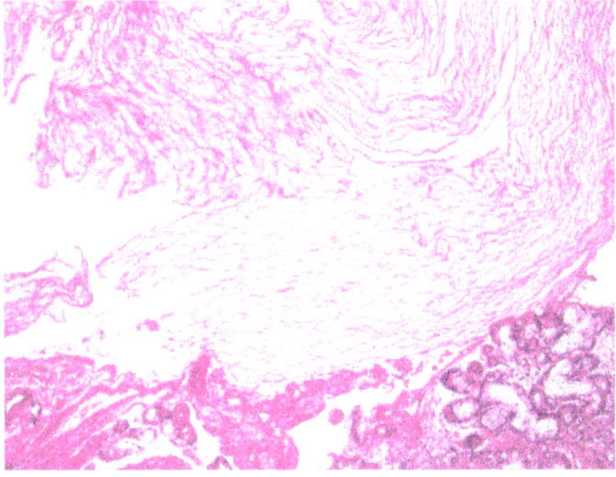

Figure 2. The specimen shows aggregation of keratin debris and normal seromucinous glands (HE, ×100).

3. Discussion

Cholesteatomas can develop in the skin, breast, kidney, central nervous system, and inside the cranium [4]-[6]. Cholesteatomas of the head and neck mostly involve the ears. Dead cells abnormally accumulate behind the damaged tympanic membrane from repeated infections or injuries and form a pearl-colored mass. Cholesteatomas within the paranasal sinus are extremely rare compared to those in the temporal bone [4] [5]. Cholesteatomas occur most frequently in the frontal nasal sinus, which was still lower frequency. Thus, cholesteatomas in MS are even less common and have been rarely reported. One case of maxillary sinus cholesteatoma was reported in 1999, in which the cholesteatoma was accompanied by tooth extraction in the maxillary sinus [7]. The inner layer of the paranasal sinuses consists of respiratory epithelium with pseudostratified ciliated columnar epithelium. If this respiratory epithelium is replaced partially or entirely with keratinized squamous epithelium, it would form a cholesteatoma [1].

There are several hypotheses explaining the development of cholesteatomas inside the paranasal sinuses. The theory of "congenital epithelial rest" is widely recognized and suggests that cholesteatomas can originate from the remaining epithelial tissues after the embryonic developmental process. If the division of the two ectodermal surfaces near the 5th week of embryo development is incomplete, the neural groove closure will not occur normally. Therefore, some portion of the epithelial tissues remains in between these two surfaces, leading to cholesteatoma development [2] [3] [8] [9]. Further theories include "the implantation theory", contending that epithelial tissues are directly injected due to injuries such as surgery [4] [9]; the "immigration theory" that hyperkeratinized squamous epithelium in a normal position moves inside the sinus through the sinus opening [1] [9]; and the "metaplasia theory" that chronic infection causes metaplasia of the normal membrane in the sinus [1] [9]-[11]. Although none of these theories clearly explain the development of cholesteatomas, they provide insight into the general understanding of cholesteatoma formation in the nasal sinus.

In this case, the patient had no history of surgery or previous sinus inflammation; therefore, the cholesteatoma appeared to originate from the remnant epithelial tissue and grew from the lateral wall of the retromaxillary sinus [2] [3] [8]. As intranasal sinus cholesteatomas are rare, it is difficult to diagnose them without histopathological examination of samples obtained through surgery. However, medical history, physical examination findings, and imaging studies can provide reasonable suspicion [2].

Symptoms develop as the cholesteatoma expands into the nasal sinus, and the symptoms themselves may vary according to the location of the cholesteatoma. If the cholesteatoma expands towards the ostiomeatal complex, rhinorrhea and sinusitis may occur. If it infiltrates into the nasal vestibule, nasal obstruction may be possible. When the cholesteatoma invades the anterolateral wall of the antrum, facial swelling and tenderness on palpation could appear, while invasion into the inferior part of the antrum may lead to palate swelling. If it extends into the upper part of maxillary sinus, exophthalmos, conjunctival swelling, and oculomotor dysfunction could develop [2] [4].

In CT images, the characteristic intra-sinus cholesteatoma shows a relatively homogeneous, expansile lesion with osteoclasia in the surrounding area. If the image shows an enhancing cystic mass involving the paranasal sinuses and infiltrating the paranasal bone, it may indicate a cholesteatoma of the paranasal sinus. Although this feature has limited diagnostic value because intra-maxillary sinus mucocele or fungal sinusitis present with similar findings, such an examination is relatively convenient and provides an easy approach to detect the lesion characteristics [9] [12]. Thus, it could be an appropriate procedure for preliminary diagnosis and follow-up examinations [7].

Magnetic resonance imaging (MRI) is helpful in the diagnosis and decision making due to the excellent soft tissue projection. However, MRI examinations are costly and therefore only performed if paranasal sinus cholesteatoma is suspected [7]. Treatment of cholesteatoma involves complete removal of the cholesteatoma and the wrapping sac [6]. There are no established treatment guidelines for intranasal cholesteatoma. Several researchers recommended the Caldwell-Luc operation for complete removal of intra-sinus cholesteatoma [1] [9] [13]. The Caldwell-Luc operation would have been a consideration in this case if the cholesteatoma was larger and had further expanded into the medial side. Fortunately, the cholesteatoma in this case was not huge and did not extend inside the sinus and showed minimal bony erosion. This made lesion removal by an endoscopic sinus operation possible. However, to ensure complete removal and easier follow-up in the outpatient clinic, a large antrostomy was performed. Postoperative relapse has not been reported yet. In this case, the cholesteatoma seemed to originate from the retromaxillary space and was diagnosed as cholesteatoma. Further follow-up observations are necessary to determine the natural course of this retromaxillary cholesteatoma.

4. Conclusion

Retromaxillary sinus cholesteatoma is extremely rare and may have no specific symptoms until it grows near the surrounding structures. It may show an enhancing cystic mass involving the paranasal sinuses and infiltrating the paranasal bone in PNS CT. Paranasal cholesteatoma should be removed completely by surgery because of its expansile characteristics.

Conflicts

The authors have no conflicts of interest to declare in relation to this article.

References

[1] Pogorel, B.S. and Budd, E.G. (1965) Cholesteatoma of the Maxillary Sinus. *Archives of Otolaryngology*, **82**, 532-534. http://dx.doi.org/10.1001/archotol.1965.00760010534016

[2] Hartman, J.M., Stankiewicz, J.A. and Maywood, I.L. (1991) Cholesteatoma of the Paranasal Sinuses: Case Report and Review of the Literature. *Ear, Nose & Throat Journal*, **70**, 719-725.

[3] Sadoff, R.S. and Pliskin, A. (1989) Cholesteatoma (Keratoma) of the Maxillary Sinus: Report of a Case. *Journal of Oral and Maxillofacial Surgery*, **47**, 873-876. http://dx.doi.org/10.1016/S0278-2391(89)80052-7

[4] Hopp, M.L. and Montgomery, W.W. (1984) Primary and Secondary Keratomas of the Frontal Sinus. *Laryngoscope*, **94**, 628-632. http://dx.doi.org/10.1288/00005537-198405000-00010

[5] Paaske, P.B. (1984) Cholesteatoma of the Maxillary Sinus. *Journal of Laryngology and Otology*, **98**, 539-541. http://dx.doi.org/10.1017/S0022215100147048

[6] Puttamadaiah, G.M., Vijayashree, M.S., Viswanatha, B. and Kaur, J. (2014) Cholesteatoma of Maxillary Sinus Mimicking Malignancy. *Research in Otolaryngology*, **3**, 57-59.

[7] Sang, H.P., Seung, H.B., Tae, H.S. and Young, J.C. (1999) Cholesteatoma of the Maxillary Sinus. *Korean Journal of Otolaryngology-Head and Neck Surgery*, **42**, 522-525.

[8] Baxter, J.J.R. (1966) Cholesteatoma of the Maxillary Antrum. *Journal of Laryngology and Otology*, **80**, 1059-1061. http://dx.doi.org/10.1017/S002221510006638X

[9] Viswanatha, B., Nayak, L.K. and Karthik, S. (2007) Cholesteatoma of the Maxillary Sinus. *Ear, Nose & Throat Journal*, **86**, 351-353.

[10] Mills, P.C. and Sycamore, E.M.K. (1958) Cholesteatoma of the Maxillary Antrum. *Journal of Laryngology and Otology*, **72**, 580-583. http://dx.doi.org/10.1017/S0022215100054347

[11] Das, S.K. (1971) Cholesteatoma of the Maxillary Antrum. *Journal of Laryngology and Otology*, **85**, 397-400. http://dx.doi.org/10.1017/S0022215100073588

[12] Valvassori, G.E. (2003) Imaging of the Temporal Bone. In: Glasscock, M.E. and Gulya, A.J., Eds., *Shambaugh's Surgery of the Ear*, 5th Edition, B C Decker, Hamilton, 227-259.

[13] Yağci, A.B., Kara, C.O., Karabulut, N., *et al.* (2003) Horseshoe Maxillary Sinus: CT of a Unique Case with Cholesteatoma. *European Journal of Radiology Extra*, **48**, 5-7. http://dx.doi.org/10.1016/S1571-4675(03)00078-6

30

Augmentation Grafts in Septorhinoplasty: Our Experience

R. V. Nataraj, Jagade Mohan, Chavan Reshma, Parelkar Kartik, Hanawte Reshma, Singhal Arpita, Kulsange Kiran, Rengaraja Dev, Rao Kartik, Gupta Pallavi

Department of Ear, Nose & Throat and Head and Neck Surgery, Grant Government Medical College, Mumbai, India

Email: nataraj.rv@gmail.com

Abstract

Augmentation of nasal tip and/or dorsum forms the keystone of any Septorhinoplasty surgery. The grafts available for augmentation are numerous and varied. Choice of the graft depends upon the type of augmentation required, patient characteristics and, most importantly, the surgeon. In this article, we would like to present our experience with various augmentation grafts. In our experience, autografts are best grafts for augmentation. But in cases of revision surgeries or deficiency of autografts, allografts can be used. Our choice of allograft is Poly Diaxone Sheath or PDS.

Keywords

Septorhinoplasty, Augmentation Grafts, Poly Diaxone Sheath

1. Introduction

Because of its prominent position in the face, many people are self-conscious regarding the shape and size of nose.

Septorhinoplasty is amongst the most frequently performed surgeries in recent times. However this surgery may also be perceived as the most technically demanding of all cosmetic surgeries.

Augmentation in a Septorhinoplasty surgery serves numerous purposes:

1) In case of a flattened dorsum, it helps in raising and straightening the dorsum by augmenting the underlying skeleton-muscular frame work.

2) For projection or definition of nasal tip.

3) For correction of nasal obstruction caused by incompetent nasal valve(s).

4) Volume augmentation.

An ideal nasal implant, however, does not exist. Although some implant choices exhibit many of the qualities of the ideal implant, no implant satisfies all requirements. The ideal nasal implant should be readily available, inexpensive, inert, nontoxic, non-carcinogenic, sterilizable, easy to sculpt, easily camouflaged, and able to provide volume and mechanical support. Furthermore, the ideal implant should interact favorably with surrounding tissues, maintain its form over time, resist trauma, infection and extrusion, and remain easy to remove [1].

2. Discussion

There are various types of implants available. The final choice of the implants depends upon the surgeon. The types of implants can be classified according to the source of origin:

2.1. Autografts

These types of grafts are harvested from the same patient and bear closest resemblance to an ideal graft- biocompatible and low rate of rejection & extrusion, no risk of disease transmission and minimal inflammatory reaction seen. The major limitation with autografts is limited availability and morbidity associated with their harvesting. The types of autografts may include cartilage, bone and soft tissues like fascia and skin.

2.2. Cartilage

"***THE CARTILAGE IS TO A RHINOPLASTIC SURGEON WHAT WOOD IS TO CARPENTER***".

Cartilage is most preferred amongst the autografts available as it can provide both support & volume and can also be easily cut & molded into desired shape and size. However, the tendency of the cartilage to warp over a period of time remains its greatest drawback.

2.2.1. Septal Cartilage

It is the preferred graft for nasal reconstruction as it can be harvested from the same surgical field. However it cannot be used in cases where a large amount of graft is required (**Figure 1** and **Figure 2**).

2.2.2. Conchal Cartilage

It is the second most preferred autologus graft. It can be harvested by anterior incision, posterior incision or inferior incision. The two different parts of conchal cartilage used are Concha Cavum and Concha Cymba. Concha Cavum, as the name suggests, is concave in shape and thus finds its use as tip graft or dorsal graft. Whereas Concha Cymba resembles the lateral crura of lower lateral cartilage and therefore is used in cases of deficient or lost (**Figure 3** and **Figure 4**).

2.2.3. Coastal Cartilage

It is preferred when abundant cartilage or also a bone is required. This type of graft can be harvested from 5th to 9th ribs, but 7th rib is preferred. Harvesting of coastal cartilage presents with two chief limitations, both of which can be minimized with proper handling techniques. First being the tendency of the cartilage to wrap over time. This drawback can be minimized by separating the cartilage from the perichondrium and carving the cartilage equally from all sides so as to use the central portion of cartilage which has lower tendency to wrap. Second drawback is significant donor site morbidity including pain, incision scar and, in rare cases, pneumothorax. Lastly calcification of the cartilage in elderly may render the graft unsuitable for carving (**Figure 5**).

2.2.4. Composite Graft

A composite graft is a combination of more than one material, typically skin and cartilage with or without bone and fascia. This graft is most commonly harvested from the ear. This graft is used in patients with alar retraction and correct vestibular stenosis.

TYPES OF GRAFTS FOR TIP AND DORSAL AUGMENTATION

Shield or Sheen graft

Shield grafts are useful Rhinoplasty surgeries to provide a better tip definition. The name is derived from the shield like shape of the graft. It is placed over the medial crura of the Lower Lateral Lartilages (LLC) extending to the domes or even above (**Figure 6**).

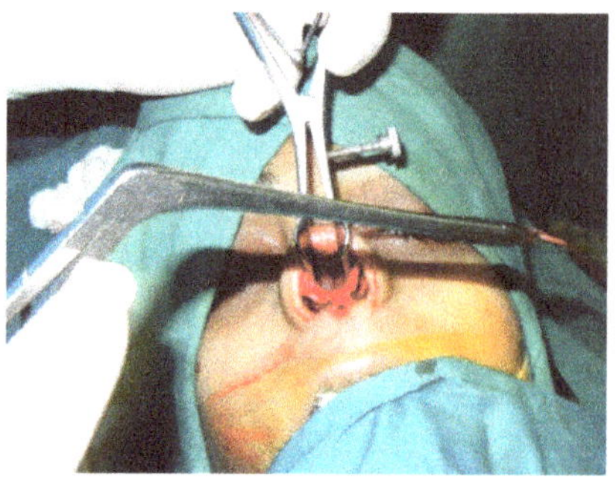

Figure 1. Septal cartilage being harvested.

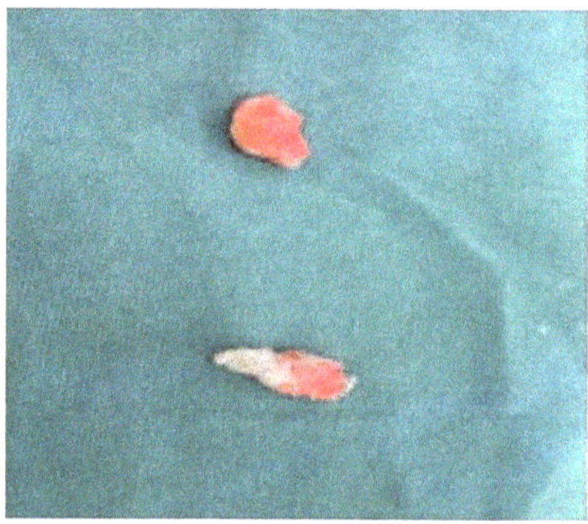

Figure 2. Septal cartilage being harvested.

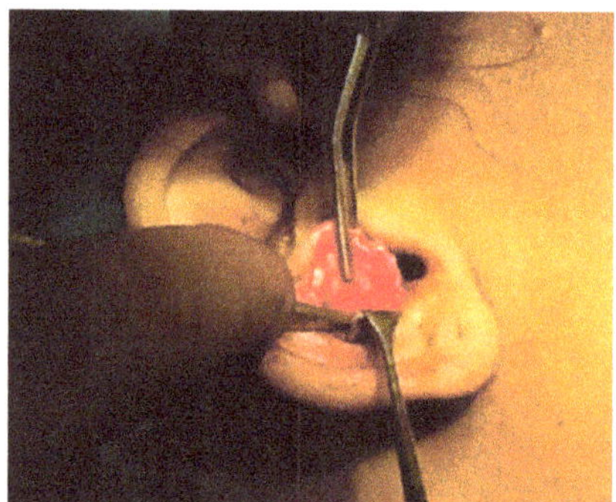

Figure 3. Conchal Cartilage being harvested through anterior approach.

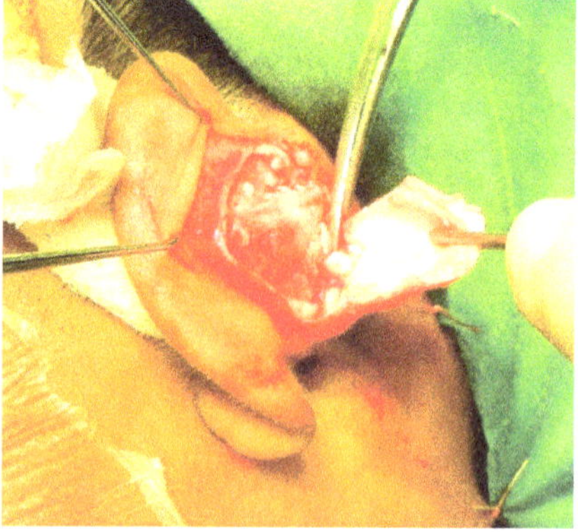

Figure 4. Conchal Cartilage being harvested through anterior approach.

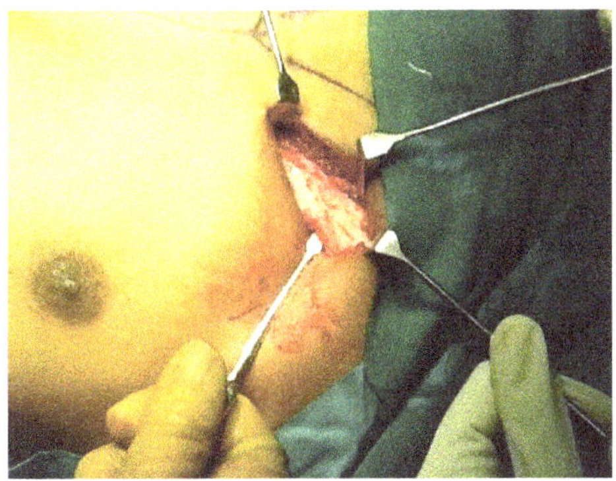

Figure 5. Harvesting of costal cartilage.

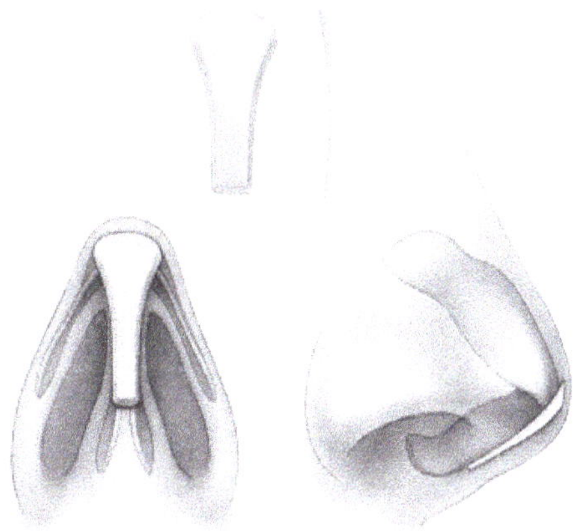

Figure 6. Diagrammatic representation of sheen graft.

Columellar strut graft [2]

Columellar struts are a type of cartilage graft used for tip augmentation in Rhinoplasty. Named so because, in addition to providing better tip definition, it also helps in resizing the columella. It is placed in between the medial crurae of the Lower Lateral Cartilages (LLC) (**Figure 7**).

Septal extension graft (SEG)

It is a type of cartilage graft which is placed to lengthened the septum and nose. Usually this graft is taken from thick septum, rib cartilage and double layer ear cartilages. It is usually fixed to the nasal septum and provides a better tip definition [3] (**Figure 8**).

Spreader graft

Spreader grafts are used to correct the middle vault of the nose and are placed between the upper lateral cartilage and the dorsal septum [4] [5] (**Figure 9** and **Figure 10**).

Umbrella Graft

These kinds of grafts were first described by Peck in 1989 in his book titled "Techniques in Aesthetic Rhinoplasty". It mainly consists of a vertical cartilaginous strut placed between the medial crura for better definition and elevation of the tip. It is usually used in conjuncture with a Dorsal Onlay Graft or Dorsal Augmentation Graft [6] (**Figure 11**).

Dorsal Onlay Graft or Dorsal Augmentation Graft

This is a kind of graft that is used to augment the entire dorsum. It's especially useful in cases of depressed or flattened septum. The most preferred cartilage for carving of a Dorsal Augmentation Graft is rib cartilage [7] [8] (**Figure 12**).

Sandwich Graft

In the type of Sandwich Graft, that is used in our institute; an allograft (for example Poly Diaoxone Sheet) is

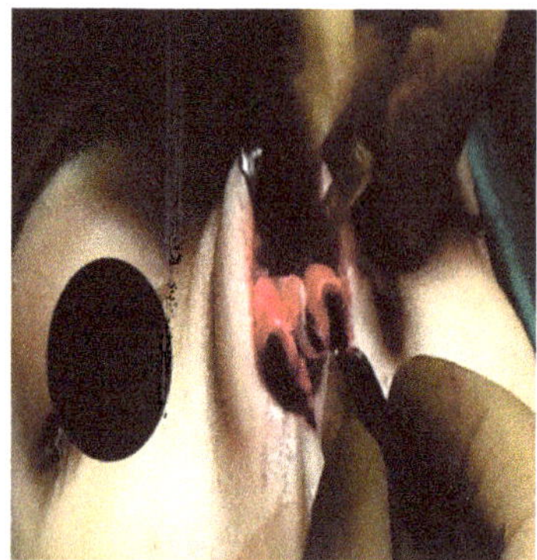

Figure 7. Columellar strut graft bei-ng placed.

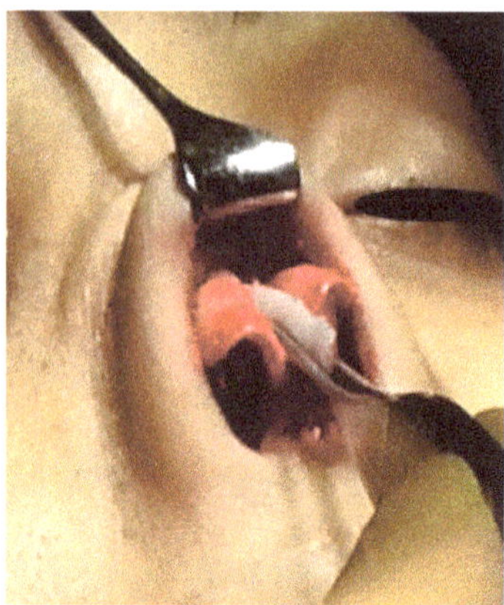

Figure 8. Septal extension graft being placed.

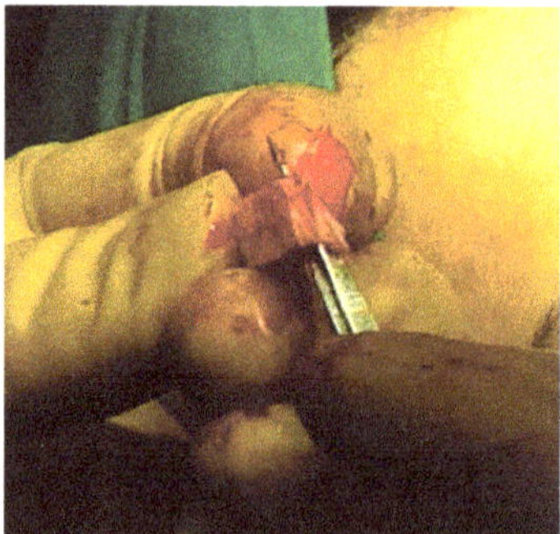

Figure 9 Spreader graft being carved.

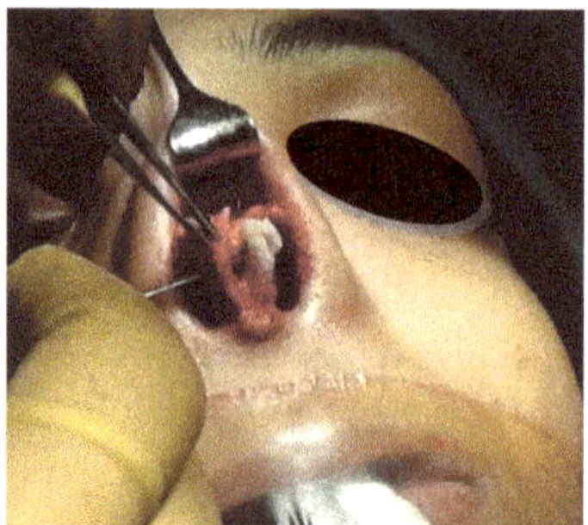

Figure 10. Septal extension graft being placed.

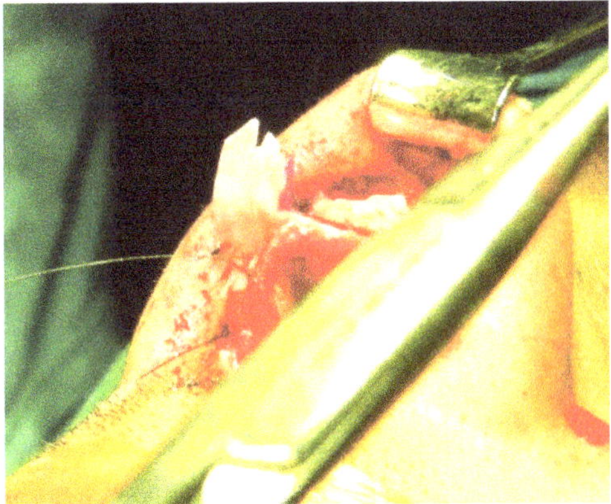

Figure 11. Umbrella graft.

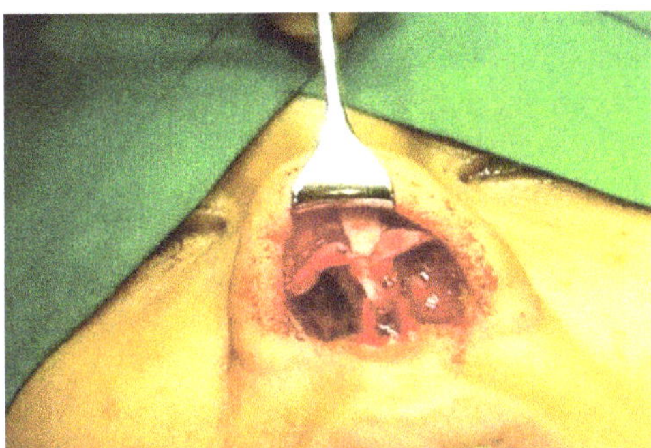

Figure 12. Dorsal augmentation graft.

sandwiched between two autografts like septal cartilage or conchal cartilage. This enables the surgeon to judiciously use the cartilage available at hand in cases of Revision Septorhinoplasty or in cases of cartilage deficiency [7] [8] (**Figure 13**).

2.3. Bone

The most common indication for the use of bone in nose surgery is for dorsal on lay grafting with or without columellar support. Membranous bones (ex-Calvarium) are preferred over endochondral bones (ex-Olecranon process and Iliac crest) because of lower rates of resorption. Chief limitations associated with use of bone as a graft include greater susceptibility to fracture, stiff infrastructure which makes carving difficult and prolonged period of immobilization required for graft fixation [1] [9].

2.4. Soft Tissue

Use of soft tissue grafts in dorsal augmentation is very limited because they fail to provide structural support which is vital for dorsal augmentation. Chief use of soft tissue grafts include, camouflaging minor irregularities of skin and adding volume. Most popular amongst the soft tissue grafts is Temporalis fascia graft.

- **Homografts**

This kind of graft is derived from soft tissue of a member of the same species. Most commonly used homografts include Irradiated Costal Cartilage (ICC) and Purified human acellular dermal graft [1] [10].

Irradiated Costal Cartilage (*ICC*)

This type of graft is harvested from the costal cartilage of cadavers and is irradiated with 30,000 to 40,000 Gy of ionizing radiation to decrease the risk of transmission of diseases. The advantages of using ICC graft include low risk of disease transmission, minimal immunogenic reactions and thereby very low rates of extrusion. The chief limitations associated with this kind of graft include tendency to wrap over time and resorption. As described previously for autologous rib cartilage grafting, to decrease the risk of warping, the perichondrium and outer cortex of rib should be removed and the technique of symmetric carving should be employed.

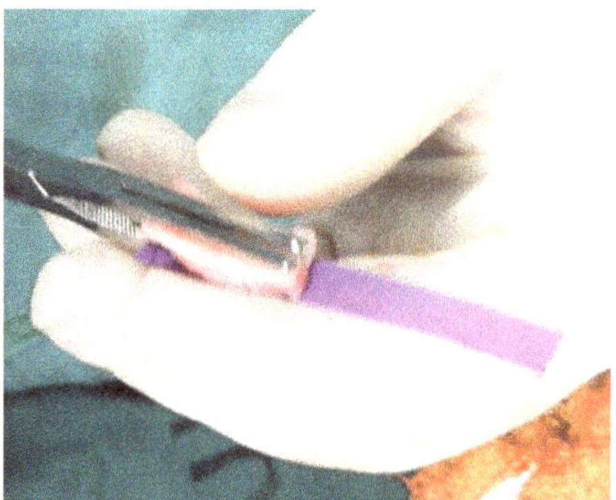

Figure 13. PDS being used to carve sandwhich graft.

Purified Human Acellular Dermal Graft

The dermis harvested from cadavers is subjected to a process that removes the epidermis and dermal cellular matrix but keeps the extracellular architecture of the dermis intact to facilitate regeneration. The principal uses of this graft are in form of overlay graft, to camouflage over implants, and as volume filling material. Limitations include inability to provide structural support and high rates of resorption.

- **Allografts**

These are synthetic grafts which are chemically composed of polymers *i.e.* repeating units of macromolecules. The unique characteristics required in a nasal implant include pores, malleability and consistency. Pores allow in-growth of the host tissue which decreases the dead space and prevents colonization of bacteria. This also helps in stabilization of the implant [1] [10].

- **Silicon**
- **Medpore**
- **Goretex**
- **PDS**
- **Fillers**

Out of which PDS is most commonly used and fillers are used for touch up.

PDS

PDS is and absorbable implant which is made up of an aliphatic polyester poly-p-dioxanone. PDS is degraded by hydrolysis and is completely absorbed by 25 weeks. It has many unique properties which makes it conducive for nasal surgeries [11] (**Figure 14** and **Figure 15**).

1) Absorbability—PDS plate remains intact during the critical healing process of the first 10 weeks after implantation but is absorbed completely within 25 weeks, leaving no residue and minimal fibrous scar tissue.

2) Structure & Support—Clinical studies show; PDS Plate provides non-warping support during healing. PDS Plate supports the graft pieces as a guide, bridging and supporting the nasal structure and preventing overlap and bending.

3) Cartilage Management—Patients who have undergone multiple nasal surgeries risk graft depletion. PDS Plate offers a highly versatile and reliable way of making maximal use of many cartilage fragments otherwise discarded, and may reduce the need for secondary cartilage donor site surgery.

4) Versatile—PDS Plate is available in a number of sizes and configurations, one of which is perforated. The product can be trimmed to suit a variety of anatomical conditions and surgical needs including Rhinoplasty and Septoplasty procedures, and the temporary scaffold can be used to construct Columellar Struts, Septal Extension Grafts, Alar Battens, and Upper Lateral Replacement grafts.

3. Conclusion

In any nasal reconstructive procedure, the final aesthetic outcome is determined by the graft or implant. An ideal graft does not exist. However Autografts bear closest resemblance to an ideal graft but their availability is limited. In cases of Revision Septorhinoplasty and in cases of limited availability of autografts, allografts play an important role. Amongst all the allograft available at our institute, PDS is the most preferred, as it bears a very

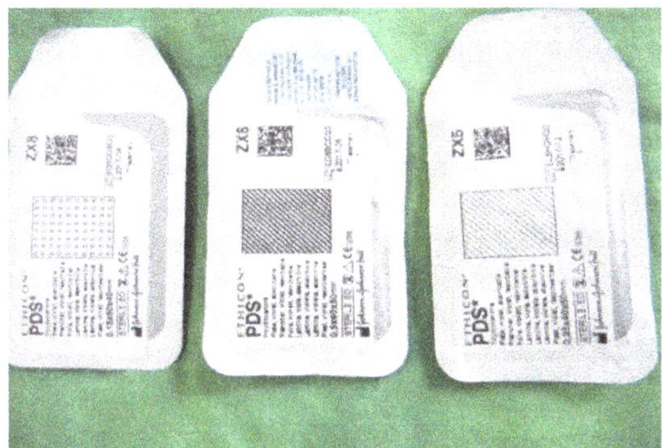

Figure 14. PDS and Introperative use of PDS.

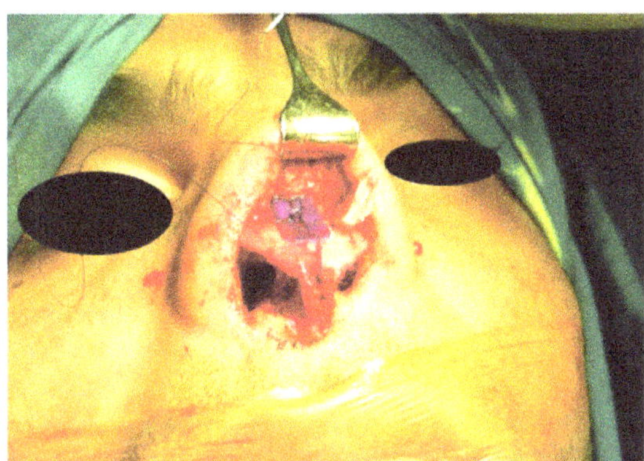

Figure 15. PDS and introperative use of PDS.

close resemblance to an ideal graft.

References

[1] Romo III, T. and Pearson, J.M. (2008) Nasal Implants. *Facial Plastic Surgery Clinics of North America*, **16**, 123-132. http://dx.doi.org/10.1016/j.fsc.2007.09.004

[2] Sadeghi, M., Saedi, B., Sazegar, A.A. and Amiri, M. (2009) The Role of Columellar Struts to Gain and Maintain Tip Projection and Rotation: A Randomized Blinded Trial. *American Journal of Rhinology and Allergy*, **23**, e47-e50. http://dx.doi.org/10.2500/ajra.2009.23.3392

[3] Kim, J.H., Song, J.W., Park, S.W., Oh, W.S. and Lee, J.H. (2014) Effective Septal Extension Graft for Asian Rhinoplasty. *Archives of Plastic Surgery*, **41**, 3-11.

[4] Roofe, S.B. (2004) Surgery of the Nasal Valve. *Archives of Facial Plastic Surgury*, **6**, 167-171. http://dx.doi.org/10.1001/archfaci.6.3.167

[5] Teymoortash, A., Fasunla J.A. and Sazgar, A.A. (2012) The Value of Spreader Grafts in Rhinoplasty: A Critical Review. *European Archives of Oto-Rhino-Laryngology*, **269**, 1411-1416. http://dx.doi.org/10.1007/s00405-011-1837-y

[6] Menick, F.J. (1999) Anatomic Reconstruction of the Nasal Tip Cartilage in Secondary and Reconstructive Rhinoplasty. *Plastic and Reconstructive Surgery*, **104**, 2187-2201.

[7] Scattolin, A. and D'Ascanio, L. (2013) Grafts in "Closed" Rhinoplasty. *Acta Otorhinolaryngologica Italica*, **33**, 169-176.

[8] Bussi, M., Palonta, F. and Toma, S. (2013) Grafting in Revision Rhinoplasty. *Acta Otorhinolaryngologica Italica*, **33**, 183-189.

[9] Saeed, M., Hussain, Z. and Mian, F.A. (2012) Augmentation Rhinoplasty with Autologus Iliac Crest Bone Graft. *A.P.M.C*, **6**, 18-21.

[10] Breitbart, A.S. and Ablaza, V.J. (2006) Implant Materials. In: Thorne, C.H., Bartlett, S.P., Beasley, R.W., Aston, S.J., Gurtner, G.C. and Spear, S.L., Eds., *Grabb and Smith's Plastic Surgery*, 6th Edition, Lippincott Williams & Wilkins, Philadelphia, Chapter 7, 58-65.

[11] www.pdsflexibleplate.com

The Impact of Age on Cochlear Implant Performance

Brian Schwab, Michele Gandolfi, Erica Lai, Erin Reilly, Lorie Singer, Ana H. Kim

Department of Otolaryngology, New York Eye and Ear Infirmary of Mount Sinai, New York, USA
Email: bschwab@nyee.edu

Abstract

Objective: Cochlear implantation is the emerging treatment of choice for severe and profound sensorineural hearing loss, yet there are conflicting data on outcomes in adults. There is significant variability in the literature concerning the exact effect of age on cochlear implant outcomes. We sought to evaluate the outcomes of cochlear implant performance stratified by age. Study Design: Retrospective review. Methods: Audiologic preoperative and postoperative evaluation consisted of word recognition scores (Consonant-Nucleus-Consonant). Complications were retrospectively collected after each cochlear implantation. A sub-analysis was performed comparing patients implanted at a younger (21 - 64 years) and older (65 and above) age. Results: A total of 240 patients were evaluated. Patients experienced a significant improvement in audiologic performance as seen with word recognition scores ($p < 0.00001$). The mean post-implant score was 44.6% (at 3 months) and 53.5% (at 24 months) at 50 dB compared to average pre-implantation aided score of 6%. There was no significant difference between postoperative performances in younger versus older patient groups. Multiple regressions showed no correlation with duration of deafness at time of implantation or age and performance. There was no significant difference in performance based on side of implantation. Conclusion: This is one of the largest series to date on hearing outcomes in adults who receive a cochlear implant. No statistical differences were noted between the younger and older groups or based on side of implantation. The audiologic benefit in the adult population is clearly demonstrated.

Keywords

Cochlear Implantation, Age, Duration of Deafness

1. Introduction

According to the World Health Organization, 328 million adults have disabling hearing loss. Globally, hearing loss is the third leading cause of disability [1]. The demand for treatment is high, and for some patients, traditional methods of amplification are no longer sufficient. Cochlear implantation (CI) is the emerging treatment of choice for severe and profound sensorineural hearing loss, yet there are conflicting data on outcomes in adults [2]. There is significant variability in individual outcomes and benefits, and little data exist regarding the exact effect of age on CI outcomes. With the increasing prevalence of hearing loss, understanding patient outcomes after CI in adults is imperative.

A number of different factors have been suggested as having prognostic value for implantation benefit, and several predictive models have been designed [3]-[5]. Duration of deafness has been quoted as being the most important prognostic indicator with an inverse relationship to speech performance after implantation. It has been postulated that this may be a result of neuronal reorganization in favor of visual processing secondary to auditory deprivation [6]. Leung *et al.* found that a shorter percentage of life spent with hearing loss and residual speech recognition carried a greater predictive value in determining postoperative performance than age [7]. Numerous studies have corroborated the prognostic value of shorter duration of deafness and improved outcome [8]-[10]. Yet, there have been other papers proposing that these factors are not exclusively predictive of word recognition scores post cochlear implantation [11]. Though duration of deafness seems to be one potential influencing component for post-implant outcomes, the literature advocates that many factors may potentially influence an individual's speech understanding with a CI. For example, Green *et al.* reported duration of deafness to be an independent predictor of performance, accounting for 9% of the variability in a retrospective study examining 117 postlingually-deaf patients [12]. They concluded that, apart from duration of deafness, "Other factors must influence implant performance".

Furthermore, the relationship between duration of deafness and age has not been thoroughly investigated to the extent of providing a definitive conclusion. A study by Roberts *et al.* found that older patients significantly improved their speech recognition abilities after implantation but to a lesser degree than younger recipients [13]. This was confirmed by Lin *et al.* who reported that the magnitude of gain in the speech scores was negatively associated with age at implantation. Lin *et al.* noted that a 60-year old would expect a 75 percentage point improvement in speech scores, compared to a 50 point improvement in an 80-year old adult [14]. These results suggest that elderly recipients do not improve to the extent of their younger counterparts. However, other studies have failed to conclusively demonstrate a direct correlation between age and decreased outcome within the adult population with respect to word scores or pure-tone audiometry [10] [15]. Evidence to the contrary by Alice *et al.*, for example, showed there was no statistical difference in improvement between older and younger age groups [16].

This study seeks to shed further light on the body of research regarding CI performance in adults. It was hypothesized that older participants would show significant improvement in hearing outcomes after CI, but it was expected that this benefit would be less than in younger CI recipients. Furthermore, it was hypothesized that duration of deafness would have a stronger correlation with hearing outcomes than age at implantation.

2. Materials and Methods

2.1. Study Design

This is a retrospective review of medical records of postlingually deafened patients greater than 21 years who met the criteria for cochlear implantation from April 1993 to December 2013. Institutional review board exemption was obtained for this study (#E-13.19). Patients were included in the review of medical records if they were aged 21 and older at time of implantation without cochlear anomalies precluding complete electrode insertion. Exclusion criteria included any patient failing to perform standardized testing through one year postoperatively. Complications were not considered part of the exclusion criteria. Patients were divided into two groups: "younger" CI recipients were defined as people who underwent cochlear implantation between the ages of 21 and 64 whereas "older" CI recipients underwent surgery after the age of 65.

2.2. Diagnostic Tests

All tests were performed in an IAC standard double-wall booth audiometry room under conditions meeting ANSI and ISO standards, including calibration, noise levels, and sounds levels. Speech perception materials were presented preoperatively and postoperatively in the IAC standard double-wall booth. The Consonant-

Nucleus-Consonant (CNC) test in quiet at 50 dB was performed pre- and postoperatively. This test was developed to provide lists of monosyllabic words with equal phonemic distribution across lists with each list exhibiting approximately the same phonemic distribution as the English language. When patients performed above 80 percent on CNC testing, AzBio sentence testing in quiet was also tested.

2.3. Statistical Analysis

The Mann-Whitney nonparametric U test was used to compare age groups with respect to preoperative SRT and audiological testing data. The Mann-Whitney nonparametric U test was also used to compare groups postoperatively. All reported P-values were calculated as two-sided with a level < 0.05 being considered statistically significant. Multiple regression was performed for correlation between age, duration of deafness, and CNC score at a given postoperative time period. All statistical analyses were performed using Excel (Microsoft, Redmond, W.A.). A multiple regression model was also used to fit the data to a polymetric equation.

3. Results

3.1. Patient Demographics

There were 119 patients in the younger age group and 121 patients in the older group. There was a similar gender distribution in the two groups: 65 (54.6%) were female and 54 (45.4%) were male in the younger group; 61 (50.4%) were female and 60 (49.6%) were male in the older group. The average age of the younger group was 46 (range 21 - 64 years at age of implantation). The average age of the older group of patients was 72 (range 65 - 88 years). The mean duration of hearing loss was 19.3 years ± 14.2 in the younger group (range 0.2 - 50.7 years) and 23.4 ± 16.6 years in the older group (range 0.5 - 63.0 years). The right ear was implanted in 70 (58.8%) younger patients and 60 (49.6%) older patients and the left ear in 47 (39.5%) younger and 58 (47.9%) older patients. Five patients were implanted bilaterally (2 younger patients and 3 older patients). Of the younger patients, 79 lost their hearing because of idiopathic hearing loss; 18 had familial or genetic hearing loss; 8 had an infectious etiology; 7 lost their hearing due to a physical or noise-induced trauma; and 7 had Meniere's disease. Of the older patients, 66 lost their hearing because of idiopathic hearing loss; 28 had familial or genetic hearing loss; 14 lost their hearing due to a physical or noise-induced trauma; 8 had an infectious etiology; and 5 had Meniere's disease. Demographic data is summarized in **Table 1**. There were very few surgical complications overall, consisting of two wound infections and six patients with dizziness or hyperacusis. Five patients had the implant removed and were re-implanted due to device failure.

Table 1. Patient demographics.

Demographic Characteristics	
Number of patients	240
Age range at the time of implantation (mean), years	21 - 88 (56 ± 16.8)
Duration of deafness range (mean), years	0 - 63 (21 ± 15.4)
Sex (Male, Female)	114, 126
Side (Left, Right, Bilateral)	105, 130, 5
Etiology:	
Idopathic	145
Familial or genetic	46
Infectious	16
Physical or noise-induced	21
Meniere's	12

3.2. Audiologic Performance and Regression

There was no significant difference in preoperative speech perception scores between the younger and older groups ($p = 0.27$). The average aided CNC score pre-implant was 5.3% for the younger group and 6.7% for the older group.

Average CNC scores in quiet post-implant in the younger age group at 3, 12 and 24 months post-implant were 45.7%, 55.2% and 55.7%, respectively, compared to 43.5%, 52.5% and 51.3% in the older age group, respectively (**Figure 1**).

There were no statistical differences in postoperative performance data between the younger and older groups at 3 months ($p = 0.46$), 12 months ($p = 0.86$), or 24 months ($p = 0.64$). AZBio scores in quiet were also analyzed (results not included in full analysis) to verify results and showed similar trends with no significant differences at 3 months ($p = 0.62$), 12 months ($p = 0.12$), or 24 months ($p = 0.50$).

At 24 months, multiple regressions showed very weak correlation between age, duration of deafness, and CNC with a multiple regression coefficient of 0.27. Duration of deafness did not seem to have a significant impact (**Figure 2**).

For verification, a simple regression and correlation factor were calculated and found to be non-significant. After 24 months, 27.9% of data points show correlation with age and duration; at 12 months, 16.7% of data points show correlation with age and duration; at 6 months, 16.27% of data points show correlation with age and

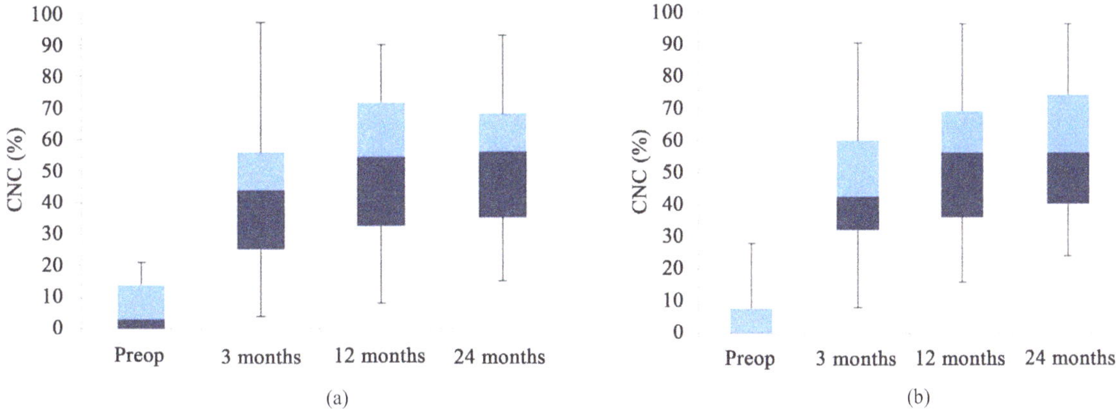

Figure 1. Box whisker plot of pre- and postoperative CNC speech perception in quiet scores in Younger (a) and Older (b) patients. The light light blue bars represent upper quartile and dark blue the lower quartile. (a) CNC data in younger patients; (b) CNC data in older patients.

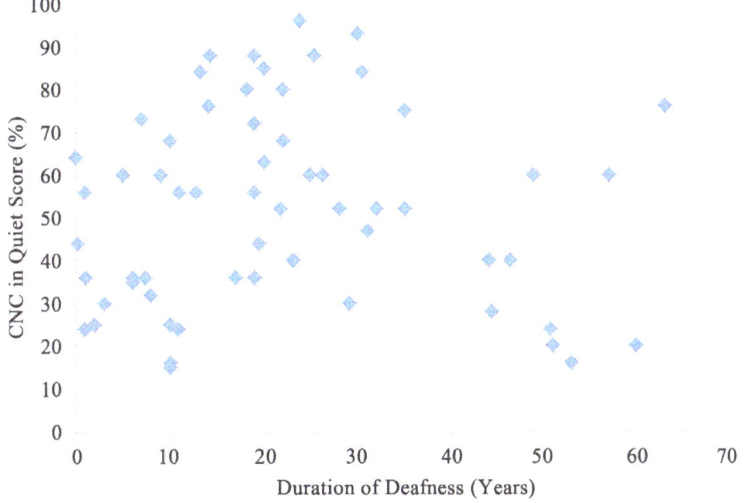

Figure 2. CNC in quiet scores two years after implantation as a function of duration of deafness at the time of implantation.

duration; at 3 months, 13.9% of data points show correlation with age and duration (**Figures 3(a)-(d)**). A multiple regression equation was used to fit the data to a predictive polymetric model and showed an R2 value of 0.931 (**Figure 3(e)**).

A sub-analysis was performed to examine the differences in postoperative performances in patients implanted in the left ear against patients implanted in the right ear (**Figure 4**).

There were no significant differences in average CNC scores at two years: those implanted in the left had an average CNC score of 52.4% whereas those implanted on the right had an average CNC score of 51.5% (p = 0.73).

4. Discussion

Patients in this study experienced a significant improvement in audiologic performance post-CI as seen with CNC word scores ($p < 0.05$). This is in accordance with data from other studies showing significant improvement in both speech and word scores in the adult population [17]-[25]. The complication rate was similar to that reported in other studies with only two wound infections and other minor complications; there have been multiple prior studies demonstrating that surgical complications are a rarity even in this adult age group [19] [26] [27].

There has been much deliberation about the effect of age at implantation versus duration of hearing loss on speech perception scores after CI [7] [14] [28]-[31]. Previous data show that age at implantation is significantly associated with poorer CI outcomes [14]. The reason is thought to be the association with cognitive processing required for auditory processing and decoding of the input supplied by the CI [32]. The cognitive ability to pro-

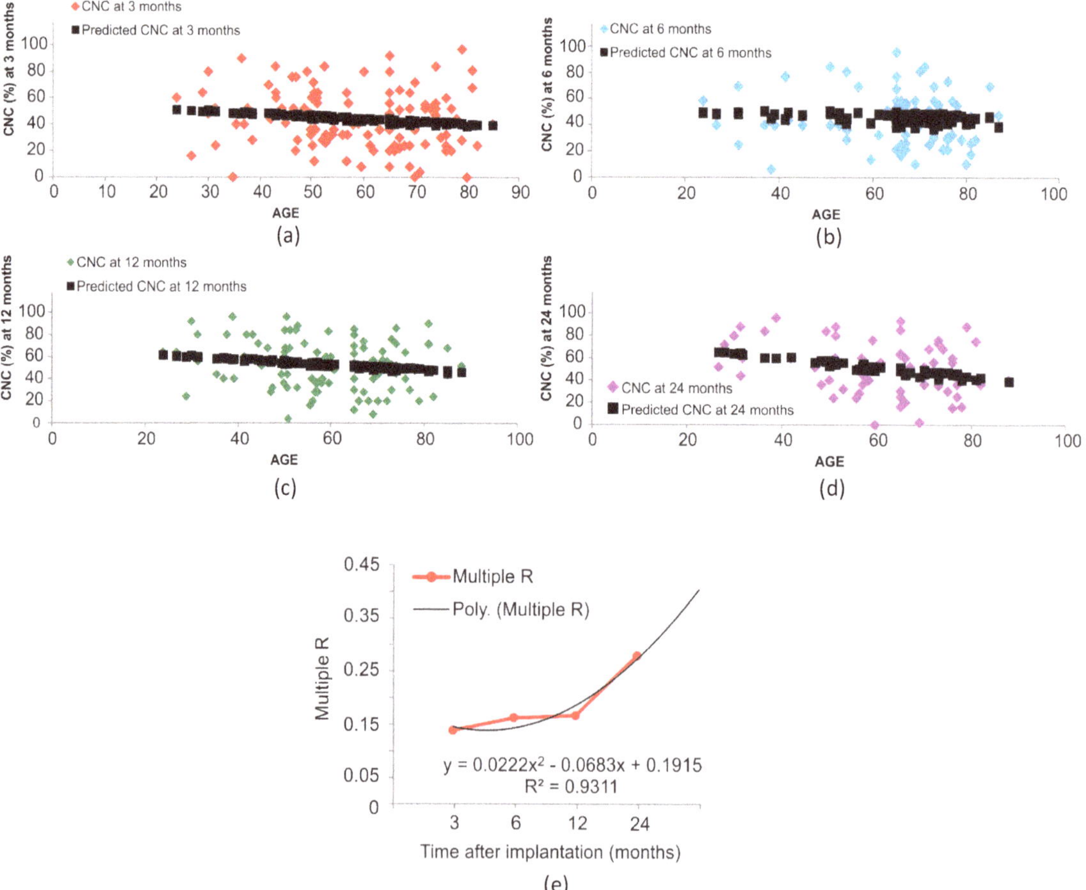

Figure 3. Multiple regression with (a) correlation between age and CNC at 3 months; (b) correlation between age and CNC at 6 months; (c) correlation between age and CNC at 12 months; (d) correlation between age and CNC at 24 months; and (e) trend curve.

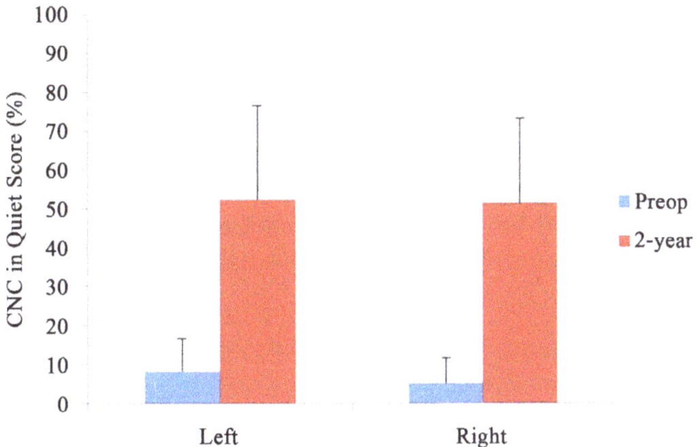

Figure 4. Pre- and 2-year postoperative speech perception scores in quiet for patients implanted in the left versus right ear.

cess and decode is thought to decline with age [33] [34]. When we stratified our age groups into younger (ages 21 – 64) and older (65+), there was no statistical difference in CNC word scores at 3, 12, or 24 months post-operative. This suggests that the older group did not require a prolonged time to acclimate to the cochlear implant technology as predicted in prior studies. Perhaps there is a correlation between cognitive ability and outcomes, but older adults with good cognitive function and close follow up seemed to have significant improvement in this study. There was no mention of cognitive decline, dementia, Alzheimer's or other similar diagnoses in the charts of any of the patients that were implanted in our study.

The prior studies reporting older adult recipients attaining poorer speech perception scores compared with younger patients postoperatively were based on testing in noise [35]-[37]. This problem most likely reflects a complementary interaction between the auditory and cognitive systems. This complex environment is when cognitive decline can show its effect on outcomes. However, our study focused on CNC testing in quiet, so this was unable to be elucidated. Leung *et al.* found that a shorter percentage of life spent with hearing loss and residual speech recognition carry a greater predictive value in determining postoperative performance than age [7]. In contrast, we did not observe such a clear correlation between duration of deafness and outcomes post-implant, as has other studies [25] [38] [39]. However, this can also be due to the fact that this was a retrospective study relying on self-reported duration of hearing loss. Authors have used a variety of methods to delineate the time-frame of hearing loss in retrospective studies. For example, Rubinstein *et al.* asked patients when they stopped being able to use the telephone in the ear to be implanted [9]. This is one unfortunate limitation for retrospective reviews of charts. It should be clarified, as well, that studies in the literature tend to emphasize duration of profound hearing loss as opposed to duration of any form of hearing loss. Patients typically are able to remember more accurately the transition to a profound hearing loss wherein they lose functionality such as being able to talk on the telephone.

Duration of deafness has been shown to have a negative correlation with post-implant performance in a number of studies [40]. Multiple authors and institutions have contributed predictive models for post-implant outcomes, typically using duration of deafness as a primary variable. Several other authors, however, have found no correlation or only a weak correlation between duration of deafness and postoperative performance [40]-[42]. For example, Waltzman *et al.* studied the relationship between preoperative factors and two-year postoperative performance in 82 patients at the Department of Veterans Affairs and noted only a weak correlation with length of deafness and postoperative performance [41]. Hamzavi *et al.* drew a similar conclusion, noting duration of deafness did not appear to have relevant effects on the final outcome [42]. Moreover, there is high variability in the coefficient of determination and correlation coefficient (*i.e.*, R^2 and r) data seen in prior studies that attempt to support duration of deafness as being significant.

Our data similarly hint at a weak correlation between outcome and duration of deafness. The correlation coefficient of 0.27 indicates that there was no definitive connection between variables at all. It is difficult to draw universal conclusions about duration of deafness across studies because information is typically acquired via patient report, which relies on patient memory for historical accuracy. This is (like in most reports) a limitation of our study and data set. It appears the literature is not conclusive as to the clinical significance that duration of deafness plays in CI, and our data support the notion that a lengthy duration of deafness in postlingually deafened adults is not a contraindication for implantation.

This study has clinical implications in the setting of counseling postlingually deafened adults regarding the therapeutic options for hearing restoration. While hearing aid amplification may be appropriate for people with mild to moderate hearing loss, adults with severe to profound sensorineural hearing loss should be made aware of the benefits along with potential risks of CI. Most clinicians now agree that age should not be an excluding factor when choosing candidates for cochlear implantation. The fact that this type of surgery is well-tolerated requires a short operative time, and causes minimal blood loss is advantageous to the senior population. Rather than basing the decision of surgery on years of life or duration of deafness, a multidisciplinary approach to adequately assess eligibility should be employed. Indeed, further studies are needed to better understand how this multifactorial process is impacted by the numerous factors to predict postoperative outcomes.

5. Conclusion

Our findings suggest that cochlear implantation in both age groups is equally effective in improving speech scores. We did not observe a clear correlation between duration of deafness and post-implant speech outcomes. However, further research using a uniform definition constituting duration of deafness is needed to better understand how it affects outcomes.

Acknowledgements

We would like to thank Dr. Ksenia Varakina for her assistance with statistical analysis.

References

[1] Stevens, G., Flaxman, S., Brunskill, E., *et al.* (2013) Global and Regional Hearing Impairment Prevalence: An Analysis of 42 Studies in 29 Countries. *The European Journal of Public Health*, **23**, 146-152. http://dx.doi.org/10.1093/eurpub/ckr176

[2] Semenov, Y.R., Martinez-Monedero, R. and Niparko, J.K. (2012) Cochlear Implants: Clinical and Societal Outcomes. *Otolaryngologic Clinics of North America*, **45**, 959-981. http://dx.doi.org/10.1016/j.otc.2012.06.003

[3] Blamey, P., Artieres, F., Başkent, D., *et al.* (2012) Factors Affecting Auditory Performance of Postlinguistically Deaf Adults Using Cochlear Implants: An Update with 2251 Patients. *Audiology and Neurotology*, **18**, 36-47. http://dx.doi.org/10.1159/000343189

[4] Roditi, R.E., Poissant, S.F., Bero, E.M., *et al.* (2009) A Predictive Model of Cochlear Implant Performance in Postlingually Deafened Adults. *Otology & Neurotology*, **30**, 449-454. http://dx.doi.org/10.1097/MAO.0b013e31819d3480

[5] Lazard, D.S., Vincent, C., Venail, F., *et al.* (2012) Pre-, Per- and Postoperative Factors Affecting Performance of Postlinguistically Deaf Adults Using Cochlear Implants: A New Conceptual Model over Time. *PloS ONE*, **7**, e48739. http://dx.doi.org/10.1371/journal.pone.0048739

[6] Hirschfelder, A., Gräbel, S. and Olze, H. (2008) The Impact of Cochlear Implantation on Quality of Life: The Role of Audiologic Performance and Variables. *Otolaryngology—Head and Neck Surgery*, **138**, 357-362. http://dx.doi.org/10.1016/j.otohns.2007.10.019

[7] Leung, J., Wang, N., Yeagle, J.D., *et al.* (2005) Predictive Models for Cochlear Implantation in Elderly Candidates. *Archives of Otolaryngology—Head & Neck Surgery*, **131**, 1049-1054. http://dx.doi.org/10.1001/archotol.131.12.1049

[8] Blamey, P., Pyman, B., Gordon, C., *et al.* (1992) Factors Predicting Post-Operative Sentence Scores in Postlingually Deaf Adult Cochlear Implant Patients. *Annals of Otology, Rhinology and Laryngology*, **101**, 342-348. http://dx.doi.org/10.1177/000348949210100410

[9] Rubinstein, J.T., Parkinson, W.S., Tyler, R.S. and Gantz, B.J. (1999) Residual Speech Recognition and Cochlear Implant Performance: Effects of Implantation Criteria. *American Journal of Otology*, **20**, 445-452.

[10] UK Cochlear Implant Study Group (2004) Criteria of Candidacy for Unilateral Cochlear Implantation in Postlingually deafened Adults I: Theory and Measures of Effectiveness. *Ear and Hearing*, **25**, 310-335. http://dx.doi.org/10.1097/01.AUD.0000134549.48718.53

[11] Gantz, B.J., Tyler, R.S., Rubinstein, J.T., Wolaver, A., Lowder, M., Abbas, P., *et al.* (2002) Binaural Cochlear Implants Placed during the Same Operation. *Otology & Neurotology*, **23**, 169-180. http://dx.doi.org/10.1097/00129492-200203000-00012

[12] Green, K.M.J., Bhatt, Y.M., Mawman, D.J., O'driscoll, M.P., Saeed, S.R., Ramsden, R.T. and Green, M.W. (2007) Predictors of Audiological Outcome Following Cochlear Implantation in Adults. *Cochlear Implants International*, **8**, 1-11. http://dx.doi.org/10.1179/cim.2007.8.1.1

[13] Roberts, D.S., Lin, H.W., Herrmann, B.S. and Lee, D.J. (2013) Differential Cochlear Implant Outcomes in Older Adults. *The Laryngoscope*, **123**, 1952-1956. http://dx.doi.org/10.1002/lary.23676

[14] Lin, F.R., Chien, W.W., Li, L.S., Clarrett, D.M., Niparko, J.K. and Francis, H.W. (2012) Cochlear Implantation in Older Adults. *Medicine*, **91**, 229-239. http://dx.doi.org/10.1097/MD.0b013e31826b145a

[15] Friedman, D.R., Green, J., Fang, Y.X., Ensor, K., Roland, J.T. and Waltzman, S.B. (2015) Sequential Bilateral Cochlear Implantation in the Adolescent Population. *Laryngoscope*, **125**, 1952-1958. http://dx.doi.org/10.1002/lary.25293

[16] Alice, B., Silvia, M., Laura, G., Patrizia, T. and Roberto, B. (2013) Cochlear Implantation in the Elderly: Surgical and Hearing Outcomes. *BMC Surgery*, **13**, S1. http://dx.doi.org/10.1186/1471-2482-13-S2-S1

[17] Skarzynsky, P.H., Olszewsky, L., Skarzynsky, H., *et al.* (2012) Cochlear Implantation in the Aging Population. *Audiology and Neurotology*, **17**, 15-17.

[18] Luntz, M., Yehudai, N., Most, T., *et al.* (2012) Cochlear Implantation in the Elderly: Surgical and Hearing Outcomes. *Audiology and Neurotology*, **17**, 14-15.

[19] Huarte, A., Lezaun, R. and Manrique, M. (2014) Quality of Life Outcomes for Cochlear Implantation in the Elderly. *Audiology and Neurotology*, **19**, 36-39. http://dx.doi.org/10.1159/000371608

[20] Poissant, S.F., Beaudoin, F., Huang, J., Brodsky, J. and Lee, D.J. (2008) Impact of Cochlear Implantation on Speech Understanding, Depression, and Loneliness in the Elderly. *Journal of Otolaryngology—Head & Neck Surgery*, **37**, 488-494.

[21] Migirov, L., Taitelbaum-Swead, R., Drendel, M., Hildesheimer, M. and Kronenberg, J. (2010) Cochlear Implantation in Elderly Patients: Surgical and Audiological Outcome. *Gerontology*, **56**, 123-128. http://dx.doi.org/10.1159/000235864

[22] Chatelin, V., Kim, E.J., Driscoll, C., Larky, J., Polite, C., Price, L. and Lalwani, A.K. (2004) Cochlear Implant Outcomes in the Elderly. *Otology & Neurotology*, **25**, 298-301. http://dx.doi.org/10.1097/00129492-200405000-00017

[23] Eshraghi, A.A., Rodriguez, M., Balkany, T.J., Telischi, F.F., Angeli, S., Hodges, A.V. and Adil, E. (2009) Cochlear Implant Surgery in Patients More than Seventy-Nine Years Old. *Laryngoscope*, **119**, 1180-1183. http://dx.doi.org/10.1002/lary.20182

[24] Francis, H.W., Chee, N., Yeagle, J., Cheng, A. and Niparko, J.K. (2002) Impact of Cochlear Implants on the Functional Health Status of Older Adults. *Laryngoscope*, **112**, 1482-1488. http://dx.doi.org/10.1097/00005537-200208000-00028

[25] Kelsall, D.C., Shallop, J.K. and Burnelli, T. (1995) Cochlear Implantation in the Elderly. *American Journal of Otolaryngology*, **16**, 609-615.

[26] Jeppesen, J. and Faber, C.E. (2013) Surgical Complications Following Cochlear Implantation in Adults Based on a Proposed Reporting Consensus. *Acta Oto-Laryngologica*, **133**, 1012-1021. http://dx.doi.org/10.3109/00016489.2013.797604

[27] Cohen, N.L. and Hoffman, R.A. (1991) Complications of Cochlear Implant Surgery in Adults and Children. *Annals of Otology, Rhinology & Laryngology*, **100**, 708-711. http://dx.doi.org/10.1177/000348949110000903

[28] Carlson, M.L., Breen, J.T., Gifford, R.H., Driscoll, C.L., Neff, B.A., Beatty, C.W., *et al.* (2010) Cochlear Implantation in the Octogenarian and Nonagenarian. *Otology & Neurotology*, **31**, 1343-1349.

[29] Chan, V., Tong, M., Yue, V., Wong, T., Leung, E., Yuen, K. and van Hasselt, A. (2007) Performance of Older Adult Cochlear Implant Users in Hong Kong. *Ear and Hearing*, **28**, 52S-55S.

[30] Migirov, L., Taitelbaum-Swead, R., Drendel, M., Hildesheimer, M. and Kronenberg, J. (2010) Cochlear Implantation in Elderly Patients: Surgical and Audiological Outcome. *Gerontology*, **56**, 123-128.

[31] Vermeire, K., Brokx, J.P., Wuyts, F.L., Cochet, E., Hofkens, A. and Van de Heyning, P.H. (2005) Quality-of-Life Benefit from Cochlear Implantation in the Elderly. *Otology & Neurotology*, **26**, 188-195.

[32] Tun, P.A., McCoy, S. and Wingfield, A. (2009) Aging, Hearing Acuity, and the Attentional Costs of Effortful Listening. *Psychology and Aging*, **24**, 761-766.

[33] Salthouse, T.A. (2000) Aging and Measures of Processing Speed. *Biological Psychology*, **54**, 35-54.

[34] Salthouse, T.A. (1996) The Processing-Speed Theory of Adult Age Differences in Cognition. *Psychological Review*, **103**, 403-428.

[35] Sanchez-Cuadrado, I., Lassaletta, L., Perez-More, R.M., Zernotti, M., Di Gregorio, M.F., Boccio, C. and Gavilán, J. (2013) Is There an Age Limit for Cochlear Implantation? *Annals of Otology, Rhinology, & Laryngology*, **122**, 222-228.

http://dx.doi.org/10.1177/000348941312200402

[36] Schneider, B.A., Pichora-Fuller, K. and Daneman, M. (2010) Effects of Senescent Changes in Audition and Cognition on Spoken Language Comprehension. In: Gordon-Salant, S., *et al.*, Eds., *The Aging Auditory System*, Springer, New York, 167-210. http://dx.doi.org/10.1007/978-1-4419-0993-0_7

[37] Holden, L.K., Finley, C.C., Firszt, J.B., Holden, T.A., Brenner, C., Potts, L.G., *et al.* (2013) Factors Affecting Open-Set Word Recognition in Adults with Cochlear Implants. *Ear & Hearing*, **43**, 342-360. http://dx.doi.org/10.1097/AUD.0b013e3182741aa7

[38] Sterkers, O., Mosnier, I., Ambert-Dahan, E., Herelle-Dupuy, E., Bozorg-Grayeli, A. and Bouccara, D. (2004) Cochlear Implants in Elderly People: Preliminary Results. *Acta Oto-Laryngologica*, **124**, 64-67. http://dx.doi.org/10.1080/03655230410017184

[39] Lachowska, M., Pastuszka, A., Glinka, P. and Niemczyk, K. (2013) Is Cochlear Implantation a Good Treatment Method for Profoundly Deafened Elderly? *Clinical Interventions of Aging*, **8**, 1339-1346. http://dx.doi.org/10.2147/CIA.S50698

[40] Van Dijk, J.E., van Olphen, A.F., Mens, L.H., Brokx, J.P., van den Broek, P. and Smoorenburg, G.F. (1995) Predictive Factors for Success with a Cochlear Implant. *Annals of Otology, Rhinology & Laryngology*, **166**, 196-198.

[41] Waltzman, S.B., Fisher, S.G., Niparko, J.K. and Cohen, N.L. (1995) Predictors of Postoperative Performance with Cochlear Implants. *Annals of Otology, Rhinology & Laryngology*, **165**, 15-18.

[42] Hamzavi, J., Baumgartner, W.D., Pok, S.M., Franz, P. and Gstoettner, W. (2003) Variables Affecting Speech Perception in Postlingually Deaf Adults Following Cochlear Implantation. *Acta Oto-Laryngologica*, **123**, 493-498. http://dx.doi.org/10.1080/0036554021000028120

32

Reversible Paclitaxel-Induced Bilateral Vocal Fold Paresis

Jeffrey Hsu, Melin Tan-Geller

Montefiore Medical Center, New York, USA
Email: jeffreyvhsu@gmail.com

Abstract

Introduction: Chemotherapy is a rare cause of iatrogenic vocal fold dysfunction. It has been reported in three main classes of chemotherapy agents and often occurs during the treatment interval. We present a case of bilateral vocal cord paresis with delayed presentation after completion of chemotherapy. Methods: One case, managed with observation and serial exams, is presented. A review of previous case reports of chemotherapy-induced vocal cord paresis and possible mechanisms of injury was performed. Results: Patient improved both symptomatically and through objective findings over the one-year course of observation. Conclusion: Diagnosis of chemotherapy-induced vocal cord paresis is dependent on a thorough history and physical exam. Management is predicated in that the dysfunction is often dose dependent and reversible, necessitating both cessation of the offending agent and the knowledge that any treatment is likely needed for only a temporary time. Chemotherapy-induced vocal fold paresis should be in the differential for patients presenting with hoarseness, dysphonia, stridor and a positive chemotherapy history.

Keywords

Vocal Cord Paralysis, Chemotherapy

1. Introduction

The most common cause of vocal fold paralysis is iatrogenic injury from surgical intervention or intubation. Thyroid and parathyroid surgery as well as cardiothoracic surgery defines a large percentage of surgical vocal fold paralysis etiology. A much less common iatrogenic source of injury is chemotherapy. While several chemotherapeutic drugs such as vincristine and vinblastine are known to be neurotoxic, few are known to affect vocal fold function.

Paclitaxel (Taxol) is a common chemotherapeutic drug originally developed from the Pacific yew tree (*Taxus brevifolia*) and has been used in the treatment in multiple malignancies including lung, ovarian, and breast cancers. While neurotoxicity is its biggest limit in application, currently there is only one case of vocal fold palsy reported in the literature to date [1]. It was diagnosed during active treatment and found to be reversible upon cessation of drug administration. We presented a case of delayed presentation of bilateral vocal fold paresis in a patient who completed a neo adjuvant chemotherapy regimen including paclitaxel for breast cancer. It was the second case of its kind, but distinguishable in that onset of symptomatic vocal fold paresis starting well after completion of treatment.

2. Case Report

A 62-year-old female with history of left invasive ductal carcinoma presented in April 2013 with several months of loss of the high vocal range and increased vocal strain. She is a classically trained singer who sings in a choir and at that time, noticed decreased range in her highest singing frequencies with need for increased straining. She denied any issues with her speaking voice, dysphagia, stridor or respiratory difficulty. Her oncologists noted her to have grade 1 fatigue and neuropathy, manifesting as upper extremity weakness and lower extremity paresthesias.

She underwent 12 treatments of neoadjuvant therapy of Paclitaxel, Herceptin and Vorinostat for her clinically staged cT3N3MO breast cancer from July 2012 to October 2012. Besides an episode of febrile neutropenia, no complications were described. Further treatments for her breast cancer included left mastectomy with a negative axillary lymph node dissection in January 2013 and subsequent intensity modulated radiotherapy along with maintenance Herceptin.

Her initial otolaryngologic exam was significant for mobile but paretic vocal folds bilaterally and near complete glottic closure. She was treated with multiple sessions of voice therapy where she learned exercises on how to compensate for her vocal fold paresis. Repeat endoscopic exam two months later revealed full mobility of the left fold with residual mild paresis of the right true fold and complete glottic closure (**Figure 1**). One year after her initial presentation, she was without voice complaints and laryngoscopy revealed completely normal vocal fold mobility.

As is the custom in our institution, no signed informed consent was necessary due to the deidentification of the patient's exam and clinical course but verbal consent was obtained from the patient prior to publication.

3. Discussion

Vocal fold paresis often presents with symptoms such as dysphonia, hoarseness, dysphagia or aspiration. The four most common etiologies have been cited to be malignancy, iatrogenic, idiopathic, and neck trauma [2]. Common iatrogenic causes include surgeries in the head and neck region as well as endotracheal intubations. One less common iatrogenic cause is neurotoxicity from chemotherapeutic agents.

Neurotoxicity is a common side effect of chemotherapy drugs, mostly seen with vinca alkaloids and taxanes. Historically, the dose limiting effects have been peripheral neuropathies but have also been known to affect the motor and autonomic nervous systems. Symptoms typically manifest with increased dose dependency, increased infusion rates and with onset within close proximity of consumption. Cranial nerve palsies have been a very rare presentation of chemotherapy-induced neurotoxicity [3]-[5]. Though rare, there are at least three different chemotherapeutic classes known to cause vocal fold paresis.

Since its introduction, there have been over 43 case reports of vinca alkaloids induced vocal fold paresis [5]-[9]. Vinca alkaloids function through prevention of tubulin polymerization, disrupting microtubule formation and halting cell division. Though the pathophysiology of neurotoxicity has not been clearly defined, it is hypothesized that the vinca alkaloids disrupts axonal transport and nerve conductance. Clinical manifestations have included hoarseness, dysphagia, cough, and stridor with patients being diagnosed with both unilateral and bilateral vocal fold paresis. Vincristine has been found to be the most neurotoxic, followed by vinblastine, and vinorelbine [10]. In the Pediatric Otolaryngology Group study, four cases of vincristine-induced laryngeal paralysis were seen over five and half years among 293 children. In their literature search, only 10 pediatric cases had been previously reported since 1966, likely revealing an underreporting of cases [11]. Though symptoms are often reversible with cessation of use, patients can undergo a phenomenon called coasting where symptoms worsen before they improve [5] [10]. Treatment has ranged from observation to tracheotomy to address airway compromise.

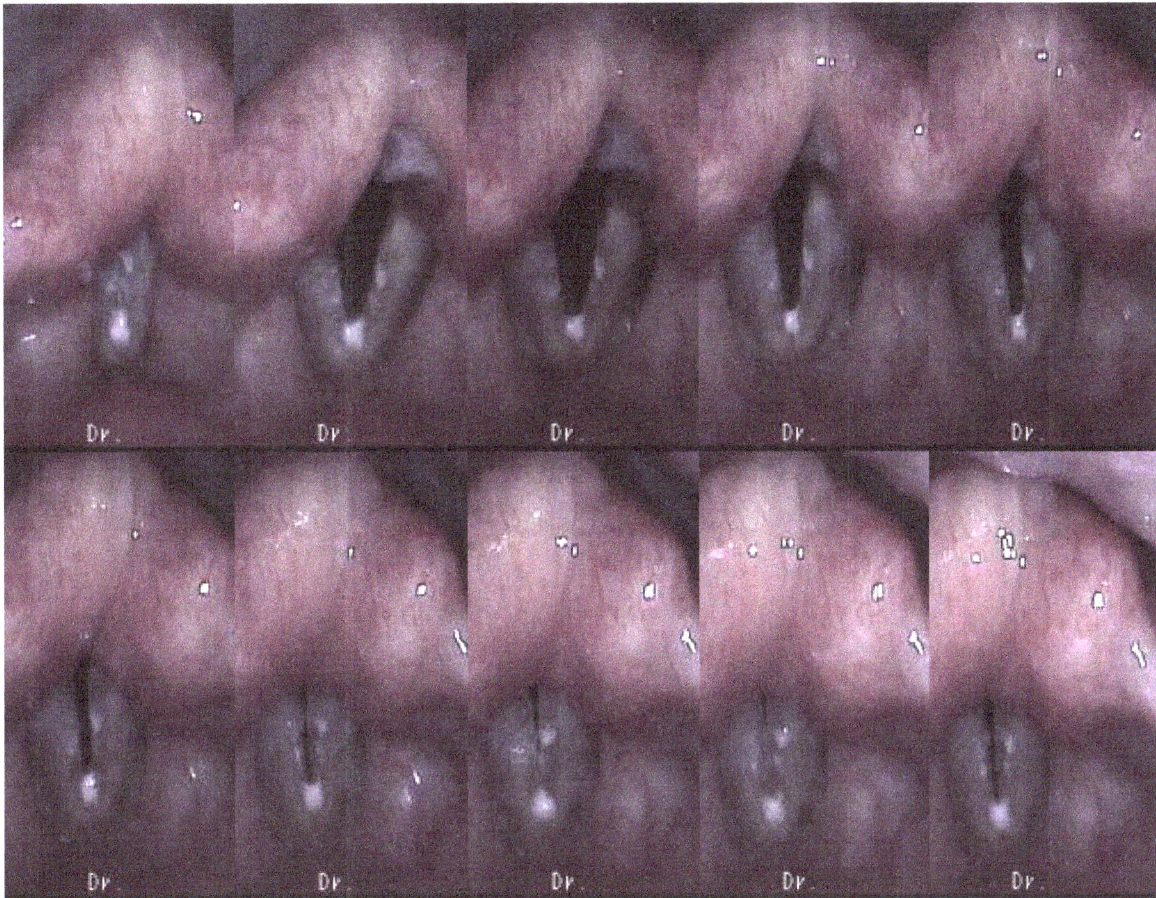

Figure 1. Fiberoptic laryngeal exam. Sequential still images of patient's fiberoptic laryngeal exam during one of the serial follow up exams. From right to left, the left vocal fold is seen to be in varying position while the patient is abducting and adducting her vocal fold while the right vocal fold remains in similar position throughout the exam. Here, we are able to see the partial recovery of the left vocal fold while the right is still paretic.

Cisplatin is a platinum derivative who mechanism involves the inhibition of DNA synthesis by forming crosslinks of DNA molecules. Its neurotoxic effects normally affect the sensory system and occur with accumulating doses. In most patients it is often reversible, though incomplete [10]. Again, while the exact neuropathic mechanism is not known, it is hypothesized that injury occurs at the dorsal root ganglion for sensory nerves while also causing axonopathy in other nerve types. There has been one previously cited case involving a patient receiving cisplatin for small cell lung cancer presenting with stridor and bilateral vocal fold paralysis [12]. The patient required an urgent tracheotomy but was ultimately able to bedecannulated with return of vocal fold function.

Paclitaxel is a part of many chemotherapy regimens for a wide range of cancers. Its chemotherapeutic effects are due to its ability to promote the formation and stabilization of polymerized microtubules, disrupting cell mitosis. [10] It, like many other chemotherapeutic drugs, is limited by neurotoxicity. This manifests itself most often as a sensory peripheral neuropathy in a stocking-glove presentation [10], but has also been reported to cause other, more unusual presentations including vocal fold palsy [1] and facial nerve palsy [3]. With paclitaxel, neurotoxic symptoms usually manifest in first 24 - 72 hours [13], which are dose dependent [14], and often associated with prior neurotoxic agents and underlying neuropathy [13] [14].

There has been one reported case of paclitaxel induced vocal fold paresis. The patient developed unilateral vocal fold paresis after her 3rd dose of paclitaxel which was reversed upon cessation of the drug [1]. Paclitaxel binds to the B-tubulin subunit, preventing of microtubule disassembly which leads to inability for a cell to divide and then its death. Like the vinca alkaloids, its toxic effects have been postulated though impairment of axoplasmic transport via its disruption of normal microtubule function [10]. In our case, like the previously cited cranial nerve neuropathies [3], neurotoxicity was reversible. Most instances of neuropathy have showed recovery within six months of drug cessation.

In contrast to the previously described case involving paclitaxel, our patient presented nearly six months after the completion of therapy as opposed to during the course of receiving paclitaxel. On exam, both vocal folds appeared paretic compared to the previously seen unilateral injury. Our patient's symptoms resolved with vigilant observation and no further treatment. It appears that from comparisons to the previously cited case, there can be a varied manifestation of paclitaxel-induced toxicity of the recurrent laryngeal nerve in both respects to time of presentation and clinical findings. This could imply that like vinca associated toxicity, many other patients might have undiagnosed paclitaxel mediated vocal fold injury and this phenomenon is underreported [11].

Other known neurotoxic chemotherapeutic drugs include ixabepilone, bortezomib, thalidomide, eribulin, nelarabine, cytarabine, procarbazine, and teoposdie. Though there have been no reports of vocal fold paresis with their use, patients on any of these chemotherapeutic drugs have the possibility of recurrent laryngeal nerve injury.

In our case, management of the bilateral vocal cord paresis was conservative, with the use of voice therapy and serial follow up. From the previously reported literature cases, patients with vocal fold paresis treatment ranged from observation to tracheotomy [5] [10] [11]. Ultimately, the magnitude of intervention is correlated to the level of airway obstruction and functional deficits that result from the vocal fold dysfunction.

4. Conclusion

While trauma, malignancy, and iatrogenic factors are common causes of vocal fold paresis, history of neurotoxic chemotherapeutic drugs should be part of any evaluation. This importance lies in the experience that it is often dose dependent and reversible, necessitating both cessation of the offending agent and the knowledge that any treatment is likely needed for only a temporary time. Though it is a diagnosis of exclusion, chemotherapy-induced vocal fold paresis should be in the differential for patients presenting with hoarseness, dysphonia, stridor and a positive chemotherapy history.

Conflict of Interest

The authors declare that they have no conflict of interest.

References

[1] Choi, B.S. and Robins, H.I. (2008) Reversible Paclitaxel-Induced Vocal Cord Paralysis with Later Recall with Vinorelbine. *Cancer Chemotherapy and Pharmacology*, **61**, 345-346. http://dx.doi.org/10.1007/s00280-007-0453-4

[2] Benninger, M.S., Gillen, J.B. and Altman, J.S. (1998) Changing Etiology of Vocal Fold immobility. *The Laryngoscope*, **108**, 1346-1350. http://dx.doi.org/10.1097/00005537-199809000-00016

[3] Lee, R.T., Oster, M.W., Balmaceda, C., Hesdorffer, C.S., Vahdat, L.T. and Papadopoulos, K.P. (1999) Bilateral Facial Nerve Palsy Secondary to the Administration of High-Dose Paclitaxel. *Annals of Oncology*, **10**, 1245-1247. http://dx.doi.org/10.1023/A:1008380800394

[4] Lash, S.C., Williams, C.P.R., Marsh, C.S., Crithchley, C., Hodgkins, P.R. and MacKie, E.J. (2004) Acute Sixth-Nerve Palsy after Vincristine Therapy. *Journal of American Association for Pediatric Ophthalmology and Strabismus*, **8**, 67-68. http://dx.doi.org/10.1016/j.jaapos.2003.07.010

[5] Abdul Latiff, Z., Azlin Kamal, N., Jahendran, J., Alias, H., See Goh, B., Zulkifli Syed Zakaria, S., *et al.* (2010) Vincristine-Induced Vocal Cord Palsy: Case Report and Review of the Literature. *Journal Pediatric Hematology Oncology*, **32**, 407-410. http://dx.doi.org/10.1097/MPH.0b013e3181e01584

[6] Burns, B.V. and Shotton, J.C. (1998) Vocal Fold Palsy Following Vinca Alkaloid Treatment. *The Journal of Laryngology and Otolaryngology*, **112**, 485-487.

[7] Ahmed, A., Williams, D. and Nicholson, J. (2007) Vincristine-Induced Bilateral Vocal Cord Paralysis in Children. *Pediatric Blood & Cancer*, **48**, 248. http://dx.doi.org/10.1002/pbc.20850

[8] Anghelescu, D., De Armendi, A.J., Thompson, J., Sillos, E.M.A., Pui, C.-H. and Sandlund, J. (2002) Vincristine-Induced Vocal Cord Paralysis in an Infant. *Paediatric Anaesthesia*, **12**, 168-170. http://dx.doi.org/10.1046/j.1460-9592.2002.00816.x

[9] Bacon, L.C., Barnett, M.J. and Abou Mourad, Y.R. (2012) Vincristine-Induced Vocal Cord Paralysis in a Patient with Acute Lymphoblastic Leukemia. *Annals of Hematology*, **91**, 971-972. http://dx.doi.org/10.1007/s00277-011-1348-3

[10] Miltenburg, N.C. and Boogerd, W. (2014) Chemotherapy-Induced Neuropathy: A Comprehensive Survey. *Cancer Treatment Reviews*, Published Online. http://dx.doi.org/10.1016/j.ctrv.2014.04.004

[11] Kuruvilla, G., Perry, S., Wilson, B. and El-Hakim, H. (2009) The Natural History of Vincristine-Induced Laryngeal Paralysis in Children. *Archives of Otolaryngology and Head and Neck Surgery*, **135**, 101-105. http://dx.doi.org/10.1001/archoto.2008.514

[12] Taha, H., Irfan, S. and Krishnamurthy, M. (1999) Cisplatin Induced Reversible Bilateral Vocal Cord Paralysis: An Undescribed Complication of Cisplatin. *Head and Neck*, **21**, 78-79. http://dx.doi.org/10.1002/(SICI)1097-0347(199901)21:1<78::AID-HED11>3.0.CO;2-7

[13] Lipton, R.B., Apfel, S.C., Dutcher, J.P., Rosenberg, R., Kaplan, J, Berger, A., Einzig, A.I., Wiernik, P. and Schaumburg H.H. (1989) Taxol Produces a Predominantly Sensory Neuropathy. *Neurology*, **39**, 368-373. http://dx.doi.org/10.1212/WNL.39.3.368

[14] Postma, T.J., Vermorken, J.B., Liefting, A.J.M., Pinedo, H.M. and Heimans, J.J. (1995) Paclitaxel Induced Neuropathy. *Annals of Oncology*, **6**, 489-494.

33

Online Case Based Self-Study Modules as an Adjunct Learning Tool in Otorhinolaryngology: A Pilot Study

Vijayalakshmi Subramaniam[1*], Rashmi Jain[2], Sivan Yegnanarayana Iyer Saraswathy[3], Varun Mishra[4]

[1]Department of Otorhinolaryngology, Yenepoya Medical College, Yenepoya University, Mangalore, India
[2]Department of Ophthalmology, Yenepoya Medical College, Yenepoya University, Mangalore, India
[3]Department of Community Medicine, PSG Institute of Medical Sciences & Research, Coimbatore, India
[4]Information Technology Consultant, Bangalore, India
Email: [*]vijayalakshmi.s@yenepoya.edu.in, [*]vijisubbu@gmail.com

Abstract

Background/Need for innovation: Undergraduate students in Otolaryngology are on the lookout for easy modes of learning which can help them understand concepts better as well as score more in examinations. A need was hence felt to introduce a new learning resource to supplement traditional teaching-learning methods. Methods: Digital, case based self–study modules were prepared using all open source technology and validated by experts in the specialty. The modules were uploaded on a website specifically created for the purpose. They were pilot tested on twenty consenting third year undergraduate (MBBS) students using a crossover design. Post test comprising of multiple choice questions was administered to the students after a period of two weeks. Feedback was obtained from faculty and students. Results: Test scores were found to be significantly higher amongst students who used the learning modules as a supplement to regular bedside teaching ($p < 0.001$; Wilcoxon signed rank test). Majority of students agreed that the modules helped them gain confidence during internal assessment examinations and would help revision. Conclusions: Online, case based, self-study modules helped students to perform better when used as a supplement to traditional teaching methods. Students agreed that it enabled easy understanding of subject and helped them gain confidence.

Keywords

Self-Study Modules, Teaching-Learning Methods, Web-Based Instruction, Online Learning

[*]Corresponding author.

1. Introduction

The undergraduate student is overburdened with information and is on the lookout for easier modes of learning for concept enhancement and better performance in examinations. Information Technology based (IT) applications have permeated through almost every field and medical education is no exception. Undergraduate training in Otolaryngology (ORL) is mainly imparted through traditional classroom based teaching, bedside clinics and operating room teaching. The combination of a web based forum with traditional methods would provide for a blended learning environment. While, bed side clinics continue to be the best setting in which the skills of history taking, physical examination, clinical reasoning, decision making, empathy and professionalism can be taught as a whole to medical students, online learning when combined with traditional methods is easily repeatable and can thus increase the effectiveness of teaching. As a facilitator in ORL, the first author felt the need to introduce a new learning resource to revive student interest in the subject of ORL and to promote active self-directed learning. This project was undertaken to develop case oriented self-study modules in ORL, evaluate the impact of these modules on student learning as well as assess student and faculty feedback on these online self learning modules.

2. Methodology

This study was done in a private medical college affiliated to a Deemed University in South India. Approval was obtained for the project from the University ethics committee. Discussions were initiated with IT experts in the university. Department faculty was apprised of the proposed project. Specific learning objectives for four "**MUST KNOW**" cases (Deviated Nasal septum, Antrochoanal polyp, Ethmoidal polyposis and Chronic Tonsillitis) were written. Digital self learning modules comprising interlinked history, clinical examination, investigations, diagnosis and patient management were developed. Videos and images were used. Flash player was used as a container for all videos. Hot Potatoes™ Version 6 (Free software for creating interactive multiple-choice, short-answer, jumbled-sentence, crossword, matching/ordering and gap-fill exercises for the World Wide Web; http://hotpot.uvic.ca/) was used for creating the quizzes, crosswords, matching and gap fill exercises (**Figure 1**). Feedback questionnaire for was designed using SurveyMonkey® (Online questionnaire and survey software; http://www.surveymonkey.com/). The modules were validated by experts in the specialty and uploaded on a dedicated website created for the purpose. The learning modules were pilot tested on 20 third year undergraduate (MBBS) students who gave consent to participate in the study. A cross over design was adopted and the students were randomly divided into two groups of 10 each. Access to two modules was secured to each group respectively. Both the groups were taught all the 4 cases during the bed side clinics as well.

After a period of two weeks, a post test comprising 40 multiple choice questions (10 questions pertaining to each module) was administered to both the groups. Student feedback on the modules was obtained using a 5-point Likert Scale questionnaire (5 = Very strongly agree 4 = Strongly agree 3 = Agree 2 = Strongly disagree 1 = Very strongly disagree). Faculty perceptions were assessed using a questionnaire. Post test scores obtained were statistically analyzed using Wilcoxon signed rank test. Internal consistency of the student feedback questionnaire was estimated by Cronbach alpha calculated using MS-Excel calculator. Likert scale responses were interpreted using Consensus measure [1].

3. Results

The Cronbach alpha of the student feedback questionnaire was 0.92. Mean rating for items analyzed in the student feedback ranged between 1.6 - 3.4 (1-strong agreement and 5-strong disagreement). The student feedback responses represented as Consensus measure are depicted in **Figure 2**. Majority (85%) of students agreed that the modules helped them gain confidence during internal assessment examinations and would help revision. They also felt that the quality of the modules with respect to audiovisual material was good but further improvements could be made with respect to resolution. Most students (95%; n = 19) also said that such modules should be prepared for all other topics in the subject and also the same should be replicated in other subjects as well. They also found the quizzes and crosswords embedded in each module to be interesting and agreed that such self study modules increased their understanding of the subject matter and its clinical application. Most of the students mentioned that the website was slow and videos took very long to load. This was also noted by the faculty. The strengths and weaknesses as described by the students and faculty in their feedback responses are

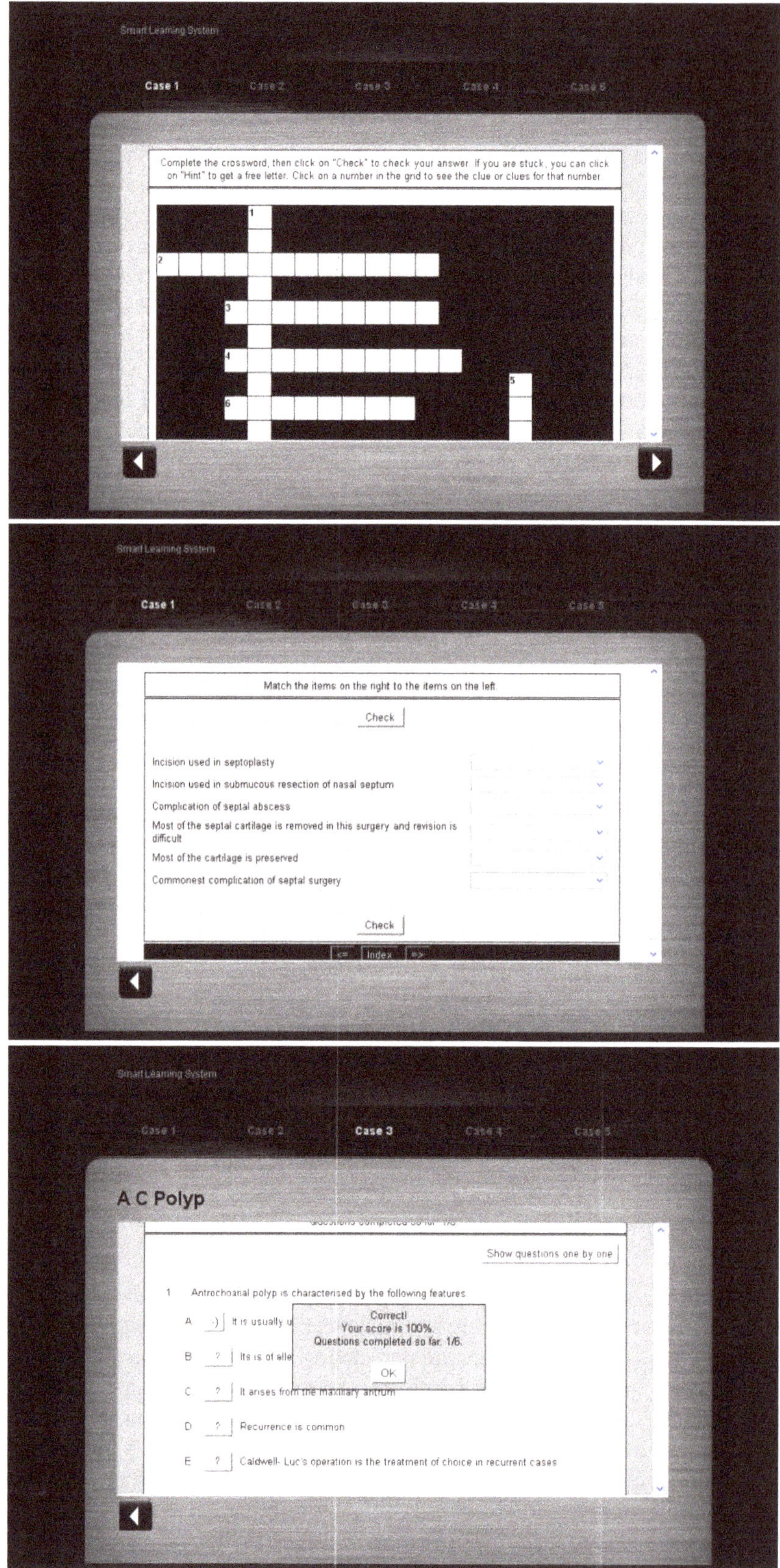

Figure 1. Screen shot of the crosswords, matching and gap fill exercises.

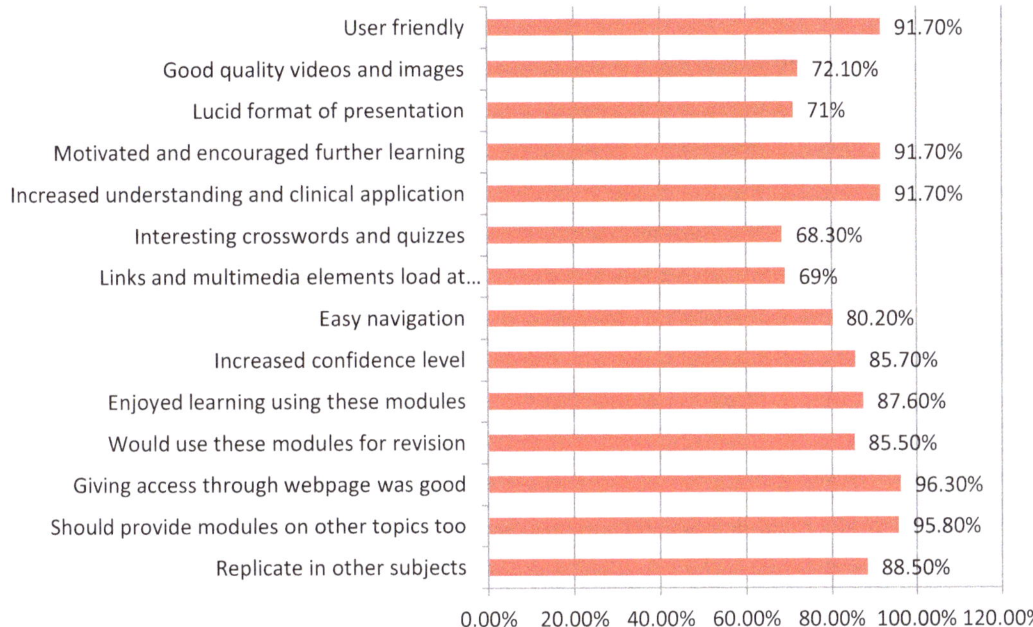

Figure 2. Students feedback-consensus measure (Values closer to 100 indicate greater agreement and values greater indicate greater disagreement).

summarised in **Table 1**. Post test scores were found to be significantly higher amongst students who used the learning modules as a supplement to traditional teaching ($p < 0.001$ as calculated by Wilcoxon signed rank test).

4. Discussion

Web based instruction has been gaining popularity in medical education in recent years. The combination of online instruction with traditional teaching methods has been observed to enhance learning outcomes [2]-[5]. Otorhinolaryngology (ORL) is one of the subjects taught to medical students during the third year medical undergraduate (MBBS) course in India. Teaching is accomplished through lectures, seminars and patient demonstrations. The internet offers an enriching platform and permits students to learn at their own pace. Online self study modules are an effective and inexpensive tool that could be used to enhance learning. They are easily repeatable and promote self-directed learning.

Online learning modules have been introduced in specialties such as emergency medicine, and pediatric and adolescent gynecology and increase in knowledge as well as test scores has been demonstrated [4] [5]. A pilot study done in the field of dermatology suggested that interactive IT based self learning modules could be combined effectively with a "play area concept". Although these did not improve student performance in their written examinations, the authors have opined that these modules would promote self-directed learning among students and thus enhance the quality of teaching and learning in dermatology [6]. Similarly, in a study where free online otolaryngology educational modules were provided to residents, quantifiable improvement in examination scores was not noted. However, it was recommended as an inexpensive way to enhance learning opportunities. The ease of access alone without the need to carry a textbook or journal made these modules a valuable learning resource [2].

The results of this study showed improved student performance when these modules were used as a supplement to traditional teaching methods as evidenced by better post test scores. Since the modules were case based, students opined that they were practical and increased their understanding of the subject. They also agreed strongly that they would use these modules to revise for exams. They found some of the crosswords tough for which they are being given more practice time. Both students and faculty remarked that the website was slow and videos took long to load. This aspect is being looked into by the IT experts. This was a pilot study and hence had the limitations of being tried on a small sample of students. The number of topics covered was also limited. However, the results are encouraging and gave us confidence that such modules could be prepared using open source technology even in resource limited settings like ours.

Table 1. Summary of strengths and weaknesses of learning modules as described by students and faculty.

STUDENTS		FACULTY	
Strengths	Weaknesses	Strengths	Weaknesses
Simple and clear explanation, easy to revise	Slow website—some videos don't load, no home/back button	Practical oriented, systematic approach to case	Slow website—videos don't load
Good videos, each module has small videos of short duration	Information overload	Fun filled interactive quizzes and crosswords	Doesn't cover entire course content, more modules need to be developed
The quizzes and crosswords were fun	Some crosswords were very tough to crack	Good audiovisuals, short videos, can be watched multiple times and hence improved retention	Few unclear images
Practical oriented	Resolution should be bigger	Clarity of presentation, caters to slow learners	Repetition is needed for difficult information

Future Plans

We plan to improve the existing modules based on the feedback received from students and make them more interactive. We also plan to develop more modules to cover the entire otolaryngology curriculum in future.

5. Conclusion

Online case based self learning modules increased students performance when used as an adjunct to traditional teaching methods for undergraduate teaching in ORL. They enabled easy understanding of subject among students and fostered confidence in them. These would help in revision for examinations. They serve as an efficient means of enhancing self-directed learning. It is therefore suggested that a virtual repository of case oriented self learning modules is created and used for training and assessment of students.

Source(s) of Support

This study was done as part of the Education Innovation Project during the FAIMER Fellowship Program at PSG-FAIMER Regional Institute, Coimbatore, India.

Conflicting Interest

Nil.

Acknowledgements

This study was done as part of the Education Innovation Project during the FAIMER Fellowship Program at PSG-FAIMER Regional Institute, Coimbatore, India. The authors acknowledge the support of Dr. Ghulam Jeelani Qadiri, Principal, Yenepoya Medical College, Mangalore, Dr. Thomas V. Chacko, Director, PSG-FRI and fellows and faculty of PSG-FAIMER Regional Institute, Coimbatore, India.

References

[1] Tastle, W.J., Russell, J. and Wierman, M.J. (2008) A New Measure to Analyze Student Performance Using the Likert Scale. *Information Systems Education Journal*, **6**. http://isedj.org/6/35/

[2] Cabrera-Muffly, C., Bryson, P.C., Sykes, K.J. and Shnayder, Y. (2015) Free Online Otolaryngology Educational Modules: A Pilot Study. *JAMA Otolaryngology—Head & Neck Surgery*, **141**, 324-328. http://dx.doi.org/10.1001/jamaoto.2015.41

[3] Kandasamy, T. and Fung, K. (2009) Interactive Internet-Based Cases for Undergraduate Otolaryngology Education. *Otolaryngology—Head and Neck Surgery*, **140**, 398-402. http://dx.doi.org/10.1016/j.otohns.2008.11.033

[4] Burnette, K., Ramundo, M., Stevenson, M. and Beeson, M.S. (2009) Evaluation of a Web-Based Asynchronous Pediatric Emergency Medicine Learning Tool for Residents and Medical Students. *Academic Emergency Medicine*, **16**, S46-S50. http://dx.doi.org/10.1111/j.1553-2712.2009.00598.x

[5] De Silva, N.K., Dietrich, J.E. and Young, A.E. (2010) Pediatric and Adolescent Gynecology Learned via a Web-Based Computerized Case Series. *Journal of Pediatric and Adolescent Gynecology*, **23**, 111-115. http://dx.doi.org/10.1016/j.jpag.2009.09.008

[6] Kaliyadan, F., Manoj, J., Dharmaratnam, A.D. and Sreekanth, G. (2010) Self-Learning Digital Modules in Dermatology: A Pilot Study. *Journal of the European Academy of Dermatology and Venereology*, **24**, 655-660. http://dx.doi.org/10.1111/j.1468-3083.2009.03478.x

34

Prognostic Significance of Vascular Endothelial Growth Factor-A (VEGF-A) and Ki-67 Expression in Head and Neck Cancer Patient with Negative Neck

Vipa Boonkitticharoen[1], Boonchu Kulapaditharom[2], Noppadol Larbcharoensub[3], Phurich Praneetvatakul[2], Thongchai Bhongmakapat[2]

[1]Department of Diagnostic and Therapeutic Radiology, Ramathibodi Hospital, Mahidol University, Bangkok, Thailand
[2]Department of Otolaryngology, Ramathibodi Hospital, Mahidol University, Bangkok, Thailand
[3]Department of Pathology, Ramathibodi Hospital, Mahidol University, Bangkok, Thailand
Email: vipa.bon@mahidol.ac.th

Abstract

Background: Management of N0 neck in patients with head and neck squamous cell carcinoma (HNSCC) remains a subject of continued debate. Prognostic biomarkers might provide useful information for treatment selection and adjustment. Objective: To evaluate the prognostic relevance of VEGF-A and Ki-67 expression to types of neck management. Methods: This prospective study included 140 patients with HNSCC. Tumor expression of VEGF-A and Ki-67 was measured by immunohistochemistry. Based on tumor size and site criteria, 88 patients with N0 neck were categorized as high, intermediate and low risk of subclinical neck diseases and accordingly treated by elective neck dissection (END), irradiation (ENI) and observation. Adjuvant treatment was given to tumor with close or positive margins. A multivariate Cox regression model was used to identify prognostic factors. Impact of biomarker expression, treatment type and risk category on disease-specific survival (DSS) in the setting of N0 neck were evaluated by Kaplan-Meier survival and adjusted hazard ratio (HR). Results: Coexpression of VEGF-A and Ki-67 (HR = 2.351, $p = 0.021$) and positive node (HR = 2.301, $p = 0.009$) were independent prognostic factors for HNSCC. In the setting of N0 neck, marker coexpression has an HR of 4.97 ($p = 0.004$) independent of treatment modalities ($p = 0.069$) and risk categories ($p = 0.971$). Alternatively, neither marker expression was predictive of a better treatment outcome for END compared to ENI, as suggested by the odds of patients being survived 15.4 times greater ($p = 0.01$) and the 5-year DSS rates of 85.1% versus 44.7% ($p = 0.008$). Conclusion: Coexpression of VEGF-A and Ki-67 is a suggestion of tumor micro-invasiveness in addition to risk of lymph node metastasis and may indicate the need of adjuvant

treatment despite negative tumor margins. Neither marker expression serves an indicator for the selection of END over ENI in neck management.

Keywords

Head and Neck Squamous Cell Carcinoma, Negative Neck Node, Neck Management, Prognostic Biomarkers, VEGF-A and Ki-67

1. Introduction

Head and neck squamous cell carcinoma (HNSCC) has a high propensity to invade lymph nodes in the cervical region before the development of distant metastasis [1]. The presence of nodal metastases is the most important factor for prognosis and treatment plan [2]. In patient with clinically N0 neck (cN0), there is still a high rate of occult nodal metastasis (12% - 50%) which is strongly dependent of site and T class of the primary tumor [3]. For instance, T1 cancer of the oral cavity excluding the oral tongue has the lowest rate of subclinical neck disease (<20%) as opposed to tumors of the pyriform sinus, base of tongue, supraglottic larynxes have the highest rate (>30%) despite their early T class [4] [5]. Based on a decision analysis taking into account the incidence of occult metastasis, disease control rate and treatment complications, treatment of the neck is advised for patient with a risk of subclinical neck disease ≥ 20% [6].

In management of patients with cN0 neck, there are three policies advocated: a watchful waiting policy for those with a risk < 20%; elective neck dissection (END) or elective neck irradiation (ENI) for a risk ≥ 20%; and neck treatment plus adjuvant therapy for the high risk patients [7] [8]. More than two decades since the adoption of Weiss's recommendation to treat the cN0 neck with a risk ≥ 20%, head and neck oncologists continue to debate on the appropriate strategy in neck management. Central to the debate is the issue surrounding whether a patient with cN0 neck should be treated now or be closely observed, whether the patient should be treated by END or receive ENI [9].

Pretreatment risk stratification of patients may provide information that helps selecting the appropriate modality in neck management for a particular risk category [9]. Mendenhall *et al.* [4] [5] defined risk of subclinical neck diseases on the basis of tumor T class and anatomical location to allow the stratification of patients into three risk groups: high risk > 30%; intermediate risk 20% - 30% and low risk < 20%. With an additional inclusion of prognostic markers relevant to tumor progression and metastasis, risk stratification might place the oncologist in a better position to select the most appropriate therapeutic approach for individual patients.

Recent advances in molecular biology have revealed that primary tumor is predisposed to metastasize [10]. Maintenance of primary tumor gene expression profiles in lymph node (LN) metastases [10] suggests the use of biomarkers expressing on primary tumor specimen as markers for the presence of occult LN metastases [11]. Metastasis is a highly complicated process resulting from epigenetic and genetic alterations so as to provide tumor cells with proliferative advantage, capability to evade apoptosis and to escape immune surveillance. To metastasize, tumor cells must further acquire the ability to degrade interstitial matrix, lose cell-to-cell contact, invade blood and lymph vessels and to induce angiogenesis and lymphangiogenesis [12] [13]. Proteins that have been identified as promoters of LN metastasis in HNSCC can be grouped according to their biological functions: cell cycle regulation and proliferation [e.g. epidermal growth factor receptor (EGFR), cyclin D1, Ki-67]; tumor suppressor and apoptosis [e.g. p53, p21, Bcl-2]; cell adhesion and matrix degradation [e.g. cadherins, CD44, matrix metalloproteinases (MMPs)]; tumor hypoxia [e.g. hypoxia inducible factor-1 (HIF-1), carbonic anhydrase IX (CA IX), glucose transporters (GLUT)]; angiogenesis and lymphangiogesis [e.g. VEGF-A, VEGF-C, LYE-1] [14]-[16]. Since tumor proliferation and angiogenesis are known to play important part in tumor progression and metastasis [12], VEGF-A, an angiogenesis regulator, and Ki-67, a proliferation marker, are markers of interest for their associations with LN metastasis [17]-[22] and prognosis in HNSCC [19] [21] [23]-[25]. In our previous study, increased expression of Ki-67 was associated with positive neck nodes, either expression of VEGF-A or Ki-67 was recognized in tumor with advanced T class. Coexpression of VEGF-A and Ki-67 represented an aggressive tumor phenotype for being associated to LN metastasis especially in early tumor of the oral cavity, oropharynx and hypopharynx [20].

This investigation is the continuum of a prospective study on the use of VEGF-A and Ki-67 in prediction of

LN metastasis in HNSCC [20]. The purposes of this study were two-folds, namely: 1) to assess whether combined VEGF-A and Ki-67 expression represented an independent prognostic index for this series of surgery treated HNSCC; 2) to evaluate the impact of VEGF-A and Ki-67 expression on survival of patients with N0 neck underwent various modalities of neck management from observation, ENI, END to END plus adjuvant treatment.

2. Patients and Methods

2.1. Study Overview

This prospective study cohort has been previously described [20]. A total of 147 patients diagnosed with squamous cell carcinoma (SCC) of the head and neck were consecutively included during 2001-2005 at Department of Otolaryngology, Ramathibodi Hospital. The inclusion criteria were treatment-naive patients with resectable SCC of the oral cavity, oropharynx, hypopharynx and larynx, stage I-IV. Patients with distant metastasis or recurrence disease were excluded. Pretreatment tumor specimens were obtained upon the agreement with Ramathibodi Hospital Ethics Committee in the use of tumor specimens for scientific analysis and receiving patients' written informed consents. The paraffin-embedded tumor specimens were stained for the expression of VEGF-A and Ki-67 by immunohistochemistry. The techniques of tissue staining and methods for determination of marker expression have been described in details in our previous study [20].

To evaluate whether VEGF-A and Ki-67 expression could serve as a significant prognostic indicator for the present series of patients with surgery treated tumor of the head and neck, demographic (age and gender), and clinicopathological factors (tumor grade and location, T stage and nodal status) were included in survival analysis. Of a total of 147 patients included previously, only 140 were eligible for study because of the availability of complete data for survival analysis. Of these 140 patients, 52 (37.1%) had pathologically confirmed positive neck nodes and 88 (62.9%) had negative nodes either clinically defined or pathologically confirmed. Demographic, clinicopathological characteristics and biomarker expression in patients with positive and negative necks are presented in **Table 1**.

Table 1. Demographic, clinicopathologic and biological variables in association with nodal status.

Variable	Total, n	Node negative n (%)	Node positive n (%)	*p*
Age at diagnosis				
≤64 years	73	43 (58.9)	30 (41.1)	0.40
>64 years	67	45 (67.2)	22 (32.8)	
Sex				
Male	112	73 (34.8)	39 (65.2)	0.36
Female	28	15 (46.4)	13 (53.6)	
Tumor site				
Oral cavity	57	40 (70.2)	17 (29.8)	<<0.0001
Pharynx	27	3 (11.1)	24 (88.9)	
Larynx	56	45 (80.4)	11 (19.6)	
Differentiation				
Well	89	64 (71.9)	25 (28.1)	0.014
Moderate and poor	51	24 (47.1)	27 (52.9)	
T stage				
T1, 2	62	46 (74.2)	16 (25.8)	0.021
T3, 4	78	42 (53.8)	36 (46.2)	
VEGF-A				
High > 2.74	55	25 (45.5)	30 (54.5)	0.001
Low ≤ 2.74	85	63 (74.1)	22 (25.9)	
Ki-67				
High > 58.61%	55	31 (56.4)	24 (43.6)	0.21
Low ≤ 58.61%	85	58 (68.2)	27 (31.8)	
Combined expression				
Both high	27	11 (40.7)	16 (59.3)	0.008
Either high	59	36 (61)	23 (39)	
Neither high	54	41 (75.9)	13 (24.1)	

2.2. Risk Category and Treatment of Patients with N0 Neck

Eighty-eight patients with N0 neck were grouped as high risk, intermediate risk and low risk of occult neck diseases according to risk definition defined by Mendenhall *et al.* [4] [5]. The high risk group (>30%) includes T1-4 pyriform sinus and base of tongue; T2-4 oropharynx (soft palate and tonsil), hypopharynx (pharyngeal wall) and supraglottic larynx; T3-4 oral cavity (floor of mouth, tongue, retro molar trigone, gingival, hard palate and buccal mucosa); T4 glottis. The intermediate risk group (20% - 30%) comprises T1-2 oral tongue; T1 oropharynx, hypopharynx and supraglottic larynx; T2 oral cavity and T3 glottis. The low risk group (<20%) encompasses T1 oral cavity and T1-2 glottis.

Table 2 shows the risk groups in this series.

Elective treatment of the neck was performed in patient with a risk of subclinical neck disease ≥ 20% [6]. Initially, elective neck dissection (END) was conducted for patients with cN0 neck (105 cases) at the time of primary surgery. Post-operative radiotherapy (PORT) was given to patients of the high risk group with the following features: tumor with closed surgical margins, T3-4 tumor of the oropharynx, hypopharynx and supraglottic larynx. Concomitant chemoradiotherapy (CCRT) using cisplatin was administered to patient with positive tumor margins. Patients of the intermediate risk group including T3-4 tumor with negative margins were either treated by END or elective neck irradiation (ENI). No neck treatment was given to the low risk group except for those T1 cancers of the floor of mouth and T2 glottic cancer to which ENI was prescribed. Patients (17 cases) with metastatic nodal diseases uncovered subsequently by histologic examination of the dissected lymph node specimens were excluded from this study (**Table 3**).

Table 2. Risk category according to tumor T class and location [4] [5].

Risk category	Occult neck diseases	T	Primary tumor site	n (%)
High	>30%	T3-4	Pyriform sinus and base of tongue	3 (8.3%)
n = 36		T3-4	Lip, buccal mucosa, tongue and hard palate	11 (30.6%)
		T2-4	Supraglottis	10 (27.8%)
		T4	Glottis	11 (30.5%)
		T3	Subglottis	1 (2.8%)
Intermediate	20% - 30%	T2	Lip, buccal mucosa and hard palate	3 (10.3%)
n = 29		T1-2	Tongue	18 (62.1%)
		T3	Glottis	8 (27.6%)
Low	<20%	T1	Lip and floor of mouth	8 (34.78%)
n = 23		T1-2	Glottis	14 (60.87%)
		T2	Subglottis	1 (4.35%)

Table 3. Biomarker expression profiles and types of neck management in patients with different risks of subclinical neck diseases. Data show number (percent).

	High risk	Intermediate risk	Low risk	*p*
	n = 36	n = 29	n = 23	
VEGF-A and Ki-67				0.002
Both high	2 (5.6)	5 (17.2)	4 (17.4)	
Either high	23 (63.9)	5 (17.2)	8 (34.8)	
Neither high	11 (30.6)	19 (65.5)	11 (47.8)	
Neck management				
END + Adj Tx	17 (47.2)	–	–	0.000
ENI	11 (30.6)	15 (51.7)	7 (30.4)	
END	8 (22.2)	14 (48.3)	–	
Observation	–	–	16 (69.6)	

END + Adj Tx: Elective neck dissection + adjuvant treatment; ENI: Elective neck irradiation; END: Elective neck dissection.

2.3. Follow-Up and Time-to-Event Measurement

The follow-up started after treatment completion in every 2 months during the first year, every 3 months in the second and every 6 months thereafter. Disease-specific survival (DSS) was the endpoint of outcome for this study. Time-to-event was defined as the duration since the date of diagnosis to the date of tumor-related death or the date of last follow-up for patients who were still alive. Data were censored for patients who were alive at the end of study; lost to follow-up; dead from causes not attributable to cancer. This study had a median follow-up time of 44 months (range, 1 - 102.1 months).

2.4. Biomarker Cutoffs for Prognostic Study

The expression of Ki-67 was determined by the percentage of positive tumor cells in hot spot area. For VEGF-A, a score varying from 0 to 4 was graded on the basis of stained intensity and percentage of cell stained [20]. In general, a median value is arbitrarily chosen as a cutoff for biomarker expression [19] [20]. In this prognostic study, optimal cutoff was chosen at a level yielding the most significant hazard ratio (HR) adjusted for potential confounding factors including age at diagnosis, gender, tumor site, tumor differentiation, T stage and nodal status. To this end, cutoffs for biomarker expression were step-wisely increased from the 50th percentile up to the 70th percentile with a five percentile increment. In the context of combined marker expression, the most significant HR of 2.357 ($p = 0.021$) was achieved at the 60th percentile cutoff, *i.e.* VEGF-A score of 2.74 and Ki-67 labeling index of 58.61%.

2.5. Statistical Analysis

Comparison of categorical data between groups was conducted by χ^2 or Fisher Exact test as appropriate. Survival analyses were performed using Predictive Analytics Software (PASW) statistics 18 (SPCC Inc., Chicago, IL, USA). To identify independent prognostic factors for this patient cohort, univariate and multivariate analyses were carried out using Cox proportional hazard regression model. Besides biomarker expression, the survival analysis also included factors generally known to influence survival of head and neck cancer patients. These factors are age at diagnosis, sex, tumor site, tumor differentiation, T stage and nodal status [26]. Significant prognostic factors were judged from the value of HR > 1 and the level of significance at $p < 0.05$. The final prognostic model was constructed by including variables with p values ≤ 0.1.

In the setting of N0 neck, impact of risk category, type of neck management and biomarker expression on DSS was assessed by Kaplan-Meier survival curve, and multivariate Cox regression model. All statistical tests were two-tailed and p value < 0.05 was considered significant.

3. Results

3.1. Prognostic Factors for HNSCC

The median follow-up time for this study was 44 months (range, 1 - 102.1 months). During follow-up periods, a total of 70 patients died: 60 due to HNSCC, 10 from tumor-unrelated causes such as diseases of the lung and liver, heart attack, old age, etc; 16 patients were lost to follow-up; 44 patients were alive at the time of last contact. The impact on disease-specific survival (DSS) was evaluated for a number of potential influencing factors including age at diagnosis, sex, primary tumor site, tumor differentiation, T stage, nodal status, and biomarker expression using univariate and multivariate Cox proportion hazard regression models. Results of the analyses are presented in **Table 4**. In univariate analysis, significant associations with poor DSS were observed for tumor of the oral cavity and pharynx in contrasting to the larynx (HR = 1.836, $p = 0.029$), positive lymph node (HR = 3.022, $p = 0.000$), increase expression of VEGF-A (HR = 1.932, $p = 0.001$), Ki-67 (HR = 1.744, $p = 0.032$) and coexpression of VEGF-A and Ki-67 (HR = 2.987, $p = 0.001$). In multivariate analysis, only positive lymph node (HR = 2.301, $p = 0.009$) and biomarker coexpression (HR = 2.357, $p = 0.021$) remained significant.

3.2. Impact of Risk Category, Biomarker Expression and Modality of Neck Management on Survival of Patients with N0 Neck

In univariate survival analysis, combined marker expression ($p = 0.001$) and modality of neck management ($p = 0.014$) were significantly affecting DSS in contrasting to the nonsignificant effect of the risk category ($p = 0.618$) (**Figures 1-3**). Multivariate Cox regression analysis revealed an overall significant p level of 0.013 for VEGF-A

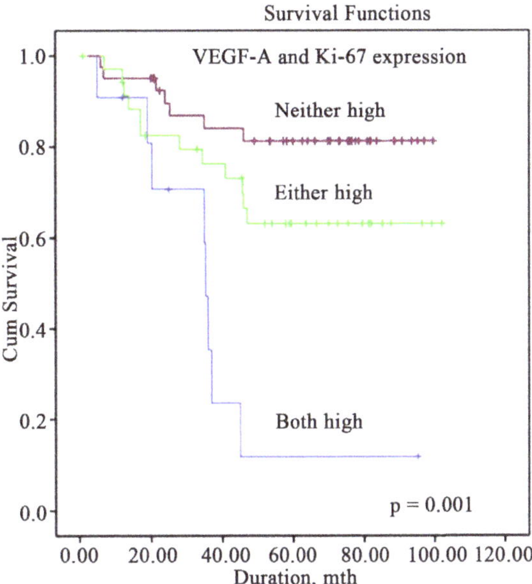

Figure 1. Kaplan-Meier survival curves for patients with tumor expressing both VEGF-A and Ki-67, either and neither markers.

Table 4. Cox proportional hazard regression analyses of prognostic factors for disease-specific survival (DSS).

Variable	Univariate		Multivariate Multivariate	
	HR (95% CI)	*p*	HR (95% CI)	*p*
Age at diagnosis				
>64 years	1.086 (0.654 - 1.801)	0.751	1.289 (0.765 - 2.173)	0.340
≤64 years	1		1	
Sex				
Male	0.848 (0.458 - 1.568)	0.599	1.253 (0.653 - 2.402)	0.498
Female	1		1	
Tumor site				
Oral and pharynx	1.836 (1.063 - 3.169)	0.029	1.650 (0.880 - 3.092)	0.118
Larynx	1		1	
Differentiation				
Moderate and poor	1.11 (0.66 - 1.869)	0.694	0.705 (0.401 - 1.238)	0.223
Well	1		1	
T stage				
T3,4	1.43 (0.85 - 2.408)	0.178	1.239 (0.701 - 2.189)	0.461
T1,2	1		1	
Nodal status				
N+	3.022 (1.809 - 5.049)	0.000	2.301 (1.231 - 4.304)	0.009
N0	1		1	
VEGF-A				
High > 2.74	1.932 (1.161 - 3.215)	0.011	1.435 (0.807 - 2.553)	0.219
Low ≤ 2.74	1		1	
Ki-67				
High > 58.61	1.744 (1.05 - 2.898)	0.032	1.559 (0.929 - 2.615)	0.093
Low ≤ 58.61%	1		1	
Combined expression				
Both high	2.987 (1.569 - 5.687)	0.001	2.357 (1.14 - 4.873)	0.021
Either high	1.241 (0.665 - 2.314)	0.498	1.187 (0.559 - 2.353)	0.624
Neither high	1		1	

HR: Hazard ratio; CI: Confidence interval.

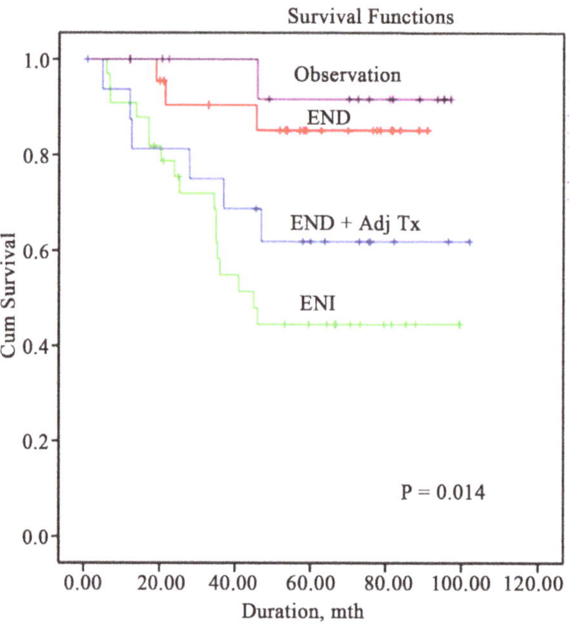

Figure 2. Kaplan-Meier survival curves for patients underwent different neck managements from elective neck dissection plus adjuvant treatment (END + Adj Tx), elective neck dissection (END), elective neck irradiation (ENI) to observation.

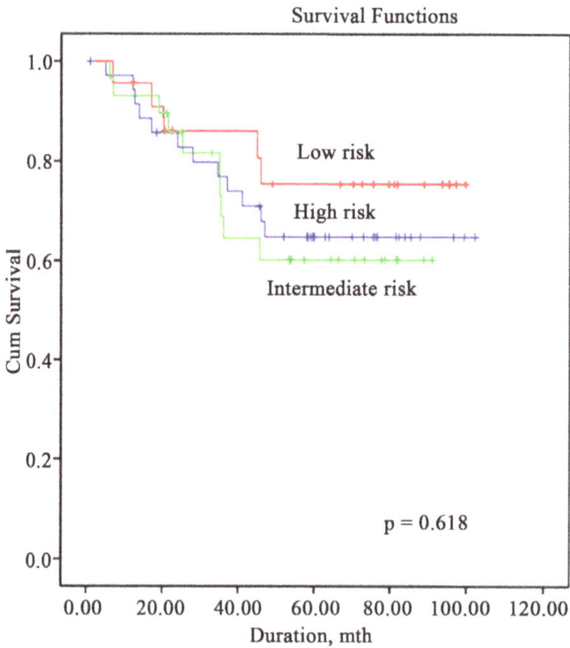

Figure 3. Kaplan-Meier survival curves for patients categorized as low, intermediate and high risks of subclinical neck diseases.

and Ki-67 expression. In relative to tumor with neither marker expression, only coexpression of VEGF-A and Ki-67 was observed with a significant HR of 4.97 ($p = 0.004$). For the modality of neck management, the impact was at a marginally significant level with a p value of 0.069. In comparing different types of neck treatment to observation, significant HR of 8.737 ($p = 0.036$) was obtained for neck treatment by ENI, and a marginally significant HR of 6.043 ($p = 0.098$) for END + adjuvant treatment (**Table 5**).

Table 5. Multivariate Cox regression analysis of the impact of biomarker expression and neck management on disease-specific survival.

Variable	HR	95% CI		*p*
		Lower	Upper	
VEGF-A and Ki-67				0.013
Both high	4.97	1.669	14.804	0.004
Either high	1.659	0.651	4.41	0.28
Neither high	1	–	–	–
Neck management				0.069
END + Adj Tx	6.043	0.717	50.911	0.098
ENI	8.737	1.152	66.263	0.036
END	2.621	0.269	25.504	0.407
Observation	1	–	–	–

HR: Hazard ratio; CI: Confidence interval; END + Adj Tx: Elective neck dissection + adjuvant treatment; ENI: Elective neck irradiation; END: Elective neck dissection.

3.3. Dependence of Treatment Outcomes on Biomarker Expression and Type of Neck Management

Table 6 shows how different types of neck management and patterns of combined marker expression influencing the treatment outcomes in patients with different risks of occult neck diseases. Mutual dependence among treatment outcomes, types of neck treatment and patterns of combined marker expression were tested using a 2 × 2 × 3 three-dimensional contingency table. By pair-wise comparison, results of χ^2 analyses of contingency tables are presented in **Table 7** along with log-rank test of the Kaplan-Meier survival curves.

There were two important observations according to data shown in **Table 6**. Patients with coexpression of VEGF-A and Ki-67 had a great chance (8/11 = 72.7%) to die regardless the type of neck management. On the other hand, tumors expressing neither marker were better controlled by END (with and without adjuvant treatment) than those treated by ENI. The odds of patients being alive/censored in END group were 15.4 times greater than the ENI group ($p = 0.01$). This offered an explanation why the survival for patients in the END treated group was superior to the ENI group (**Figure 2**). Five-year DSS rates for END and ENI given to patients with similar risks of occult neck diseases, *i.e.* intermediate to high risks, were 85.1% and 44.7%, respectively (p = 0.008). Radio-biologically, dividing cells are more radiosensitive than the nondividing cells. Therefore, ENI was less effective in eradicating the nondividing metastatic cells disseminated from tumor expressing neither markers. This was in contrasting to END which involved surgical removal of lymph nodes with occult metastases regardless their radiobiological property. Equivalent treatment outcomes between END and observation would implicate the effectiveness of END in removal of the subclinical neck diseases to achieve an outcome comparable to that of the observation group with low risk of occult neck diseases. This was further supported by the treatment outcome in END + adjuvant treatment group. Despite the unfavorable biomarker expression profiles similar to those of the ENI group ($p = 0.165$) and the clinicopathologically severe features in this group (*i.e.* high risk anatomical location and close or positive tumor margins), effective removal of subclinical neck diseases by END particularly in patients expressing neither markers helped improving patient survival. Pair-wise comparison of Kaplan-Meier survival curves between END + adjuvant treatment versus END or observation were nonsignificant, with *p* values of 0.099 and 0.052, respectively. Five-year DSS rates among these groups were 61.9% for END + adjuvant treatment, 85.1% for END and 91.7% for observation.

4. Discussion

Management of the negative neck in patients with HNSCC is a subject of extensive debate. Issue central to the debate usually involves the question whether END would offer a survival advantage over the policy of watchful waiting. When there is an indication for neck treatment, should a patient be treated with END or ENI [19].

Table 6. Biomarker expression in association with treatment outcomes in patients of different risk categories underwent various types of neck management. Data show number of patients.

Neck management	VEGF-A and Ki-67	High risk			Intermediate risk			Low risk		
		Dead	Censored	Total	Dead	Censored	Total	Dead	Censored	Total
END + Adj Tx	Both	2	0	2	–	–	–	–	–	–
	Either	4	7	11	–	–	–	–	–	–
	Neither	0	4	4	–	–	–	–	–	–
	Total	6	11	17	–	–	–	–	–	–
ENI	Both	0	0	0	3	1	4	2	0	2
	Either	4	5	9	1	1	2	1	2	3
	Neither	2	0	2	3	6	9	1	1	2
	Total	6	5	11	7	8	15	4	3	7
END	Both	0	0	0	1	0	1	–	–	–
	Either	0	3	3	1	2	3	–	–	–
	Neither	0	5	5	1	9	10	–	–	–
	Total	0	8	8	3	11	14	–	–	–
Observation	Both	–	–	–	–	–	–	0	2	2
	Either	–	–	–	–	–	–	1	4	5
	Neither	–	–	–	–	–	–	0	9	9
	Total	–	–	–	–	–	–	1	15	16

END + Adj Tx: Elective neck dissection + adjuvant treatment; ENI: Elective neck irradiation; END: Elective neck dissection.

Table 7. Pair-wise comparison between treatment outcomes in terms of Kaplan-Meier survival or frequency data presented in a 2 × 2 × 3 three-dimensional contingency table. Data show p values of the tests.

	Analysis	END + Adj Tx	ENI	END	Observation
END + Adj Tx	Kaplan-Meier survival	–	0.308	0.099	0.052
	Contingency table	–	0.165	< 0.001	0.013
ENI	Kaplan-Meier survival	0.308	–	0.005	0.005
	Contingency table	0.165	–	0.002	0.025
END	Kaplan-Meier survival	0.099	0.005	–	0.517
	Contingency table	<0.001	0.002	–	0.327
Observation	Kaplan-Meier survival	0.052	0.005	0.517	–
	Contingency table	0.013	0.025	0.327	–

END + Adj Tx: Elective neck dissection + adjuvant treatment; ENI: Elective neck irradiation; END: Elective neck dissection.

At our institute, strategy of neck management has been based on the site and T class of the primary tumor. The decision to treat the neck was made when a risk of subclinical neck disease ≥ 20% [6]. The types of neck management were in well accord with the risk categories defined by Mendenhall *et al.* [4] [5]. END + adjuvant treatment was prescribed for patients of the high risk group with unfavorable clinicopathological features: PORT was given to high stage tumor of the oropharynx, hypopharynx and supraglottic larynx, tumor with closed margins; CCRT for tumor of positive margins. Neck treatment either by END or ENI was performed in patients of the high risk group with negative tumor margins and those of the intermediate risk group. Close observation was planned for T1 tumor of the oral cavity and glottis. However, ENI was prescribed for T1 tumor of the floor of mouth and T2 glottic tumor. Five-year DSS rates for this series were 61.9% for END + adjuvant treatment, 85.1% for END, 44.6% for ENI and 91.7% for observation.

The aim of this study was to investigate whether the combined expression of VEGF-A and Ki-67 would provide prognostic information useful for treatment selection or adjustment. Previously, coexpression of VEGF-A and Ki-67 was observed to be an aggressive tumor phenotype for the high likelihood of 6.46 to observe lymph node metastases especially in early stage tumor of the oral cavity, oropharynx and hypopharynx [20]. In this study, coexpression of these markers was an independent prognostic indicator regardless the presence or absence of the nodal diseases. In the setting of N0 neck, marker coexpression was significantly associated with poor patient survival with an HR of 4.97 ($p = 0.013$). To the best of our knowledge, no other study has been reported for the prognostication of combined marker expression in the context of N0 neck management. However, combined biomarker expression in effective detection of LN metastasis in HNSCC was reported by other. A four-protein signature which was defined by gene products involving tumor growth, invasion and metastasis expressed on primary tumor was used in prediction of LN metastasis and survival of patients with oral SCC [27]. This four-protein signature was defined by epidermal growth factor receptor (EGFR), v-erb-b2 erythroblastic leukemia viral oncogene homolog 2 (HER-2/neu), laminin gamma 2 (LAMC 2) and ras homolog family membrane C (RHOC). The investigators reported that with a combined expression of any 2 or more proteins of the signature could detect LN metastases at sensitivity and specificity of 70% and 87.5%, respectively and could predict DSS with an adjusted HR of 5.506 ($p = 0.036$). For bladder cancer, a molecular grading model defined by combined VEGF and Ki-67 expression profiles has been used for predicting tumor recurrence and progression in noninvasive urothelial bladder cancer [28]. The molecular grades were scored: mG3 (both Ki-67 and VEGF were highly expressed), mG2 (either Ki-67 or VEGF was highly expressed) and mG1 (neither Ki-67 nor VEGF was highly expressed). Sensitivity and specificity of the combined markers in predicting tumor recurrence were 91.18% and 81.25%, respectively as opposed to the lower detection rates obtained by single markers, *i.e.* 73.53% for Ki-67 and 66.67% for VEGF.

In our study, 8 out of 11 patients with VEGF-A and Ki-67 coexpression died regardless the type of neck management. This raised a question whether such an expression profile reflected the microinvasiveness of the primary tumor in addition to the presence of the occult neck diseases. The 5-year DSS rate was 34.9% for patients with positive nodes in contrasting to the 11.8% for marker coexpression in the setting of N0 neck. Therefore, marker coexpression in patients with N0 neck might indicate the microinvasiveness of the primary tumor as well as the risk of occult neck disease. Furthermore, among 8 patients who failed, there were only 2 cases receiving the adjuvant treatment of the primary tumor. This led to the postulation that suboptimal treatment of patients with such an aggressive biological feature could be the cause of failure. Henceforth, VEGF-A and Ki-67 coexpression might serve an index in addition to tumor margins in identifying patients who might be benefited from the adjuvant treatment.

On the contrary, there was a question whether neither marker expression would indicate the absence of subclinical neck disease due to a favorable 5-year DSS rate of 81.2% and therefore would be used as an indicator suggesting neck management by wait-and-observe policy. In this subset of 41 patients, 19 were treated by END (with and without adjuvant treatment), 13 by ENI and 9 by observation. If the subclinical neck disease was absence, one could anticipate the nonsignificant treatment outcomes among these different modalities of neck management. But in fact, the odds of being survived for patients treated by END (with and without adjuvant treatment) were 15 times greater than those treated by ENI. The survival benefit for patients with neither marker expression was therefore due to surgical removal of lymph nodes containing nondividing disseminated tumor cells which were radioresistant.

In the use of END or ENI in treating patients of the same risk category, *i.e.* intermediate to high risks, a better survival was observed for END with a 5-year DSS rate of 85.1% as opposed to 44.7% for ENI. How was this observation compared to other studies? In general, ENI is an option for patients who are poor surgical candidates. Limited studies were conducted to allow the comparison of the effectiveness between END and ENI. In a prospective study using similar clinical criteria, *i.e.* tumor size and site, in management of cN0 neck for patients with SCC of the oral cavity, the authors reported the 3-year DSS rates of 86% for END and 67% for ENI [29]. These survival rates were comparable to those obtained in the current series. Our 3-year DSS rates estimated for END and ENI were 90.4% and 53.6%, respectively. Why patient survival from ENI treatment was poorer than

END. In the ENI treated group, despite the similarity in distributions of tumor site and T class, a few more patients with coexpression of VEGF-A and Ki-67 and the radioresistance of the subclinical neck diseases in patients with tumors expressing neither markers would be factors contributing to the lower rate of tumor control. Although the biomarker study did not provide information for whom should be spared from the neck treatment, it did suggest a treatment adjustment for patients who were originally planned for neck irradiation to consider neck dissection when their tumor expressing neither markers.

In comparison of treatment outcomes between END and observation which involved patients of different risk categories, *i.e.* intermediate to high risk for END and low risk for observation, survival equivalent between these neck management modalities should not be misjudged as similarity in treatment effects but rather the equivalence in outcomes of neck management in different clinical contexts, *i.e.* the effectiveness of END in removal of the subclinical neck diseases and the absence of the occult metastasis in close observation. In spite of the favorable treatment efficacy with END, there is still a concern on the unnecessary neck treatment for approximately 70% of patients who actually do not harbor the metastatic cells in their necks. In indentifying whom to be treated or spared from the neck treatment, we may need a sensitive and reliable method like sentinel node biopsy (SNB) [9]. Nevertheless, the SNB technique, although clinically attractive, is still in the investigational stage for cancer of the head and neck [9] and provides no information regarding to tumor biological behavior.

Head and neck cancers are heterogeneous in anatomical location and biological behavior. We acknowledge our study limitations for the inclusion of cancer arising from the oral cavity and the larynx and the small number of patients. Further study with large sample size is warranted to ascertain the consistency of the findings so as to gain acceptance of the use of these biomarkers as a complementary tool to the standard clinicopathological criteria in selecting the best treatment for individual patients.

5. Conclusion

Coexpression of VEGF-A and Ki-67 was a significant prognostic factor independent of modalities of neck management in the setting of N0 neck. Such a pattern of marker expression is a suggestion of an aggressive tumor phenotype implicating the microinvasiveness of the primary tumor in addition to the risk of lymph node metastasis defined previously [20] and may indicate the need of adjuvant treatment for tumor despite its negative margins. On the contrary, neither marker expression was associated with a better outcome of neck treatment by END than by ENI based on the odds of patients being survived 15 times greater and would suggest neck dissection for patient who was originally planned for neck irradiation.

Acknowledgements

The authors would like to acknowledge the grant support from Mahidol University, Bangkok, Thailand.

References

[1] Audet, N., Beasley, N.J., MacMillan,C., Jackson, D.G., Gullane, P.J. and Kamel-Reid, S. (2005) Lymphatic Vessel Density, Nodal Metastases, and Prognosis in Patients with Head and Neck Cancer. *Archives of Otolaryngology Head and Neck Surgery*, **131**, 1065-1070. http://dx.doi.org/10.1001/archotol.131.12.1065

[2] Teymoortash, A. and Werner, J.A. (2012) Current Advances in Diagnosis and Surgical Treatment of Lymph Node Metastasis in Head and Neck Cancer. *GMS Current Topics in Otorhinolaryngology-Head and Neck Surgery*, **11**, Article ID: Doc04. http://www.egms.de/en/journals/cto/2012-11/cto000086.shtml

[3] Hosal, A.S., Carrau, R.L., Johnson, J.T. and Myer, E.N. (2000) Selective Neck Dissection in the Management of the Clinically Node-Negative Neck. *Laryngoscope*, **110**, 2037-2040. http://dx.doi.org/10.1097/00005537-200012000-00011

[4] Mendenhall, W.M., Million, R.R. and Cassisi, N.J. (1986) Squamous Cell Carcinoma of the Head and Neck Treated with Radiation Therapy: The Role of Neck Dissection for Clinically Positive Neck Nodes. *International Journal of Radiation Oncology Biology Physics*, **12**, 733-740. http://dx.doi.org/10.1016/0360-3016(86)90030-1

[5] Mendenhall, W.M. and Million, R.R. (1986) Elective Neck Irradiation for Squamous Cell Carcinoma of the Head and Neck: Analysis of the Time-Dose Factors and Causes of Failure. *International Journal of Radiation Oncology Biology Physics*, **12**, 741-746. http://dx.doi.org/10.1016/0360-3016(86)90031-3

[6] Weiss, M.H., Harrison, L.B. and Isaac, R.S. (1994) Use of Decision Analysis in Planning and Management Strategy for the Stage N0 Neck. *Archives of Otolaryngology Head and Neck Surgery*, **120**, 699-702.

http://dx.doi.org/10.1001/archotol.1994.01880310005001

[7] Jalisi, S. (2005) Management of the Clinically Negative Neck in Early Squamous Cell Carcinoma of the Oral Cavity. *Otolaryngologic Clinics of North America*, **38**, 37-46. http://dx.doi.org/10.1016/j.otc.2004.09.002

[8] Li, X., Shen, Y., Di, B. and Song, Q. (2012) Metastasis of Head and Neck Squamous Cell Carcinoma. In: Li, X., Ed., *Squamous Cell Carcinoma*, In Tech, Shanghai, 1-31. http://www.intechopen.com/books/squamous-cell-carcinoma/metastasis-of-head-and-neck-squamous-cell-carcinoma-hnscc

[9] Ayman, F.H., Mohamed, E. and Mustafa, G.K. (2013) Management of Clinically Negative Neck in Oral Squamous Cell Carcinoma: A Systemic Review. *Journal of Cancer Research and Therapeutic Oncology*, **2**, 1-12. http://www.jscholaronline.org/full-text/JCRTO/302/Management-of-the-Clinically-Negative-Neck-in-Oral-Squamous-Cell-Carcinoma-A-Systematic-Review.php

[10] Roepman, P., de Jager, A., Groot Koerkamp, M.J.A., *et al.* (2006) Maintenance of Head and Neck Tumor Gene Expression Profiles upon Lymph Node Metastasis. *Cancer Research*, **66**, 11110-11114. http://dx.doi.org/10.1158/0008-5472.CAN-06-3161

[11] Takes, R.P. (2004) Staging of the Neck in Patients with Head and Neck Squamous Cell Cancer: Imaging Techniques and Biomarkers. *Oral Oncology*, **40**, 656-667. http://dx.doi.org/10.1016/j.oraloncology.2003.11.001

[12] Timar, J., Csuka, O., Remenar, E., Repassy, G. and Kasler, M. (2005) Progression of Head and Neck Squamous Cell Cancer. *Cancer and Metastasis Reviews*, **24**, 107-127. http://dx.doi.org/10.1007/s10555-005-5051-5

[13] Chiang, A.C. and Massague, J. (2008) Molecular Basis of Metastasis. *New England Journal of Medicine*, **359**, 2814-2823. http://dx.doi.org/10.1056/NEJMra0805239

[14] Takes, R.P., Rinaldo, A., Rodrigo, J.P., Devaney, K.O., Fagan, J.J. and Ferlito, A. (2008) Can Biomarkers Play a Role in the Decision about Treatment of the Clinically Negative Neck in Patients with Head and Neck Cancer? *Head Neck*, **30**, 525-538. http://dx.doi.org/10.1002/hed.20759

[15] Lothaire, P., de Azambuja, E., Dequanter, D., *et al.* (2006) Molecular Markers of Head and Neck Squamous Cell Carcinoma: Promising Signs in Need of Prospective Evaluation. *Head Neck*, **28**, 256-269. http://dx.doi.org/10.1002/hed.20326

[16] Oliveira, L.R. and Ribeiro-Silva, A. (2011) Prognostic Significance of Immunochemical Biomarkers of Oral Squamous Cell Carcinoma. *International Journal of Oral Maxillofacial Surgery*, **40**, 298-307. http://dx.doi.org/10.1016/j.ijom.2010.12.003

[17] Franchi, A., Gallo, O., Boddi, V. and Santucci, M. (1996) Prediction of Occult Neck Metastasis in Laryngeal Carcinoma: Role of Cell Proliferating Nuclear Antigen, MIB-1 and E-Cadherin Immunohistochemical Determination. *Clinical Cancer Research*, **2**, 1801-1808.

[18] Liu, M., Lawson, G., Delos, M., *et al.* (2003) Prognostic Value of Cell Proliferation Markers, Tumor Suppressor Proteins and Cell Adhesion Molecules in Primary Squamous Cell Carcinoma of the Larynx and Hypopharynx. *European Archive Oto-Rhinolaryngology*, **260**, 28-34.

[19] Myoung, H., Kim, M.J., Lee, J.H., Ok, Y.J., Paeng, J.Y. and Yun, P.Y. (2006) Correlation of Proliferative Markers (Ki-67 and PCNA) with Survival and Lymph Node Metastasis in Oral Squamous Cell Carcinoma: A Clinical and Histopathological Analysis of 113 Patients. *International Journal of Oral and Maxillofacial Surgery*, **35**, 1005-1010. http://dx.doi.org/10.1016/j.ijom.2006.07.016

[20] Boonkitticharoen, V., Kulapaditharom, B., Leopairut, J., *et al.* (2008) Vascular Endothelial Growth Factor-A and Proliferation Marker in Prediction of Lymph Node Metastasis in Oral and Pharyngeal Squamous Cell Carcinoma. *Archives of Otolaryngology Head and Neck Surgery*, **134**, 1305-1311. http://dx.doi.org/10.1001/archotol.134.12.1305

[21] Mineta, H., Miura, K., Orgino, T., *et al.* (2000) Prognostic Value of Vascular Endothelial Growth Factor (VEGF) in Head and Neck Squamous Cell Carcinomas. *British Journal of Cancer*, **83**, 775-781. http://dx.doi.org/10.1054/bjoc.2000.1357

[22] O-charoenrat, P., Rhys-Evans, P. and Eccles, S.A. (2001) Expression of Vascular Endothelial Growth Factor Family Members in Head and Neck Squamous Cell Carcinoma Correlated with Lymph Node Metastasis. *Cancer*, **92**, 556-568. http://dx.doi.org/10.1002/1097-0142(20010801)92:3<556::AID-CNCR1355>3.0.CO;2-Q

[23] Cordes, C., Munzel, A.K., Rudolph, P., Hoffmann, M., Leuschner, I. and Gottschlich, S. (2009) Immunohistochemical Staining of Ki-67 Using the Monoclonal Antibody Ki-S11 Is a Prognostic Indicator for Laryngeal Squamous Cell Carcinoma. *Anticancer Research*, **29**, 1459-1466.

[24] Smith, B.D., Smith, G.L., Carter, D., Sasaki, C.T. and Haffty, B.G. (2000) Prognostic Significance of Vascular Endothelial Growth Factor Protein Levels in Oral and Oropharyngeal Squamous Cell Carcinoma. *Journal of Clinical Oncology*, **18**, 2046-2052.

[25] Kyzas, P.A., Stefanou, D., Batistatou, A. and Agnantis, N.J. (2005) Prognostic Significance of VEGF Immunohisto-

chemical Expression and Tumor Angiogenesis in Head and Neck Squamous Cell Carcinoma. *Journal of Cancer Research and Clinical Oncology*, **131**, 624-630. http://dx.doi.org/10.1007/s00432-005-0003-6

[26] Cerezo, L., Millon, I., Torre, A., Aragon, G. and Otero, J. (1992) Prognostic Factors for Survival and Tumor Control in Cervical Lymph Node Metastases from Head and Neck Cancer. A Multivariate Study of 492 Cases. *Cancer*, **69**, 1224-1234. http://dx.doi.org/10.1002/cncr.2820690526

[27] Zanarudin, S.N.S., Sach, A., Yang, Y., *et al.* (2013) Four-Protein Signature Accurately Predicts Lymph Node Metastasis and Survival in Oral Squamous Cell Carcinoma. *Human Pathology*, **44**, 417-426. http://dx.doi.org/10.1016/j.humpath.2012.06.007

[28] Chen, J.X., Deng, N., Chen, X., *et al.* (2012) A Novel Molecular Grading Model: Combination of Ki-67 and VEGF in Predicting Tumor Recurrence and Progression in Non-invasive Urothelial Bladder Cancer. *Asian Pacific Journal of Cancer Prevention*, **13**, 2229-2234. http://dx.doi.org/10.7314/apjcp.2012.13.5.2229 http://www.koreascience.or.kr/article/ArticleFullRecord.jsp?cn=POCPA9_2012_v13n5_2229

[29] O'Brien, C.J., Traynor, S.J., McNeil, E., McMahon, J.D. and Chaplin, J.M. (2000) The Use of Clinical Criteria Alone in the Management of the Clinically Negative Neck Among Patients with Squamous Cell Carcinoma of the Oral Cavity and Oropharynx. *Archives of Otolaryngology Head and Neck Surgery*, **126**, 360-365. http://dx.doi.org/10.1001/archotol.126.3.360

35

Surgical Audit of Sino-Nasal Diseases in a Tertiary Care Centre—A Prospective Study

Ganesh Kumar Balasubramanian, Ramanathan Thirunavukkarasu, Ramesh Babu Kalyanasundaram, Gitanjali Narendran

Thanjavur Medical College, Thanjavur, India
Email: drganeshkumarb@gmail.com

Abstract

Aims of the study: 1) To study the distribution of various Sino-nasal diseases in our region; 2) To emphasize the significance of Functional Endoscopic Sinus Surgery. Material and methods: This surgical study was carried out in the Department of Otorhinolaryngology and Head and Neck Surgery, Thanjavur Medical College, Thanjavur. The study period was from 21st March 2014 to 20th March 2015 (267 cases). After a preliminary examination, all patients were subjected to Diagnostic Nasal Endoscopy followed by radiological examination. Based on the symptoms and the findings, patients were treated by surgery (mainly FESS), pharmacotherapy, and chemo-radiotherapy. Results: In our study, the majority of cases were deviated nasal septum with sinusitis about 62% (165 cases). The other cases were antrochoanal polyp 8% (21 cases), ethmoidal polyposis 9% (23 cases) and others 21% (51 cases). The age group vulnerable for these diseases is 20 - 40 years. Males are affected more commonly than females. Conclusion: Majority of the cases were treated by Functional Endoscopic Sinus Surgery. So we have to improve the surgical skills in this field to achieve a good outcome.

Keywords

Pure Tone Audiogram, Conductive Deafness, Sudden Sensorineural Hearing Loss, Ototoxicity, Presbyacusis, Noise Induced Hearing Loss

1. Introduction

This method of auditing the surgeries done in our department is a systematic and proper scrutiny of the quality of service provided to the society to improve our skills, to teach our postgraduates and also to create awareness among the public regarding the morbidity due to sinonasal diseases in our area. The nose is a prominent structure in the face with aesthetic and functional significance. It is commonly affected by allergy. The most common symptoms related to these sinonasal disorders are nasal obstruction followed by nasal discharge, disturbance of smell, bleeding from the nose, headache, facial swelling, change of voice, visual disturbances, epiphora and mouth breathing [1].

According to the National centre of Disease Statistics, sinusitis has become the most common chronic illness in the United States, surpassing arthritis. Sinonasal disease may exacerbate asthma and other Chronic Obstructive Pulmonary Diseases [2]. In developing countries like India, allergy is a common problem and most commonly seasonal. So assessment of the type and severity of allergy is mandatory to control the chronic allergic problems related to nose and paranasal sinus disorders.

Polyp is any mass of tissue that bulges or projects downwards from surface and is visible macroscopically. It is defined as prolapsed, pedunculated, polypoidal paranasal sinus mucosa. Hippocrates described the polyp as early as 460 - 370 B.C. He is considered as "Father of Rhinology". Mechanical obstruction produced by nasal septal deviation will produce persistent infection of the paranasal sinuses. So, septal surgery is necessary for these cases. Messerklinger highlighted that Osteo Meatal Complex (OMC) is the basic unit responsible for the development of infection in frontal, maxillary and ethmoid sinuses. Stammberger, Kennedy and Messerklinger also stated that cilia beated towards the natural ostium. Frontal and ethmoid sinuses drain into the middle meatus via anterior ethmoid and hence their physiology and pathology depend on conditions of the anterior ethmoid [3].

Rhinosporidiosis is managed by excision of the mass and diathermy cauterization of the base to reduce recurrence. Nasolabial cysts are removed by sublabial approach. Nasal bone reduction surgery is done by using Asche and Wallsham forceps. Biopsies of maxillary sinus malignancy were taken through inferior meatal antrostomy. These patients underwent maxillectomy. Nasopharyngeal carcinoma cases were subjected to radiotherapy after DNE and biopsy.

2. Materials and Methods

This prospective study was carried out in the Department of Otorhinolaryngology and Head and Neck Surgery in Thanjavur Medical College, Thanjavur. The study period was from March 21st 2014 to March 20th 2015 (one year). Total number of cases taken up for this audit was 267 cases. All these cases were examined by the consultants and subjected to diagnostic nasal endoscopy and computed tomography. We used Hopkins Rod endoscopes and Karl-Storz cold light source system for the Functional Endoscopic Sinus Surgery. We used appropriate angled scopes for the surgery of maxillary and frontal sinuses. All malignancy cases underwent biopsy first. Depending upon the histopathological report, definite treatment was planned. Post operative follow up is the mainstay for better outcome for all the endoscopic sinus surgeries. All the allergy related diseases were managed initially with systemic steroids tapered gradually and maintained with inhalational steroids.

3. Results

In our study Deviated Nasal Septum with Sinusitis cases are more in number, about 165 cases (62%). The sinusitis is mostly chronic and some are due to allergy. In cases with marked septal deviation, the opposite inferior turbinate will be hypertrophied. This is due the presence of submucosal neurovascular tissue in the inferior turbinate alone. The ethmoidal polyp cases are around 23 in number (9%). These polyps are formed due to allergy. Antrochoanal polyp cases are 21 in number (8%). Infection is the main etiology for this polyp followed by allergy. The others contribute about 21% (58 cases) (**Chart 1**).

DNS with Sinusitis is more common in the 20 - 40 years age group. These age groups are more commonly affected by allergy due to greater exposure to polluted environment. We know very well that antrochoanal polyp is more prevalent in children and adolescents. Our study also shows that 5 - 19 years is more commonly affected by antrochoanal polyp. It is rare in older age (over 50 years). But the reverse is true for ethmoidal polypi which are more common in the age group of 40 - 60 years, and very rare in younger age groups (**Table 1** and **Chart 2**).

Males are more commonly affected by DNS with Sinusitis than the females. Antrochoanal polyp more commonly involves females than the males. Ethmoidal polyp equally affects both sexes (**Table 2** and **Chart 3**).

The other cases are as follows:

Nasolabial cyst (8 cases)—5 were left sided cysts and the remaining 3 were right sided. There were 7 cases of rhinosporidiosis, 3 cases of juvenile nasopharyngeal angiofibroma, nasopharyngeal carcinoma 4 cases, 5 cases of benign tumors of the nasal cavity, 5 cases of carcinoma of the maxillary sinus, 3 cases of bleeding polypus of

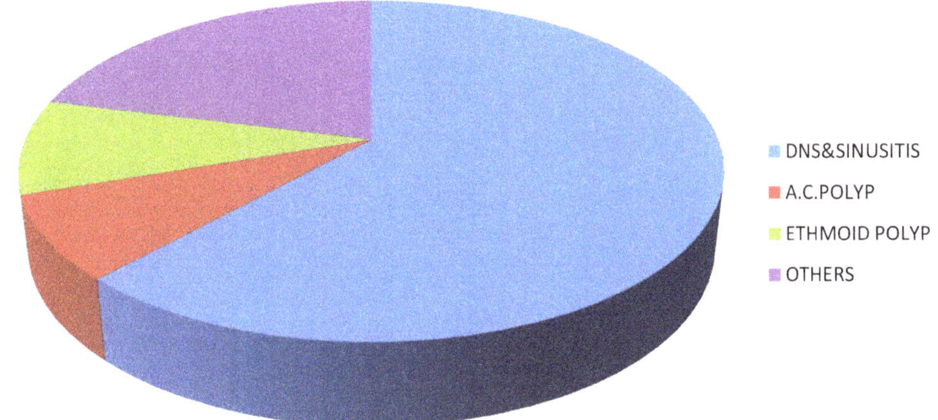

Chart 1. Distribution of common sinonasal diseases.

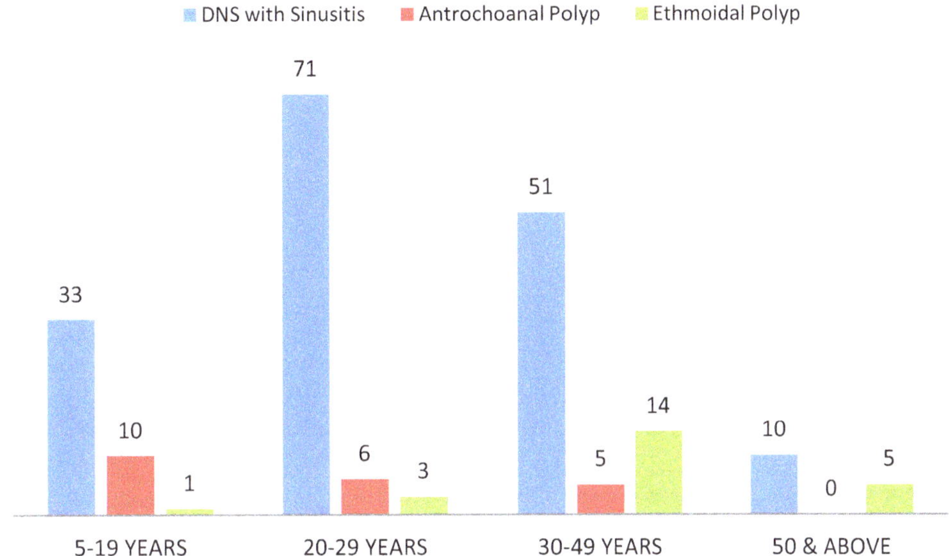

Chart 2. Common nasal pathologies in different age groups.

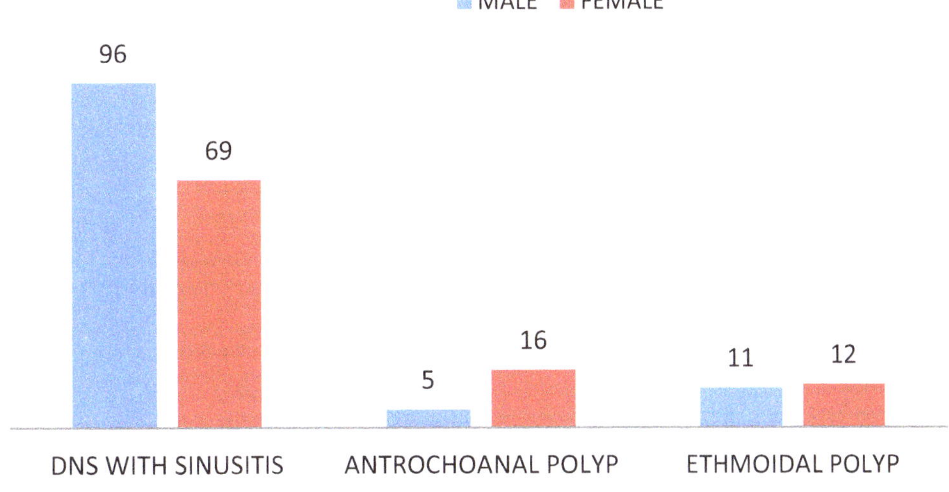

Chart 3. Sex distribution.

Table 1. Age distribution of DNS and polyp cases.

Age Group	DNS with Sinusitis	Antrochoanal Polyp	Ethmoidal Polyp	Total Cases
5 - 19 years	33	10	1	44
20 - 29 years	71	6	3	80
30 - 49 years	51	5	14	70
50 & above	10	0	5	15

Table 2. Sex distribution.

Type of Diseases	MALE	FEMALE	TOTAL
DNS with Sinusitis	96	69	165
Antrochoanal Polyp	5	16	21
Ethmoidal Polyp	11	12	23

septum, and 5 cases of fungal sinusitis, one case of cerebrospinal fluid Rhinorrhea, 3 cases of nasal myiasis, 4 cases of Rhinolith and 10 cases of fracture of nasal bone.

4. Discussion

Deviated nasal septum and sinusitis disturbs the normal function of the sinuses such as ventilation and drainage. It commonly causes nasal obstruction, epistaxis. For complete relief from sinusitis, we have to remove the disease, reduce the tissue odema, facilitate drainage and maintain permeability of ostia. Only then we can achieve normal aeration and ventilation of sinuses [4]. In the nineteenth century Caldwell-Luc surgery was the treatment of choice for Maxillary sinusitis. But nowadays it is replaced by FESS. Medical management of sinusitis has little benefit in patients with chronic refractory sinusitis with an underlying immunodeficiency, for that group we have to do combined management of surgical drainage and medical management [5].

Chronic sinusitis is increasing in number in developing countries like India. Sinusitis presents with headache, nasal discharge and postnasal drip. Treatment is initially medical management and surgery is done if there is no improvement with medicines. In 1901 Hirschmann used modified Nitze cystocsope to examine sinuses. Speilberg was the first person to use an endoscope to examine the maxillary sinus through inferior meatus. Maltz coined the term sinuscopy. The development of compact, straight and various degrees of angled endoscopes and the pioneering work of Messerklinger and Wigand et al revolutionised FESS. In 1985 William Kennedy coined the term FESS. Stammberger, Kennedy and Zinreich (1996) contributed for the widespread use of endoscopic diagnosis and management for sino-nasal diseases [6].

In our study majority of patients belong to 20 - 49 years which coincides with Rahman *et al.* but is inconsistent with Venkatachalam. The main presenting symptoms include nasal obstruction, nasal discharge, headache, facial pain, post nasal drip and recurrent sore throat. This is similar to Rice and Mathews *et al.*'s studies [7].

Sino-nasal polyps are more common in females compared to males in our study, in contrast to the Zafer *et al.* Indian study which shows male preponderance [8]. Antro choanal polyp otherwise called as Killian's polyp is common in adolescent age and in children. But ethmoidal polyp is more common in elderly. Recurrence is common in ethmoidal polyp. Malignant transformation is common in ethmoidal polyp. Nasal polyps result from chronic inflammation of the mucosa of the nose and sinuses. The symptoms are nasal obstruction, nasal discharge and change of voice. There is a strong association with asthma, aspirin sensitivity, nasal polyp (Samter's Triad) [9].

Commonest site of origin of AC polyp is floor and posterolateral wall of maxillary sinus. So it is difficult to remove it completely from its attachment in routine endoscopic sinus surgeries. In case of recurrence of AC polyp, treatment of choice is Caldwell-Luc approach, because we can easily reach the floor and posterolateral wall. All ethmoidal polyp cases were treated by oral steroids preoperatively then taken up for surgery and postoperative topical steroids were given to reduce the recurrence rate [10]. We used powered instruments like microdebrider for ethmoidal polyposis and in cases of hypertrophied inferior turbinate.

Bleeding polypus of septum is capillary haemangioma. The patient presents with epistaxis. It mostly arises from cartilaginous part of the septum. Cavernous type is rare in sino-nasal tract [11]. Inverted papilloma is a benign tumour but recurs if not treated properly and adequately. Late recurrence even after 30 years is common. Malignant transformation is about 11% (squamous cell carcinoma) [12].

Malignancy of sinonasal tract is rare. Maxillary sinus carcinoma is common. The patient complains of swelling or numbness in cheek, nasal obstruction, epistaxis, visual disturbances, facial pain, loose teeth or swelling in palate. The most common histological type is squamous cell carcinoma, commonly seen after the 4th decade. All tumours of maxillary sinus erode the lateral nasal wall [13]. Complete surgical resection of tumor followed by adjuvant radiotherapy improves survival rate [14].

In our study there were 8 cases of nasolabial cyst. Among this 5 cases were left sided cysts and the remaining 3 were right sided. They were removed in to by sublabial approach and followed up. One case recurred. There were 7 cases of Rhinosporidiosis. It was treated by excision and cauterization of the base using bipolar diathermy. We saw recurrence in 2 cases, in which the rhinosporidial mass presented in the inferior meatus, which is very difficult to remove completely due to minimal available space.

We operated 3 cases of Juvenile Nasopharyngeal Angiofibroma which was identified in the early stage and we completely removed the mass. We faced minimal bleeding only because of predominance of fibrous element. Nasopharyngeal carcinoma (4 cases) underwent DNE and biopsy taken from the fossa of rosenmuller which was obliterated in all the cases. All the cases were diagnosed as squamous cell carcinoma and sent for Radiotherapy and are under regular follow up.

There are 5 cases of benign tumors of the nasal cavity in our study. After biopsy all the cases underwent surgery for complete removal of the masses. For 2 cases we removed the mass by Lateral Rhinotomy approach and the others by trans nasal route. Around 5 cases of Carcinoma of the Maxillary sinus are presented in our study. They were subjected to biopsy after Inferior Meatal Antrostomy and after that 3 cases underwent total maxillectomy and 2 cases were sent for Brachytherapy. There are 3 cases of bleeding polypus of septum in our study which were excised. About 5 cases of fungal sinusitis are seen in our study. They were confirmed by biopsy and specific antifungals were given according to culture and sensitivity. Surgical removal of the fungal mass was done endoscopically.

Cerebrospinal fluid rhinorrhea was treated endoscopically by sandwich method using cartilage, fat, temporalis fascia, muscle, surgicel and mucosal flaps. The site of leakage was medial lamellae of cribriform plate. 3 cases of nasal myiasis were treated medically by using tincture benzoin and ether. All 3 patients were in immunocompromised state. Rhinolith were removed endoscopically. Fracture of nasal bone was treated by nasal bone reduction surgery using various forceps. Two patients underwent septorhinoplasty.

5. Conclusions

With appropriate history, nasal endoscopy and proper radiological imaging correct diagnosis can be made and proper treatment can be given. Nasal endoscopy is the best diagnostic test. FESS is a safer, efficient procedure for sinonasal diseases. Because of better illumination of the surgical field, we can achieve the best results with minimal or nil complication.

This study helps us to identify the distribution of various types of sino-nasal diseases and we can train doctors in surgical techniques and educate the patients regarding the mode of spread of certain diseases like Rhinosporidiosis. We can advise the nasal polyp cases for regular postoperative follow-up and steroid management.

References

[1] Humayun, A.H.M., Zahurul Huq, A.H.M., Ahmed, S.M.T., *et al.* (2010) Clinicopathological Study of Sinonasal Masses. *Bangladesh Journal of Otorhinolaryngology*, **16**, 15-22. http://dx.doi.org/10.3329/bjo.v16i1.5776

[2] Levine, H.C. (1990) Functional Endoscopic Sinus Surgery: Evolution, Surgery and Follow up of 250 Patients. *Laryngoscope*, **100**, 79-84.

[3] Stammberger, H. (1986) Endoscopic Endonasal Surgery Concepts in the Treatment of Recurring Rhinosinusitis. Part I. Anatomic and Patho-Physiologic Considerations. *Otolaryngology—Head & Neck Surgery*, **94**, 143-147.

[4] Park, A.H., Lau, J., Stankiewicz, J. and Chow, J. (1998) The Role of Functional Endoscopic Sinus Surgery in Asthmatic Patients. *Journal of Otolaryngology*, **27**, 275-280.

[5] Buehring, I., Friedrich, B., Schaaf, J., Schmidt, H., Ahrens, P. and Zielen, S. (1997) Chronic Sinusitis Refractory to

Standard Managements in Patients with Humoral Immunodeficiencies. *Clinical & Experimental Immunology*, **109**, 468-472. http://dx.doi.org/10.1046/j.1365-2249.1997.4831379.x

[6] Stankiewicz, J. (1991) Endoscopic Nasal and Sinus Surgery. Surgery of the Para Nasal Sinuses. 2nd Edition, W.B. Saunders Company, Philadelphia, 223-224.

[7] Mathews, B.L., Smith, L.E., Jhones, R., Miller, C. and Bookschmidt, J.K. (1991) Endoscopic Sinus Surgery: Outcome in 155 Cases. *Otolaryngology—Head & Neck Surgery*, **104**, 244-246.

[8] Zafar, U., Khan, N., Afroz, N., *et al.* (2008) Clinico Pathological Study of Non Neoplastic Lesions of Nose and Paranasal Sinuses. *Indian Journal of Pathology & Microbiology*, **51**, 26-29.

[9] Hedman, J., Kaprio, J., Poussa, T., *et al.* (1999) Prevalence of Asthma, Aspirin Intolerance, Nasal Polyposis and COPD in a Population Based Study. *International Journal of Epidemiology*, **28**, 717-722. http://dx.doi.org/10.1093/ije/28.4.717

[10] Dassonville, C., Bonfils, P., Momas, I., *et al.* (2007) Nasal Inflammation Induced by a Common Cold: Comparison between Controls and Patients with Nasal Polyposis under Topical Steroid Spray. *Acta Otorhinolaryngologica Italica*, **27**, 78-82.

[11] Pradhanaga, R.B., Adhikari, P., Thapa, N.M., *et al.* (2008) Overview of Nasal Masses. *J Inst Med*, **30**, 13-16.

[12] Barnes, L., Tse, L.L.Y. and Hunt, J.L. (2005) Schneiderian Papillomas. In: *WHO Classification of Tumours*, *Lyon*: *Pathology of Head and Neck Tumours*, IARC Press, Lyon, 28-32.

[13] Fasunla, A.J. and Lasis, A.O. (2007) Sinonasal Malignancies: A 10-Year Review in a Tertiary Health Institution. *Journal of the National Medical Association*, **99**, 1407-1410.

[14] Hoppe, B.S., Stegman, L.D., Zelefsky, M.J., *et al.* (2007) Treatment of Nasalcavity and Paranasal Sinus Cancer with Modern Radiotherapy Techniques in the Postoperative Setting-MSKCC Experience. *International Journal of Radiation Oncology • Biology • Physics*, **67**, 691-702. http://dx.doi.org/10.1016/j.ijrobp.2006.09.023

Coblation Intracapsular Tonsillectomy and Coblation Complete Tonsillectomy for Obstructive Sleep Apnea

Itzhak Braverman[1*], Alex Nemirovsky[2], Adi Klein[2], Miriam Sarid[3], Galit Avior[1]

[1]Unit of Otolaryngology-Head & Neck Surgery, Hadera, Israel
[2]Pediatric Department Hillel Yaffe Medical Center, Hadera and The Faculty of Medicine, The Technion, Haifa, Israel
[3]Western Galilee College, Acco, Israel
Email: [*]braverman@hy.health.gov.il

Abstract

Objective: Total tonsillectomy and intracapsular tonsillectomy are common procedures for the treatment of obstructive sleep apnea (OSA) in children. The objective of this study was to compare the effectiveness of coblation intracapsular tonsillectomy (ICT) and coblation complete tonsillectomy (CT) as treatments for OSA. Study design: A retrospective study of all the children ages 2 - 18 years with OSA who underwent coblation intracapsular tonsillectomy (ICT) or coblation complete tonsillectomy (CT) from January 2007 to August 2010 by the same surgeons at one institution. Methods: Data were retrieved from children's charts and from telephone interviews with children's parents, regarding pre and postoperative OSA-18 scores, postoperative pain, postoperative complications, use of analgesic drugs, and time to return to a solid food diet. Results: All 43 children who underwent ICT and 37 children who underwent CT suffered from OSA before surgery, and none did postoperatively. There were no minor complications in the ICT group, compared to 13.5% in the CT group (p = 0.01). According to parental report, 72% and 21% suffered a low level of postoperative pain, and 9% and 33% severe pain in the ICT and CT groups, respectively. For these respective groups, 49% and 73% needed analgesic drugs (p < 0.05); and 65% and 35% ate solid food during the first 3 days post surgery. Conclusions: Both ICT and CT were safe, with few complications; however recovery was faster in the ICT group, as demonstrated by less pain, and more rapid return to a solid food diet.

Keywords

Obstructive Sleep Apnea, Tonsillectomy, Coblation, Intracapsular Tonsillectomy, Pain, Adenotonsillectomy, Tonsillotomy

[*]Corresponding author.

1. Introduction

Obstructive sleep apnea (OSA) in children is characterized by a decrease or complete halt in airflow despite an ongoing effort to breath, and by upper airway collapse that disrupts normal respiratory gas exchange or causes sleep fragmentation. A systematic review concluded that 4% to 11% of children suffer from sleep-disordered breathing, ranging in severity from snoring to OSA, as assessed by parent report [1]. Consequences of untreated OSA include: failure to thrive, enuresis, attention-deficit disorder, behavior problems, poor academic performance, and cardiopulmonary disease [2] [3]. The most common etiology of OSA is adenotonsillar hypertrophy.

Tonsillar surgery is the treatment of choice for most children with OSA. Moreover, OSA, rather than chronic infection, has become the primary indication for pediatric tonsillectomy, especially in younger children [4] [5]. A large recently published randomized trial supports the beneficial effects of early adenotonsillectomy, compared with a strategy of watchful waiting, for school-age children with OSA [6]. Nevertheless, pain is a common postoperative morbidity of tonsillectomy; the degree is usually severe, and often leads to poor oral intake and dehydration.

Tonsillotomy (also known as partial tonsillectomy and as intracapsular tonsillectomy) was the most commonly performed tonsillar surgery until the 1930s, when the broad introduction and safety of general anesthesia led to a preference for tonsillectomy (also known as total or traditional tonsillectomy and as subcapsular tonsillectomy) [7]. However, tonsillectomy is associated with considerable postoperative morbidity, including long recovery, characterized by dysphagia and odinophagia due to pain, bleeding, and loss of school days. Recent years have witnessed renewed interest in tonsillotomy as treatment of OSA, by means of a variety of techniques and with positive outcomes on morbidity and postoperative pain. The advantage of tonsillotomy over conventional tonsillectomy is that it leaves a residual tonsillar tissue and capsule which protects the underlying musculature with its vessels and nerves. Microdebrider partial tonsillectomy, first described by Koltai *et al.* in 2002 [8], and coblation were two techniques employed in tonsillotomy.

Coblation technology uses the combination of radiofrequency energy with a saline solution for gently and precisely removing tonsils, preserving the capsule, and precluding damage from surrounding healthy tissue. In prospective trials comparing the two techniques, coblation and steel cold dissection, for total tonsillectomy [9] and for adenotonsillectomy [10], fewer intraoperative and postoperative complications and less postoperative pain were observed with coblation. Numerous studies and two recent reviews [11] [12] have compared recovery-related outcomes of tonsillectomy and tonsillotomy by a variety of techniques. Less pain and more rapid recovery were reported for tonsillotomy, both by microdebrider and by coblation [11] [12]; however, since different techniques were used for tonsillectomy and tonsillotomy, it was not clear if the findings were due to the technique (microdebrider, coblation) or to the intracapsular rather than subcapsular procedure. Few studies and neither of these reviews compared the effectiveness of treating OSA between the two procedures using the same technique.

The purpose of this study was to compare recovery-related outcomes and effectiveness of tonsillectomy and tonsillotomy for the treatment of OSA in children, using the same technique, namely coblation: coblation intracapsular adenotonsillectomy (ICT) and coblation subcapsular adenotonsillectomy (CT).

2. Material and Methods

This is a retrospective study of children aged 2 - 18 years old who underwent coblation intracapsular adenotonsillectomy (ICT) or coblation subcapsular adenotonsillectomy (CT) for treatment of OSA at one institution, with the same surgeons, during a five year period (2007 to 2010). The indication for ICT was OSA; and for CT, OSA together with chronic tonsillitis. OSA was clinically determined in all children before surgery. Exclusion criteria were the presence of other diseases, such as cardiac, lung or metabolic and medical treatment that influences sleep.

Data retrieved from patient charts included intraoperative complications and the number of hours postoperative that the patients consumed a fluid diet. Parents were called by telephone and asked to respond to the Obstructive Sleep Apnea Syndrome Quality of Life Survey (OSA-18) [13] regarding the period before and after surgery.

The pediatric OSA-18 questionnaire is an18-item survey that comprises 5 categories (sleep disturbance, physical symptoms, emotional distress, daytime function, caregiver concerns). Questions are scored 1 (never) to 7 (persistently) based on the frequency of symptoms. The maximum score is 126. Scores of less than 60 suggest a small impact on health-related quality of life (HRQL); scores between 60 and 80 suggest a moderate impact; and scores greater than 80 suggest a large impact.

In addition to the OSA-18 questionnaire, parents were asked to assess their children's pain for the 7 days postoperative as mild, moderate, or severe; their degree of satisfaction with the surgery, according to the visual analogue scale; the duration of time of recovery from tonsillectomy; postoperative complications; the use and frequency of analgesic drugs; and the time lapse, in days, until the start of solid food. Postoperative pain was also evaluated by the use of analgesic drugs and the timing of eating solid food, according to patients' charts.

The surgical procedure was performed as described previously [14], except for differences in the coblate settings of the surgical wand: 7 instead of 9 during ablation of the tonsils from the surface, and 7 instead of 6 during dissection.

Statistical analysis: The Chi-square test was used to compare data between the intracapsular and subcapsular groups.

3. Results

Table 1 presents demographic and clinical data according to study procedure. During the study period, 43 children, 28 boys and 15 girls, underwent ICT; and 37 children, 22 boys and 15 girls, CT. Mean OSA18 scores were 82.6 and 73.0 before surgery, in the ICT and CT groups respectively; and 25.5 and 24.6, respectively, post-operative. All the children who underwent ICT or CT with adenoidectomy were free from OSA symptoms postoperatively. Altogether, only 9% of the children were snoring post surgery, 13.5% following CT and 5% following ICT.

No intraoperative or postoperative complications were observed in the ICT group, compared to 13.5% minor complications in the CT group, most of them dehydration ($p = 0.01$).

During the first 24 hours postoperative, 67.4% in the ICT group, and 94.6% in the CT group suffered pain, according to parents' report ($p < 0.001$). Mild pain complaints during the first 3 postoperative days were 64.5% in the ICT and 28.3% in the CT group. In the ICT group, 72% of the parents rated their children's 7 days post-operative pain as mild, compared with 21% in the CT group; 9% and 33% reported severe pain following ICT and CT respectively (**Figure 1**). Fewer than half (49%) of children in the ICT group needed analgesics, compared with 73% in the CT group ($p < 0.05$). Of those who used analgesics, a higher proportion in the CT group received 3 or more doses (**Figure 2**).

In the ICT group 65% ate solid food during the first 3 days post-surgery, compared to only 35% in the CT group, despite the recommendation to eat soft food during the first week. The proportion of children who only consumed fluids for 8 or more hours postoperative was lower in the ICT group (**Figure 3**) ($p < 0.01$).

Table 1. Characteristics and outcomes of children who underwent coblation intracapsular adenotonsillectomy (ICT) and coblation subcapsular adenotonsillectomy (CT).

Characteristic	ICT	CT
Number of children	43	37
Boys	28	22
Girls	15	15
Age (years)	range 2 - 8, median 4	range 2 - 17, median 5
Mean OSA18 scores		
Before surgery	82.6	73.0
After surgery	25.5	24.6
Snoring postoperative	2 (4.7%)	5 (13.5%)
Postoperative complications	0	5 (13.5%)
Reported pain		
During 24 hours postoperative	29 (67.4%)	35 (94.6%)

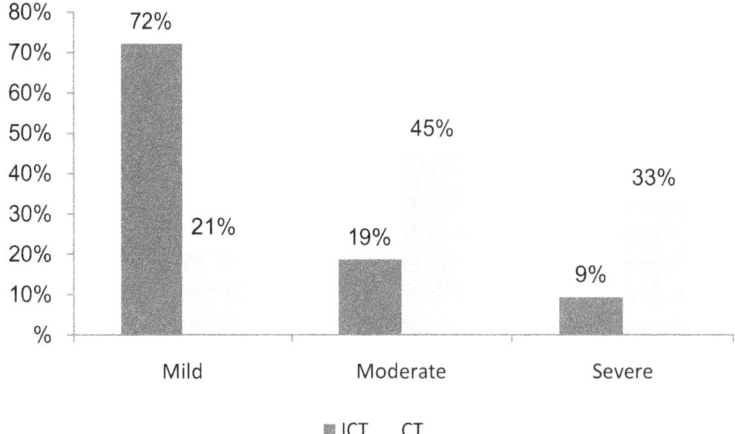

Figure 1. Pain level 7 days post surgery.

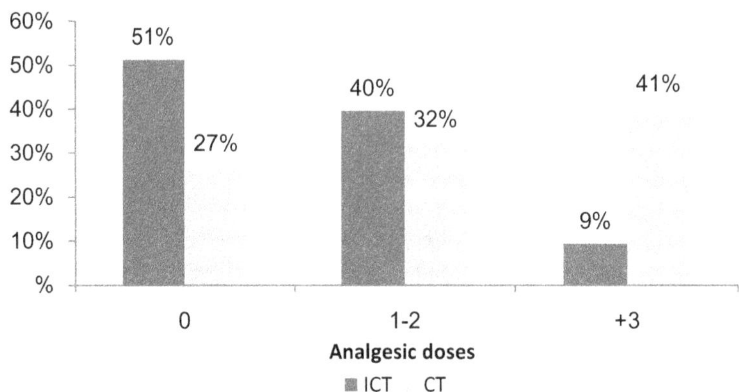

Figure 2. The number of analgesic dosages after each surgery.

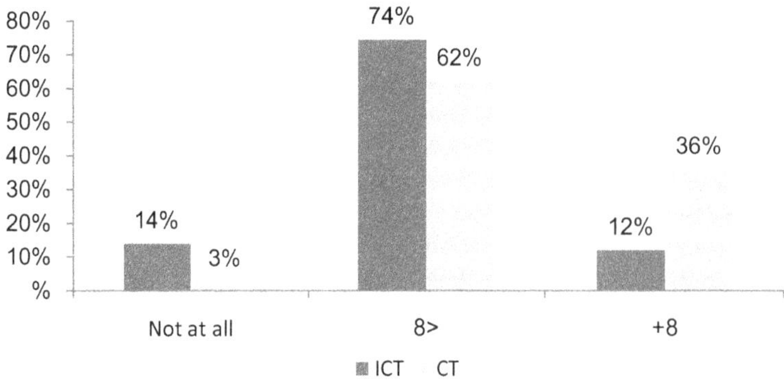

Figure 3. The number of "fluid only hours" after each surgery.

4. Discussion

This study compared subcapsular (total) (CT) and intracapsular adenotonsillectomy (ICT), both employing coblation. The two procedures demonstrated effectiveness as treatment for OSA, according to parent report, as well as safety, as assessed by few complications. The low thermal effect of coblation, 45°C - 85°C, reduces the risk of thermal injury to surrounding tissues, reducing pain and promoting healing.

Recovery from ICT was faster than from the subcapsular procedure, as demonstrated by fewer days with pain, less use of analgesic drugs, and earlier resumption of solid food ingestion. These findings support Acevedo *et al.*'s [11] subanalysis of coblation procedures, which showed a more rapid return to a regular diet and fewer days of analgesic use for tonsillotomy than tonsillectomy. However, that review included studies in which only tonsillotomies were performed by coblation, contrasting with the current study in which all tonsillectomies and tonsillotomies were performed using coblation.

The less pain experienced in the first 24 hours among children who underwent ICT compared to CT suggests less tissue injury in the former. Since the procedures were performed by the same two surgeons, such difference seems to be due to differences in the surgical techniques, and not to differences in the surgeons' skills. This is an important point since dissection skills of the surgeon has been suggested as a main factor determining the degree of tissue injury, and thus explains differences in the postoperative outcomes of different procedures [14].

In the current study, the lower level of pain reported by the ICT group after seven postoperative days is likely due to the protective effect of sparing the capsule. Similarly, in a randomized trial, significantly less pain was reported 5 and 6 days postoperative following intracapsular coblation tonsillectomy than following total coblation, despite comparable levels of pain between the groups on the first two postoperative days [14]. Likewise, in a prospective study in which coblation was used in a subcapsular approach on one side and intracapsular on the other side of the same patients, no difference in pain was reported within the first 24 hours [15].

Few studies have compared the effectiveness of tonsillar procedures for the treatment of OSA. The OSA-18 is a well-accepted questionnaire. Nevertheless, the use of parent report, and the time lapse from the surgery to the interviews, which was sometimes considerable, raises the possibility of reporting bias. To mitigate such bias, data were collected and correlated from patients' charts.

Despite the benefits of ICT, this procedure is not appropriate for patients suffering from tonsillitis in addition to OSA, due to the possible risk of infection in the tonsillar remnant and of regrowth of tonsillar tissue. Consequently, in the current study, CT, and not ICT, was performed in patients suffering from chronic tonsillitis. However, this raises the possibility of an indication bias, *i.e.* different indications for the two procedures (although all the children had OSA). In contrast, if indications were identical for the two procedures, as in randomized trials, such as those included in Walton *et al.*'s review [12], then some patients would evidently be over or undertreated. If, on the one hand, the indication for surgery was OSA without tonsillitis, then patients randomized to CT would be overtreated. If, on the other hand, the indication was tonsillitis, then those randomized to ICT would be undertreated. Thus, in contrast with the bias arising from the "real life" design of the current study, randomized trials comparing CT and ICT raise clinical and ethical questions.

Assessment of the effectiveness of CT for the treatment of chronic tonsillitis is beyond the scope of the current study. However, the fact that children who underwent CT suffered from chronic infection, in addition to OSA, is a limitation of this study, as well as of other such comparative studies [16]. Of note, greater postoperative bleeding was reported following operations in which recurrent tonsillitis, rather than non-infectious pathologies including sleep apnea, was the indication [17].

An explanation for the lower level of pain and complications in the ICT group is the sparing of the tonsillar capsule and the presence of remnant tonsillar tissue, which generates a protective effect that may achieve safer distance from vessels and nerves in the tonsillar bed. This mechanism is the major pathogenesis, in our opinion, for less morbidity in the ICT group and similar improvement in OSA. The benefits demonstrated herein of ICT in postoperative recovery and in relief from OSA are important, since OSA is currently the main indication for tonsillar surgery [4] [5]. Still, long term evaluation is necessary to assess the degree of tonsil regrowth following ICT, and the possible effect of such on OSA.

5. Conclusion

The two techniques, ICT and CT, demonstrated safety, yet there were fewer complications in the ICT group. Recovery from ICT was faster than from CT, as assessed by number of days with pain, the use of analgesic drugs and the timing to solid food ingestion. After 5 days all children in the ICT group ate solid food, while in the CT group, it took longer. In the ICT group, pain duration was shorter than in the CT group. Still, there was no significant difference in pain level between the two groups, and severe pain was not reported in either. Two thirds of the children in both groups had mild pain. The overall satisfaction from the operation and OSA symptoms was high in both groups. ICT is an effective and recommended technique for children with OSA.

Acknowledgements

The author wants to thank Ms. Cindy Cohen for her help in preparing this manuscript.

References

[1] Lumeng, J.C. and Chervin, R.D. (2008) Epidemiology of Pediatric Obstructive Sleep Apnea. *Proceedings of the American Thoracic Society*, **5**, 242-252. http://dx.doi.org/10.1513/pats.200708-135MG

[2] Kovacevic, L., Jurewicz, M., Dabaja, A., *et al.* (2013) Enuretic Children with Obstructive Sleep Apnea Syndrome: Should They See Otolaryngology First? *Journal of Pediatric Urology*, **9**, 145-150.

[3] Marcus, C.L., Brooks, L.J., Draper, K.A., *et al.* (2012) American Academy of Pediatrics. Diagnosis and Management of Childhood Obstructive Sleep Apnea Syndrome. *Pediatrics*, **130**, e714-e755. http://dx.doi.org/10.1542/peds.2012-1672

[4] Bhattacharyya, N. and Lin, H.W. (2010) Changes and Consistencies in the Epidemiology of Pediatric Adenotonsillar Surgery, 1996-2006. *Otolaryngology–Head & Neck Surgery*, **143**, 680-684. http://dx.doi.org/10.1016/j.otohns.2010.06.918

[5] Parker, N.P. and Walner, D.L. (2011) Trends in the Indications for Pediatric Tonsillectomy or Adenotonsillectomy. *International Journal of Pediatric Otorhinolaryngology*, **75**, 282-285. http://dx.doi.org/10.1016/j.ijporl.2010.11.019

[6] Marcus, C.L., Moore, R.H., Rosen, C.L., *et al.* (2013) Childhood Adenotonsillectomy Trial (CHAT). A Randomized Trial of Adenotonsillectomy for Childhood Sleep Apnea. *The New England Journal of Medicine*, **368**, 2366-2376. http://dx.doi.org/10.1056/NEJMoa1215881

[7] Koempel, J.A., Solares, C.A. and Koltai, P.J. (2006) The Evolution of Tonsil Surgery and Rethinking the Surgical Approach to Obstructive Sleep-Disordered Breathing in Children. *Journal of Laryngology and Otology*, **120**, 993-1000. http://dx.doi.org/10.1017/S0022215106002544

[8] Koltai, P.J., Solares, C.A., Mascha, E.J. and Xu, M. (2002) Intracapsular Partial Tonsillectomy for Tonsillar Hypertrophy in Children. *Laryngoscope*, **112**, 17-19. http://dx.doi.org/10.1002/lary.5541121407

[9] Omrani, M., Barati, B., Omidifar, N., Okhovvat, A.R. and Hashemi, S.A. (2012) Coblation versus Traditional Tonsillectomy: A double Blind Randomized Controlled Trial. *Journal of Research in Medical Sciences*, **17**, 45-50.

[10] Paramasivan, V.K., Arumugam, S.V. and Kameswaran, M. (2012) Randomised Comparative Study of Adenotonsillectomy by Conventional and Coblation Method for Children with Obstructive Sleep Apnoea. *International Journal of Pediatric Otorhinolaryngology*, **76**, 816-821. http://dx.doi.org/10.1016/j.ijporl.2012.02.049

[11] Acevedo, J.L., Shah, R.K. and Brietzke, S.E. (2012) Systematic Review of Complications of Tonsillotomy versus Tonsillectomy. *Otolaryngology—Head and Neck Surgery*, **146**, 871-879. http://dx.doi.org/10.1177/0194599812439017

[12] Walton, J., Ebner, Y., Stewart, M.G. and April, M.M. (2012) Systematic Review of Randomized Controlled Trials Comparing Intracapsular Tonsillectomy with Total Tonsillectomy in a Pediatric Population. *Archives of Otolaryngology—Head and Neck Surgery*, **138**, 243-249. http://dx.doi.org/10.1001/archoto.2012.16

[13] Franco Jr., R.A., Rosenfeld, R.M. and Rao, M. (2000) Quality of Life for Children with Obstructive Sleep Apnea. *Otolaryngology—Head and Neck Surgery*, **123**, 9-16. http://dx.doi.org/10.1067/mhn.2000.105254

[14] Chang, K.W. (2008) Intracapsular versus Subcapsular Coblation Tonsillectomy. *Otolaryngology—Head and Neck Surgery*, **138**, 153-157. http://dx.doi.org/10.1016/j.otohns.2007.11.006

[15] Arya, A.K., Donne, A. and Nigam, A. (2005) Double-Blind Randomized Controlled Study of Coblation Tonsillotomy versus Coblation Tonsillectomy on Postoperative Pain in Children. *Clinical Otolaryngology*, **30**, 226-229. http://dx.doi.org/10.1111/j.1365-2273.2005.00970.x

[16] Cantarella, G., Viglione, S., Forti, S., Minetti, A. and Pignataro, L. (2012) Comparing Postoperative Quality of Life in Children after Microdebrider Intracapsular Tonsillotomy and Tonsillectomy. *Auris Nasus Larynx*, **39**, 407-410. http://dx.doi.org/10.1016/j.anl.2011.10.012

[17] Khan, I., Abelardo, E., Scott, N.W., Shakeel, M., Menakaya, O., Jaramillo, M. and Mahmood, K. (2012) Coblation Tonsillectomy: Is It Inherently Bloody? *European Archives of Oto-Rhino-Laryngology*, **269**, 579-583. http://dx.doi.org/10.1007/s00405-011-1609-8

37

Effectiveness and Therapeutic Impact of CT-Guided Percutaneous Drainage for Deep Neck Abscesses

Zexing Cheng[1], Xiaoming Tang[2], Juebo Yu[1*]

[1]Department of Otolaryngology, Yangzhou First People's Hospital, Yangzhou, China
[2]Department of Computed Tomography and Interventional Radiology, Yangzhou First People's Hospital, Yangzhou, China
Email: [*]yujuebo2004@163.com

Abstract

Objective: The purpose of this study is to evaluate the effectiveness and safety of CT-guided percutaneous drainage (CPD) in the management of deep neck abscesses. Factors associated with successful treatment in patients with DNA will be identified. Methods: We retrospectively studied 29 patients who presented to the department of otolaryngology with deep neck abscesses between April 2011 and April 2015. These 29 patients were managed with CPD after antibiotic therapy or needle aspiration failed. Data on patient demographics, location of infection, existing comorbidity, duration of hospitalization, treatment received, and complications were reviewed. Results: The average age of 29 patients, including 18 men and 11 women, was 56 years old. Abscess was found in parapharyngeal space (n = 16), submandibular space (n = 7), retropharyngeal space (n = 5) and pretracheal space (n = 1). The maximum transverse diameter of abscess ranged from 4.8 cm to 8.0 cm (mean 6.03 cm). Positive cultures were found in 24 cases and the most common pathogen found was *Streptococcus viridans*. Average hospital stay was 6.7 days. Deep neck abscesses were completely removed without residual in all patients. No one had complications and no one died during and after CPD. Conclusion: CPD is a safe and highly effective procedure for treating patients with deep neck abscesses who do not respond to antibiotics therapy. This technique can also provide reliable evidence on pathogens responsible for deep neck abscesses and help otolaryngologists choose effective treatment to achieve better clinical success rate. We recommend that most deep neck abscesses should be managed initially by CPD before resorting to open surgery.

Keywords

Deep Neck Abscesses, CT-Guided Percutaneous Drainage, Abscess

[*]Corresponding author.

1. Introduction

Deep neck abscesses are defined as collections of pus contained within fascial planes and spaces of head and neck. Abscesses are likely to expand from one neck space to another. Clinical symptoms will vary, depending on the exact region and dimensions of abscess spread [1]. Simple upper respiratory infection or dental infection may ultimately progress to deep neck abscesses, with potentially life-threatening complications such as upper airway obstruction, mediastinitis, internal jugular vein thrombosis, septic shock, and death [2] [3]. Although the prevalence and complication incidence of deep neck abscesses have been diminished due to improved diagnostic techniques and widespread use of antibiotics, deep neck abscesses continue to cause significant morbidity and mortality [4]-[6].

Open surgical incision-and-drainage procedure with appropriate administration of antibiotics remains the mainstay of treatment for deep neck abscesses. However, it usually involves neck incisions and exploration, which exposes patients to a cosmetically undesirable scar and a risk of neurovascular injury. Moreover, open surgery is the most expensive treatment that usually requires general anesthesia and hospitalization. CT-guided percutaneous drainage (CPD) has been used recently to remove abscesses in patients who do not have airway compromise [1] [7]. CPD has several advantages including small point of entry, quick healing time, little or no scar formation, and lower risk of contaminating surrounding deep neck spaces. Some studies have suggested that CPD of deep neck abscesses is a less invasive and an effective alternative to open surgery in select cases [1] [7].

This study presents a four-year experience of using CPD to treat deep neck abscesses at our institution. The primary objective of this study is to evaluate the effectiveness and safety of CPD for deep neck abscesses and to determine the factors influencing clinical success.

2. Methods

2.1. Data Collection

Medical and radiological record of all patients with deep neck abscesses who underwent CPD between April 2011 and April 2015 at the department of otolaryngology of one large tertiary hospital in Yangzhou, China, were reviewed. This study was approved by Research Ethics Committee of the hospital. Patients were excluded if: they did not provide informed consent; they were pregnant; they had peritonsillar abscesses; they had superficial abscesses; they had head or neck tumors; they had multi-lobulated or ill-defined abscess; or they had recurrent neck abscesses. Altogether, 29 patients were included in this study. Information reviewed included: patient age and gender, location of infection, existing comorbidity, duration of hospitalization, treatment received and complications.

2.2. CT-Guided Percutaneous Drainage (CPD) Procedure

The decision for CPD was made if patients were in one of the following conditions: there were impending complications; no improvement was observed 48 hours after antibiotics were administered; collection of pus was found within fascial spaces or a glandular structure; lobulated abscesses were greater than 3 cm in diameter or extended into deep neck spaces.

All drainage procedures were performed with CT guidance by an interventional radiologist and an attending doctor of the ward or a resident of the department of radiology. In order to choose the safest pathway for insertion of catheter and to avoid possible injury to neighboring vital structures, radiologists with more than 10 years' experience were invited to perform the procedure.

All procedures used pigtail catheter tubes. The size of catheter, either 10F or 12F, depended on the maximum transverse diameter of patients' abscesses. The exact skin entry site was defined from the contrast-enhanced CT (CECT). A trocar-type pigtail catheter, consisting of a pigtail drainage catheter and an appropriately sized two-part trocar needle, was inserted into the abscess cavity after the puncture site was sterilely prepared and anesthetized. The catheter was secured in place by suturing. Immediately after insertion of the pigtail catheter, a 20 ml syringe was mounted on the catheter and the abscess contents were aspirated from the abscess cavity. The pus was sent for gram stain and cultures in order to identify the pathogenetic organism responsible for abscess. Then, the pigtail catheter was connected to a vacuum suction ball for continuous drainage. Flushing the tube with 15 ml of sterile saline and metronidazole once daily was usually prescribed to assure patency of the tube. It should be noted that complete evacuation by aspiration of the abscess cavity was not performed on CT table because it may result in severe hemoptysis from carotid artery rupture.

2.3. Follow-Up after CPD Procedure

CT images were taken repeatedly to confirm the correct catheter placement. Patients were firstly administered empiric parenteral antibiotics and then specific antibiotics with or without intravenous steroids based on their drug sensitivity results. Day to day follow-up of patients was done by the referring physician, including clinical observations, daily catheter output measurements, and repeated ultrasound examination and repeated CECT when necessary. Catheter was left in place until drainage of pus from the catheter stopped or decision of surgery was taken due to non-closure of the abscess cavity. After discharge from hospital, patients were asked to take oral antibiotics tailored to their antibiograms for at least 14 days. All patients were followed up regularly by clinical presentation or imaging for at least 6 months.

Technical success was defined as appropriate placement of pigtail catheter into the target abscess cavity, with confirmation by means of subsequent aspiration of pus and CT scan control. Clinical treatment success was recorded when the following criteria were met: control of sepsis, resolution of abscess cavity on imaging, and no requirement for open surgical incision-and-drainage.

3. Results

Demographics, medical history and clinical outcomes of all patients reviewed are summarized in **Table 1**. Among 29 patients with uniloculated neck abscesses, 16 of them had abscesses located in the parapharyngeal space (**Figure 1**), 7 in retropharyngeal space (**Figure 2**), 5 in submandibular space (**Figure 3**) and 1 in the pretracheal space. CECT findings revealed airway compression in 8 patients. The maximum transverse diameter of abscess ranged from 4.8 cm to 8.0 cm.

Of 29 patients undergoing CPD, immediate technical success was achieved in all patients with precise placement of catheter in deep neck abscess cavities. Direct trocar technique was applied in all cases. 10F pigtail catheter was used in 16 patients whose abscess diameter was between 3 cm and 6 cm. 12F pigtail catheter was used

Table 1. Patient demographics, medial history and clinical outcomes.

Variables	CT-guided percutaneous drainage (n = 29)
Demographics	
Mean age	56 (13.4)
Male sex (%)	18 (62.1)
Underlying diseases	
Diabetes mellitus (%)	7 (24.1)
Clinical outcomes	
Mean maximum transverse diameter of abscess (cm)	6.03 (0.79)
Mean catheter period (days)	4.8 (1.22)
Mean hospital stay (days)	6.7 (1.52)
Pathogen isolated	
Aerobic	
Streptococcus viridans	9
Staphylococcus aureus	5
Klebsiella pneumoniae	4
Escherichia coli	3
Haemophilus influenzae	2
Anaerobic	
***Peptostreptococcus* sp.**	3
***Bacteroides* sp.**	1

Data are number (SD) except where otherwise specified. SD = standard deviation.

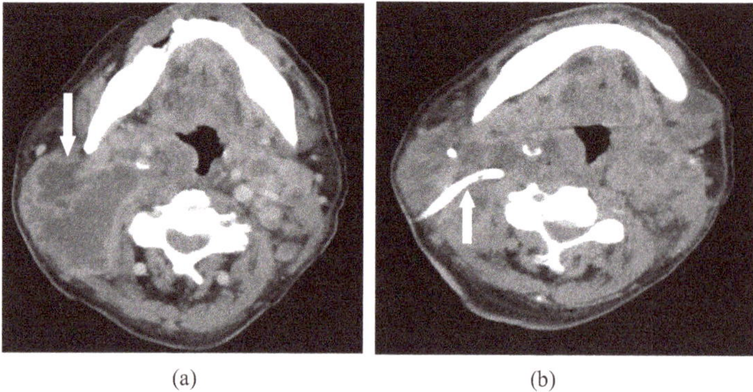

(a) (b)

Figure 1. Images from a 48-year-old man with right a paralaryngeal abscess measuring 6.5 cm × 7.5 cm × 8.0 cm, successfully treated with catheter drainage. (a) Right parapharyngeal space low attenuation abscess with contrast enhancing rim and internal septation lying deep to edematous sternocleidomastoid muscle with vascular structures lying anteromedial (arrowhead); (b) Cervical CT without contrast enhancement demonstrated the right paralaryngeal abscess with the pigtail catheter in situ (arrowhead).

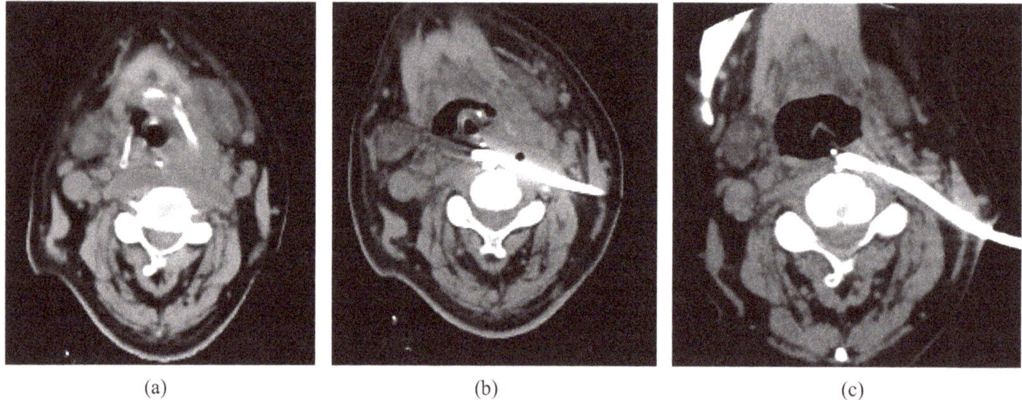

(a) (b) (c)

Figure 2. Images from a 67-year-old man with a retropharyngeal abscess measuring 2.2 cm × 6.2 cm × 8.0 cm, successfully treated with catheter drainage. (a) Contrast-enhanced neck CT reveals a uniloculated abscess (arrowhead) extending from the retropharyngeal space anterior laterally into the parapharyngeal space; (b) The trocar pigtail catheter (arrowhead) has been inserted into the abscess cavity; (c) Cervical CT without contrast enhancement taken 4 days after initial catheter drainage. An 12-F pigtail catheter (arrows) is seen within a retropharyngeal abscess cavity successfully draining the deep retropharyngeal component. No obvious pus is seen.

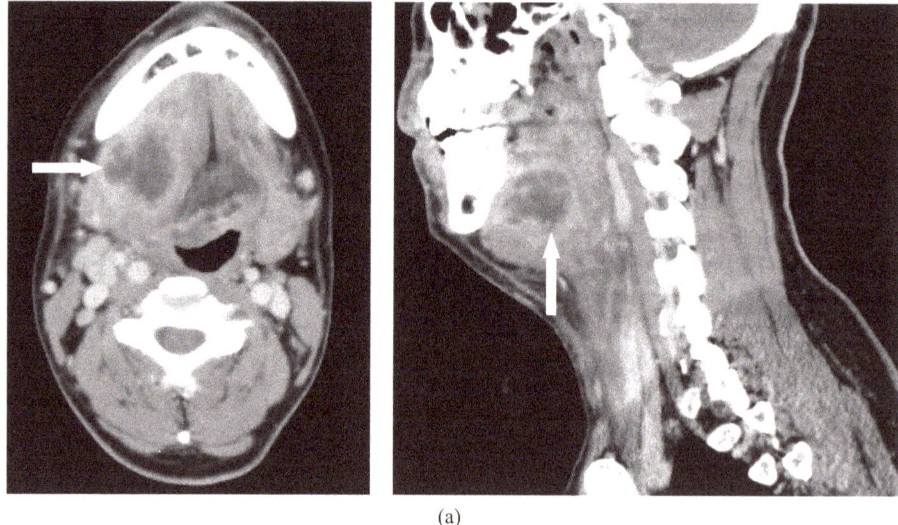

(a)

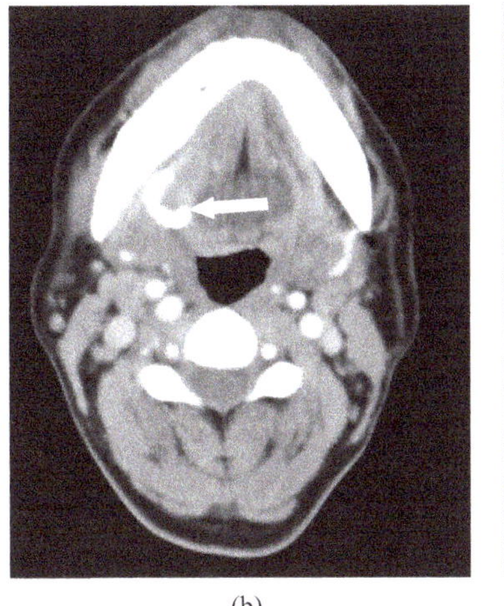

(b)

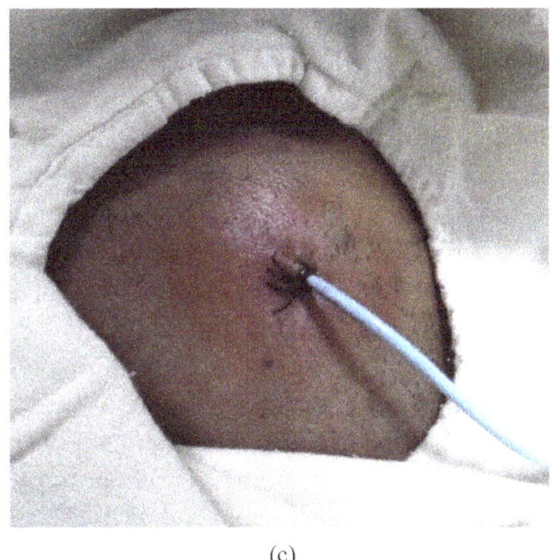

(c)

Figure 3. (a) Cervical CT (axial and sagittal reconstruction) showing a right submandibular abscess measuring 5.5 cm × 5.5 cm × 5.0 cm, located on the right side and reaching the midline, which also compressed and displaced the airway at the level of the oropharynx; (b) Percutaneous catheter in place there day after evacuation of the right parapharyngeal abscess and antibiotic treatment. No obvious pus is seen; (c) The patient after positioning of the catheter.

in 13 patients whose abscess diameter was greater than 6 cm. The procedure was well tolerated by all patients. The mean procedure time was 20 minutes. None of those patients required open incision-and-drainage surgery afterwards. Clinical success was achieved in all patients as well. After CPD, no patient required surgical treatment for uncontrolled infections, or died of infections.

At follow-up CT scan, all 29 patients who underwent CPD showed complete drainage of abscesses. The indwelling catheter period ranged from 3 to 7 days. Patients spent 6.7 days in hospital on average. Patients with diabetes mellitus (DM) had longer hospital stay than those without DM (8.6 days vs. 6.1 days) and the difference between two groups was significant ($p < 0.05$). Catheters were removed when the abscess cavity had been completely drained and symptoms such as a swollen neck, fever and pain had disappeared.

Cultures of aspirated pus were positive in 24 out of 29 patients (82.8%). Pathogens found in aspirated pus were either aerobic or anaerobic (**Table 1**). Multiple pathogens were found in four samples of abscesses.

After treatment, all patients were cured of their disease completely and no complications were detected. After discharge from hospital, no patient showed symptoms or signs of relapse at ultrasound follow-up.

4. Discussion

The widespread availability of antibiotics has reduced the incidence of deep neck abscesses drastically [2] [3]. However, deep neck abscesses remains a severe condition as it may potentially lead to life-threatening situations, especially when there is a delay in diagnosis or treatment. Surgery such as incision-and-drainage procedure bears the risk of neurovascular injury and leaving a scar. As a result, less invasive procedure has been investigated for its effectiveness and safety. In this study, we performed a retrospective study on patients who underwent CPD for deep neck abscesses. The results showed that CPD was both technically and clinically successful for all patients. No complications or relapse were reported after patients were discharged from hospital.

Clinical diagnosis of deep neck abscesses was mainly based on clinical examination and imaging examination. CT scan, especially CECT, is an important tool for evaluation of the lesion. It can be used in all patients to establish diagnosis and provide valuable information to help disclose the origin, location (also in relation to the major vascular structures and the airway), and extent of deep neck abscesses. CECT is essential in distinguishing an abscess from cellulitis or a phlegmon [8]. CECT provides a wider field of view and is more useful than ultrasound scan in defining the extent of neck abscesses as ultrasound scan cannot always identify small or deep abscess and cannot provide the specific anatomical information necessary for surgical intervention [9].

Therapeutic management of deep neck abscesses includes rational antibiotic treatment, drainage (surgical or percutaneous), repeated needle aspiration, and open surgery [1]. Recent studies have shown that, in select cases, uncomplicated deep neck abscesses can be effectively treated with antibiotics and careful monitoring, without surgical drainage [10] [11]. However, Surgical or percutaneous drainage is required in 10% to 83% of patients who presented with deep neck space infections [12] [13], as medical therapy could fail due to virulence of the responsible pathogens or inadequate concentration of antibiotics within the abscess cavity [10] [14]. The open surgical drainages are effective but have some significant disadvantages. The patients are required to have an operating room and team and a general anesthetic, which may also necessitate securing of airway fiber optically or with a tracheotomy. The open neck wounds may also add the risk of neurovascular injury and result in a cosmetically undesirable scar.

CPD has been proved to be safe and effective with less morbidity and mortality than surgical resection [15] [16]. It can improve the accuracy in reaching the involved site and decrease costs for a non-operating room procedure. Other advantages of CT-guided percutaneous drainage are rapid clinical and radiological improvement of pyogenic abscess which may avoid complications that can occur with prolonged, improved cosmetic results and conservative treatment. Therefore, it can be used as an alternative to surgical drainage.

Although ultrasound and CT scanning guidance were the most common techniques used for placement of needles or catheters, CT-guided drainage was chosen in this study. There are several reasons. First of all, CT scan is a useful diagnostic tool to detect and establish the treatment plan for deep neck abscesses. CECT is able to identify impeding airway complications before they present clinically [17]. Second, CT can differentiate abscess from carotid artery aneurysm, cellulitis or phlegmon, which is important since catheter drainage has a higher complication rate. Third, CT is optimal in determining the wall thickness of an abscess, contents of an abscess and its relationship to the adjacent neck vital structures. Moreover, any obstructing foreign body or head and neck neoplasms can also be visualized. Finally, when a deeper abscess is encountered, CT-guided needle aspiration is more feasible than ultrasound guidance [16].

Previous studies have demonstrated that CPD showed high success rate for infection treatment and saved patients from more invasive surgical intervention. In our study, none of the patients required any further surgical intervention without any complications related to drainage procedures. In addition, clinical success rate was extremely high (100%, n = 29), which is similar to prior studies, and no complications occurred. These results are comparable to the results of the largest series published to date. Cole *et al.* [7] reported successful CPD in 2 patients without complications, and surgery was avoided in these 2 patients (100% success rate). Thanos *et al.* [1] also reported successful CT-guided percutaneous catheter drainage of potentially life-threatening neck abscesses in 15 patients and surgery was avoided in 14 patients (93% success rate). Surgery was performed in one patient because of the presence of multiple internal septation that could not be drained via percutaneous catheters. No complications were reported in their study.

In this study, we used the trocar technique for pigtail catheters insertion in all cases. Although some other literature suggested that the Seldinger technique with placement of catheter might decreases the likelihood of complications [16], we believed that the choice of technique depended on the ability, experience and preference of the interventional radiologist performing the procedure. In our study, we used 10F and 12F catheters for drainage based on the size of deep neck abscesses and irrigated the abscess cavities with metronidazole and saline solution until the wash out was clear. The duration of purulent discharge varied from 3 to 9 days. We used a vacuum suction ball for continuous drainage to facilitate the evacuation of residual pus which is similar to Chang *et al.* study [18]. The main advantages of this closed drainage system are the superior and persistent negative pressure for drainage, prevention of contamination in the surgical dressing, and easy management for nursing [19]. We obtained positive cultures in 82.8% of cases, which is consistent with other studies where positive cultures ranged from 56.3% - 85.7% of deep neck abscesses cases [1] [11] [20]. Streptococcus species were found in the majority of cases (48.2%), which is also consistent with other studies of deep neck abscesses [21] [22]. Our study results suggest that CPD with bacteria cultures can help us make more rational decision on treatment for infections.

5. Limitation

The limitation of this study should be acknowledged. First of all, we included a very small sample of patients in our review. Besides, retrospective studies may be less reliable in terms of data collection. Prospective study and more cases are required to further examine the effectiveness of CPD in the future.

Conflict of Interest

The authors declare no conflict of interest.

References

[1] Thanos, L., Mylona, S., Kalioras, V., *et al.* (2005) Potentially Life-Threatening Neck Abscesses: Therapeutic Management under CT-Guided Drainage. *CardioVascular and Interventional Radiology*, **29**, 196-199. http://dx.doi.org/10.1007/s00270-004-0003-y

[2] Eftekharian, A., Roozbahany, N.A., Vaezeafshar, R., *et al.* (2009) Deep Neck Infections: A Retrospective Review of 112 Cases. *European Archives of Oto-Rhino-Laryngology*, **266**, 273-277. http://dx.doi.org/10.1007/s00405-008-0734-5

[3] Hasegawa, J., Hidaka, H., Tateda, M., Kudo, T., Sagai, S., Miyazaki, M., *et al.* (2010) An Analysis of Clinical Risk Factors of Deep Neck Infection. *Auris Nasus Larynx*, **10**, 356-361.

[4] Ridder, G.J., Technau-Ihling, K., Sander, A., *et al.* (2005) Spectrum and Management of Deep Neck Space Infections: An 8-Year Experience of 234 Cases. *Otolaryngology—Head & Neck Surgery*, **133**, 709-714. http://dx.doi.org/10.1016/j.otohns.2005.07.001

[5] Huang, T.T., Liu, T.C., Chen, P.R., Tseng, F.Y., Yeh, T.H. and Chen, Y.S. (2004) Deep Neck Infection: Analysis of 185 Cases. *Head & Neck*, **26**, 854-860. http://dx.doi.org/10.1002/hed.20014

[6] Bottin, R., Marioni, G., Rinaldi, R., *et al.* (2003) Deep Neck Infection: A Present-Day Complication. A Retrospective Review of 83 Cases (1998-2001). *European Archives of Oto-Rhino-Laryngology*, **260**, 576-579. http://dx.doi.org/10.1007/s00405-003-0634-7

[7] Cole, D., Bankoff, M. and Carter, B. (1984) Percutaneous Catheter Drainage of Deep Neck Infections Guided by CT. *Radiology*, **152**, 224. http://dx.doi.org/10.1148/radiology.152.1.6729120

[8] Marioni, G., Castegnaro, E., Staffieri, C., *et al.* (2006) Deep Neck Infection in Elderly Patients. A Single Institution Experience (2000-2004). *Aging Clinical and Experimental Research*, **18**, 127-132. http://dx.doi.org/10.1007/BF03327427

[9] Smith II, J.L., Hsu, J.M. and Chang, J. (2006) Predicting Deep Neck Space Abscess Using Computed Tomography. *American Journal of Otolaryngology*, **27**, 244-247. http://dx.doi.org/10.1016/j.amjoto.2005.11.008

[10] McClay, J.E., Murray, A.D. and Booth, T. (2003) Intravenous Antibiotic Therapy for Deep Neck Abscesses Defined by Computed Tomography. *Archives of Otolaryngology—Head & Neck Surgery*, **129**, 1207-1212. http://dx.doi.org/10.1001/archotol.129.11.1207

[11] Lee, Y.Q. and Kanagalingam, J. (2011) Deep Neck Abscesses: The Singapore Experience. *European Archives of Oto-Rhino-Laryngology*, **268**, 609-614. http://dx.doi.org/10.1007/s00405-010-1387-8

[12] Mayor, G.P., Milan, J.M. and Martinez-Vidal, A. (2001) Is Conservative Treatment of Deep Neck Space Infections Appropriate? *Head & Neck*, **23**, 126-133. http://dx.doi.org/10.1002/1097-0347(200102)23:2<126::AID-HED1007>3.0.CO;2-N

[13] Ridder, J.G., Eglinger, C.F., Technau-Ihlinge, K., *et al.* (2000) Deep Neck Abscess Masquerading Hypopharyngeal Carcinoma. *Otolaryngology—Head and Neck Surgery*, **123**, 659-660. http://dx.doi.org/10.1067/mhn.2000.110613

[14] Oh, J.-H., Kim, Y. and Kim, C.-H. (2007) Parapharyngeal Abscess: Comprehensive Management Protocol. *ORL*, **69**, 37-42. http://dx.doi.org/10.1159/000096715

[15] Poe, L.B., Petro, G.R. and Matta, I. (1996) Percutaneous CT-Guided Aspiration of Deep Neck Abscesses. *AJNR—American Journal of Neuroradiology*, **17**, 1359-1363.

[16] Cottrell, D.A., Bankoff, M. and Norris, L.H. (1992) Computed Tomography-Guided Percutaneous Drainage of a Head and Neck Infection. *Journal of Oral and Maxillofacial Surgery*, **50**, 1119-1121. http://dx.doi.org/10.1016/0278-2391(92)90505-T

[17] Cmejrek, R., Coticchia, J. and Arnold, J. (2002) Presentation, Diagnosis, and Management of Deep-Neck Abscesses in Infants. *Archives of Otolaryngology—Head & Neck Surgery*, **128**, 1361-1364. http://dx.doi.org/10.1001/archotol.128.12.1361

[18] Chang, K.P., Chen, Y.L., Hao, S.P. and Chen, S.M. (2005) Ultrasound-Guided Closed Drainage for Abscesses of the Head and Neck. *Otolaryngology—Head and Neck Surgery*, **132**, 119-124. http://dx.doi.org/10.1016/j.otohns.2004.08.004

[19] Peckitt, N.S., Fields, M.J. and Gregory, M.C. (1990) A Closed Drainage System for Head and Neck Sepsis. *Journal of Oral and Maxillofacial Surgery*, **48**, 758-759. http://dx.doi.org/10.1016/0278-2391(90)90068-D

[20] Asai, N., Ohkuni, Y., Yamazaki, I., *et al.* (2013) Therapeutic Impact of CT-Guided Percutaneous Catheter Drainage in Treatment of Deep Tissue Abscesses. *The Brazilian Journal of Infectious Diseases*, **17**, 483-486. http://dx.doi.org/10.1016/j.bjid.2012.12.008

[21] Duszak Jr., R.L., Levy, J.M., Akins, E.W., Bakal, C.W., *et al.* (2000) Percutaneous Catheter Drainage of Infected Intra-

Abdominal Fluid Collections. American College of Radiology. ACR Appropriateness Criteria. *Radiology*, **215**, 1067-1075.

[22] Van Sonnenberg, E., Wittich, G.R., Edwards, D.K., Casola, G., von Waldenburg, H.S., *et al*. (1987) Percutaneous Diagnostic and Therapeutic Interventional Radiologic Procedures in Children: Experience in 100 Patients. *Radiology*, **162**, 601-605. http://dx.doi.org/10.1148/radiology.162.3.2949336

38

Atypical Olfactory Neuroblastoma Presenting as Sinonasal Polyposis with Nasopharyngeal Extension: A Case Report

Jagdish Prasad Purohit, Chandra Bhan*, Bhoopendra Singh, Ajay Pratap Singh, Siva Selvaraj, Manish Pandey, Vijay Krishna Sharma

Department of ENT, Head and Neck Surgery, MLB Medical College, Jhansi, India
Email: *chandrabhan.prajapati@gmail.com, bhoopimedico@gmail.com, chandrabhanprajapati1@gmail.com, dr.aps27@gmail.com, drsivaselvaraj@gmail.com, selvarajk.siva@gmail.com, chandrabhan.prajapati1@gmail.com

Abstract

Background: Olfactory neuroblastoma also known as Esthesioneuroblastoma (ENB) is a tumor arising from the basal layer of olfactory epithelium in the superior recess of the nasal cavity in the region of cribriform plate. Incidence peaks once in 11 - 20 years of age and again in 50 - 60 years of age. It is equally found in men and women. Aim: The main aim of this case report is to characterize the clinical features of ENB showing nasopharyngeal involvement and its importance in the differential diagnosis of sinonasal neuroendocrine malignancies. Case presentation: Two cases are reported. The first case was a 21-year-old male with symptoms of nasal obstruction, recurrent epistaxis, nasal discharge, headache and paresthesia over the face with an evolution of 1 year with no previous history of trauma. Diagnostic nasal endoscopy revealed reddish gray mass filling bilateral nasal cavities. Posterior rhinoscopy revealed mass coming through choanae and filling the nasopharynx. Endoscopic resection of tumor was done and postoperatively all the symptoms of the patient resolved. The second case was a 62-year-old male with complaints of nasal obstruction, nasal discharge, recurrent epistaxis, anosmia and difficulty in swallowing. On computed tomography, anteriorly, the mass was extending up to external nares and posteriorly up to the nasopharynx, superiorly up to nasal roof and inferiorly up to hard palate. No obvious erosion of floor of anterior cranial fossa was seen. No intracranial extension was seen. Surgery was advised but patient refused to undergo any treatment. Conclusion: This study highlights the characteristics and clinical features of ENB showing nasopharyngeal involvement and their importance in the differential diagnosis of sinonasal neuroendocrine malignancies.

*Corresponding author.

Keywords

Esthesioneuroblastoma, Cribriform Plate, Neuroectodermal

1. Introduction

Olfactory neuroblastoma is an uncommon tumor of neuroectodermal origin, arising from basal cells of the olfactory neuroepithelium [1] [2]. Olfactory neuroblastoma represents less than 5 percent of all sinonasal malignancies. It is histologically similar to adrenal or sympathetic ganglionic neuroblastomas and retinoblastomas. The incidence of this tumor has a bimodal distribution with peaks at 20 and 50 years of age [3]. Unlike most of the sinonasal malignancies, it is equally distributed in women and men. The non-specific symptoms of nasal obstruction, recurrent epistaxis, hyposmia, headache and the special anatomical location of the tumor often lead to a diagnosis of benign paranasal disease thus delaying the correct diagnosis [4]. As the tumor grows, it tends to spread submucosally in all directions to involve the paranasal sinuses, nasal cavity, oral cavity, the orbits, and the brain [5] [6]. Tumor cells are mitotically active and developing into sustentacular and neuronal cells. There exist variable neurofibrillary materials. Neuro endocrine tumor is capable of causing paraneoplastic syndromes by secreting peptides.

Objective

This study highlights the characteristics and clinical features of ENB showing nasopharyngeal involvement and their importance in the differential diagnosis of sinonasal neuroendocrine malignancies.

2. Case Report

2.1. Case 1

A 21years old male came to our hospital complaining of nasal obstruction, recurrent epistaxis, nasal discharge, headache and paresthesia over the face with an evolution of 1 year with no previous history of trauma. Diagnostic nasal endoscopy revealed reddish gray mass filling the posterior part of the bilateral nasal cavities. Posterior rhinoscopy revealed mass coming through choanae and filling the nasopharynx. In the medical history, the patient had no reports of viral infections in childhood or other systemic illness. No family history of any hereditary diseases. Patient also denied any alcohol consumption or tobacco use. Cervical lymph node enlargement was not found on palpation.

Conventional X-rays and computed tomography (CT) revealed nasal cavities, bilateral maxillary, frontal, ethmoidal and sphenoidal sinuses soft tissue opacity. Lesion was extending in the posterior nasal cavity, upper part of posterior nasal septum and nasopharynx. Severe deossification of intervening bones was found. Both osteomeatal units were blocked and lamina papyracea were intact. Crista galli was normal (**Figure 1** and **Figure 2**).

Microscopic examination of the incisional biopsy and surgical specimen showed cellular tissue consisting of uniformly small cells with round dense nuclei and scanty eosinophilic cytoplasm. Cells were arranged to form compact masses with occasional rosettes and fibrillary reticular background, separated by loose fibro-vascular stroma. Incisional biopsy suggested diagnosis towards olfactory neuroblastoma (**Figure 3**).

Patient was thoroughly evaluated; endoscopic removal of mass from the nasal cavity, maxillary, ethmoidal, sphenoidal and frontal sinuses and nasopharynx was done. Posterior part of nasal septum was removed. No adjuvant treatment was given. Patient became asymptomatic after surgery and during follow up.

2.2. Case 2

A 62 years old male patient came to our hospital with complaints of nasal obstruction, nasal discharge, recurrent epistaxis, anosmia and difficulty in swallowing for 10 years. Anterior rhinoscopy revealed reddish gray mass filling bilateral nasal cavities. Posterior rhinoscopy revealed mass coming through choanae and filling the nasopharynx. Mass was pushing hard and soft palate downwards compromising the oral cavity space (**Figure 4**). In the medical history of the patient there were no reports of trauma or other systemic illnesses. No family history of hereditary diseases was there. He gave history of alcohol consumption and smoking. Cervical lymph node enlargement was not detected on palpation.

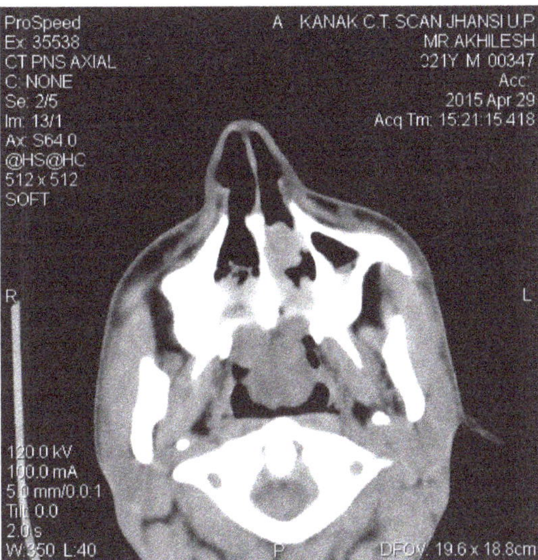

Figure 1. Case 1: CT PNS axial view showing tumor occupying the nasal cavity and extending up to nasopharynx.

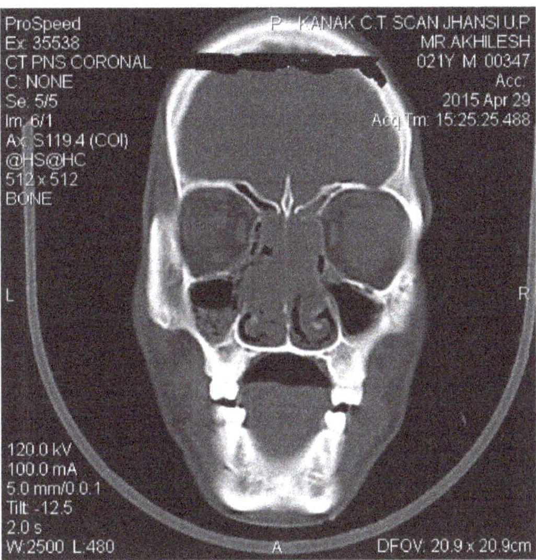

Figure 2. Case 1: CT PNS coronal view showing tumor occupying the nasal cavity with sinuses involvement.

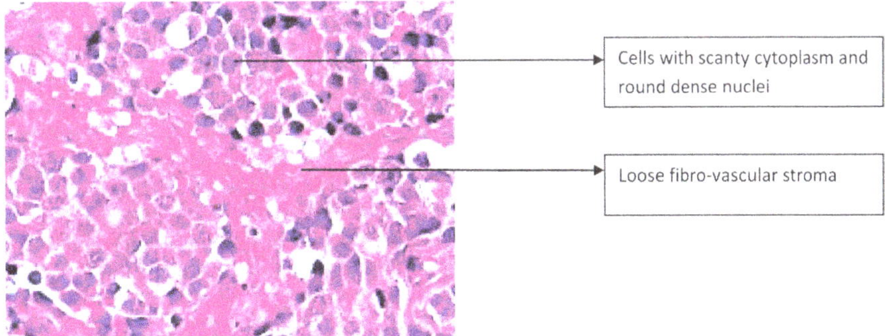

Figure 3. Case 1: Histopathological section showing cellular tissue with round dense nuclei and scanty cytoplasm. Cells are arranged in compact masses with separated by loose fibro-vascular stroma.

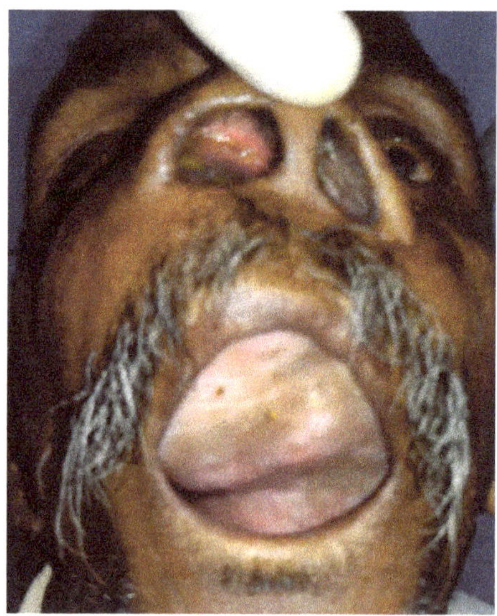

Figure 4. Case 2: Tumor occupying bilateral nasal cavity and pressing palate downwards.

Computed tomography revealed large soft tissue mass filling the entire nasal cavity. Anteriorly nasal septum was pushed towards left side; posteriorly nasal septum was not visualized. Bilateral frontal, ethmoidal and sphenoidal sinuses were opacified. Hard palate was pushed inferiorly and was thinned out. Anteriorly the mass was extending up to external nostril and posteriorly up to the nasopharynx, superiorly up to nasal roof and inferiorly up to hard palate. No obvious erosion of floor of anterior cranial fossa was seen. No intracranial extension was seen (**Figure 5**).

Microscopic examination of the incisional biopsy and surgical specimen showed highly vascular cellular tumor tissue consisting of proliferating uniformly small round to oval cells having large round hyperchromatic nucleus and scanty cytoplasm to form confluent masses, with occasional pseudorosettes separated by finely fibrillar stroma infiltrated by few inflammatory cells. Incisional biopsy suggested diagnosis towards round cell tumor (**Figure 6**).

Surgery and chemotherapy was advised to the patient but he refused any kinds of treatments.

3. Discussion

Sinonasal neuroendocrine malignancies are complex and rare with Esthesioneuroblastoma representing the most undifferentiated end of the spectrum of neuroendocrine tumors [7]. Esthesioneuroblastoma originates from olfactory epithelium in the upper nasal cavity in the region of the cribriform plate. Esthesioneuroblastoma accounts for approximately 3% to 6% of nasal cavity and paranasal sinus cancer cases, 0.3% of upper aero digestive tract malignancies and less than 1% of all head and neck cancers. This tumor is found equally in man and woman and occurs over a wide age range, though a bimodal age distribution with an early peak from 11 to 20 years and a later peak between 50 and 60 years of age has been reported [2]. Approximately 1300 cases have been identified since Berger and Luc described the first case in 1924 as esthesioneuroepithelioma olfactif.

Esthesioneuroblastoma is characterized by slow progression and locally aggressive behavior, which lead to long-term survival but very frequent late local recurrence. The aggressiveness of esthesioneuroblastoma is partly due to their complex anatomical location, close to vital structures, which is associated with non-specific symptoms that lead to delay in the patient diagnosis. The reported cases revealed atypical esthesioneuroblastoma identified by nasal symptoms, with radiographic images that suggested a polypoidal mass occupying the sinuses and nasal cavity and nasopharynx.

The diagnosis of esthesioneuroblastoma via light microscopy by itself can be difficult since the tumor tends to exhibit little or no differentiation. Pathological classification is challenging because the tumors must be differentiated from other round cell neoplasms of the nasal cavity such as Non-Hodgkin's lymphoma, Ewing's sarcoma, mucosal malignant melanoma and neuroendocrine carcinomas [8].

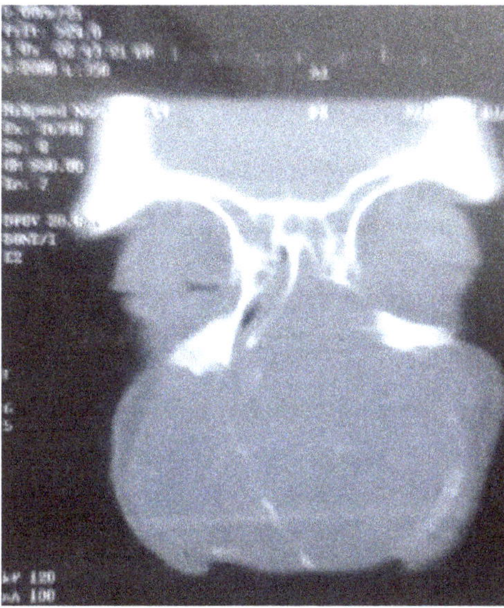

Figure 5. Case 2: CT scan showing sinuses involvement without intracranial extension.

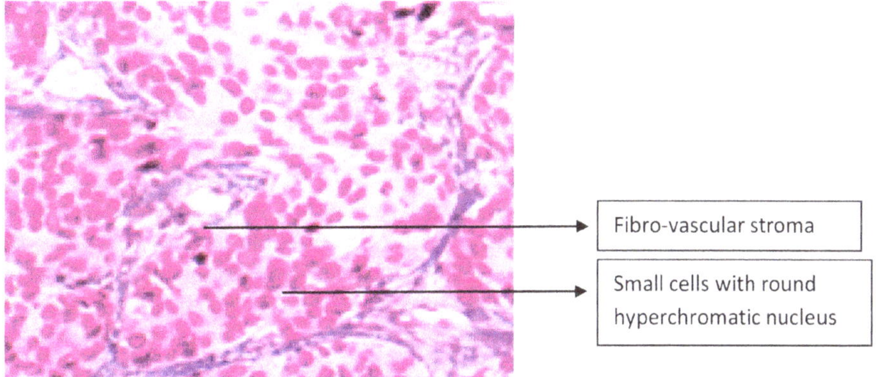

Figure 6. Case 2: Histopathological section showing highly vascular tissue consisting of proliferating small round cells having large round hyperchromatic nucleus, scanty cytoplasm, separated by finely fibrillar, stroma, infiltrated by small numbers of inflammatory cells.

The histopathological parameters that help in differentiating these tumors include the pattern of tumor cell arrangement, stroma, nuclear chromatin characteristics, presence or absence of neutrophil and rossetting. The use of a broad panel of antibodies in immunohistochemical staining may help to establish a final diagnosis. Esthesioneuroblastoma is usually positive for general neuroendocrine markers, such as neuron specific enolase (NSE), S-100 protein, synaptophysin (Syn) and chromogranin. Esthesioneuroblastoma is typically the most positive on immunohistochemical staining. ENB shows S-100 protein positive peripheral dendritic cells corresponding to Schwann cells present within the neoplasm or at the edges of tumor nests. Positivity varies in the cases reported in the literature for vimentin, keratin, glial fibrillary acidic protein, and neurofilaments [9] [10]. In the reported case the tumor showed strong positive expression of NSE, synaptophysin and vimentin. Significant correlation between CD44 expression and the stage of the disease has been suggested to help in predicting the clinical outcome. CD44s negative tumors are significantly correlated with the lack of differentiation. Thus over-expression of CD44s could be considered as a predictor of absence of infiltration of the tumor and neuroblastic tumors subtypes with favorable prognosis [11]. Staging and 5 year survival of esthesioneuroblastoma was given by Kadish in 1976 (**Table 1**). ENB was classified according to TNM system by DULGUEROV et CALCATERRA (1992) (**Table 2**).

The rates of primary tumor recurrence vary and most of the case series show local recurrence rates of approximately 14% to 30%. The mean time of recurrence is 2 years, but recurrences can occur as late as 10 years after the initial diagnosis, with approximately 50% of them occurring after 5 years [9] [10] [12].

Table 1. Clinical classifications of esthesioneuroblastoma KADISH (1976) [15].

Stage	Location	5 year survival
Stage A	Tumor localized to the nasal cavity	75%
Stage B	Spread to sinuses	68%
Stage C	Extension over paranasal sinuses	41%

Table 2. TNM classification according to DULGUEROV et CALCATERRA (1992).

T1	Tumor localized to the nasal cavity and paranasal sinuses with a space between tumor and lamina cribosa
T2	Tumor developed in nasal cavity or sinuses but in contact with cribriform lamina and/or sphenoid extension
T3	Tumor with intracranial extradural and/or orbital expansion
T4	Tumor with intracranial intradural extension
N0	No metastatic cervical nodes
N1	Metastatic cervical nodes
M0	No distant metastases
M1	Distant metastases

Craniofacial resection with definitive or adjuvant radiotherapy has been used for local control. Chemotherapy can be used in an adjuvant or neoadjuvant attempt and also in the metastatic phase or recurrent or advanced disease, although its effectiveness has still not been established. Such multimodality therapy has become the most common approach to esthesioneuroblastoma [13] [14].

According to above classification, the tumor of both the patient can be categorized as intermediate grade malignancy (T2N0M0) and along with clinical stage (Kadish B.). Endoscopic resection of tumor was done in first case and postoperatively all the symptoms of the patient resolved. Second patient refused all kinds of treatment.

4. Conclusion

This study highlights the characteristics and clinical features of ENB with nasal cavity and nasopharyngeal involvement and its importance in the differential diagnosis of sinonasal neuroendocrine malignancies.

Affiliation

Nil.

References

[1] Lund, V.J. and Milroy, C. (1993) Olfactory Neuroblastoma: Clinical and Pathological Aspects. *Rhinology*, **31**, 1-6.

[2] Elkon, D. and Hightower, S.I. (1979) Esthesioneuroblastoma. *Cancer*, **44**, 1087-1094. http://dx.doi.org/10.1002/1097-0142(197909)44:3<1087::AID-CNCR2820440343>3.0.CO;2-A

[3] Palacios & Valvassori, 1998; Hwang, *et al.*; Tamase, *et al.*, 2004; Lin, *et al.*; Ghaffar & Salahuddin, 2005; Yu, *et al.*; Iliades, *et al.*, 2002; Thompson, 2009.

[4] Dulguerov, P., Allal, A.S. and Calcaterra, T.C. (2001) Esthesioneuroblastoma: A Meta Analysis and Review. *The Lancet Oncology*, **2**, 683-690. http://dx.doi.org/10.1016/S1470-2045(01)00558-7

[5] Mills, S.E. and Frierson Jr., H.F. (1985) Olfactory Neuroblastoma: A Clinicopathological Study of 21 Cases. *The American Journal of Surgical Pathology*, **9**, 317-327. http://dx.doi.org/10.1097/00000478-198505000-00001

[6] Batsakis, J.G. (1979) Tumors of the Head and Neck. 2nd Edition, Williams and Wilkins, Baltimore, 338-349.

[7] Wenig, B.M., Prasad, M.L., Dulguerov, P., Fanburg, J.C., Kapadia, S.B. and Thomson, L.D. (2005) Neuroectodermal tumors. In: Barnes, L., Eveson, J.W., Reichart, P. and Sidransky, D., Eds., *WHO Classification of Tumors*, Pathology and Genetics, Head and Neck Tumors, IARC Press, Lyon, 65-75.

[8] Thompson, L.D. (2009) Olfactory Neuroblastoma. *Head and Neck Pathology*, **3**, 252-259. http://dx.doi.org/10.1007/s12105-009-0125-2

[9] Menon, S., Pai, P., Sengar, M., Aggarwal, J.P. and Kane, S.V. (2010) Sinonasal Malignancies with Neuroendocrine Differentiation: Case Series and Review of Literature. *Indian Journal of Pathology & Microbiology*, **53**, 28-34. http://dx.doi.org/10.4103/0377-4929.59179

[10] Zhang, M., Zhou, L., Wang, D.H., Huang, W.T. and Wang, S.Y. (2010) Diagnosis and Management of Esthesioneuroblastoma. *ORL: Journal for Oto-Rhino-Laryngology and Its Related Specialties*, **72**, 113-118. http://dx.doi.org/10.1159/000278255

[11] Tabyaoui, I., Tahiri-Jouti, N., Serhier, Z., Bennani-Othmani, M., Sibai, H., Itri, M., Benchekroun, S. and Zamiati, S. (2013) Immunohistochemical Expression of CD44s in Human Neuroblastic Tumors: Moroccan Experience and Highlights on Current Data. *Diagnostic Pathology*, **8**, 39. http://dx.doi.org/10.1186/1746-1596-8-39

[12] Gore, M.R. and Zanation, A.M. (2009) Salvage Treatment of Late Neck Metastasis in Esthesioneuroblastoma: A Meta-Analysis. *Archives of Otolaryngology—Head & Neck Surgery*, **135**, 1030-1034. http://dx.doi.org/10.1001/archoto.2009.143

[13] Kane, A.J., Sughrue, M.E., Rutkowski, M.J., Aranda, D., Mills, S.A., Buencamino, R., Fang, S., Barani, I.J. and Parsa, A.T. (2010) Post Treatment Prognosis of Patients with Esthesioneuroblastoma. *Journal of Neurosurgery*, **113**, 340-351. http://dx.doi.org/10.3171/2010.2.JNS091897

[14] Platek, M.E., Merzianu, M., Mashtare, T.L., Popat, S.R., Rigual, N.R., Warren, G.W. and Singh, A.K. (2011) Improved Survival Following Surgery and Radiation Therapy for Olfactory Neuroblastoma: Analysis of the SEER Database. *Radiation Oncology*, **6**, 41. http://dx.doi.org/10.1186/1748-717X-6-41

[15] Kadish, S., Goodman, M. and Wang, C.C. (1976) Olfactory Neuroblastoma. A Clinical Analysis of 17 Cases. *Cancer*, **23**, 1571-1676. http://dx.doi.org/10.1002/1097-0142(197603)37:3<1571::AID-CNCR2820370347>3.0.CO;2-L

39

Surgical Experience in the Management of 125 Patients with Thyroid Masses in Kashmir

M. S. Sheikh[1], S. Bunafsha[2], S. Gul Afshan[3]

[1]Associate Professor of ENT, Government Medical College Srinagar, Kashmir, India
[2]Medical Interne, Women's Medical College Hospital, Uttara Model Town, Dhaka, Bangladesh
[3]Externe, Women's Medical College, Dhaka, Bangladesh
Email: dr.sheikhms@yahoo.com

Abstract

Results of surgical treatment in 125 patients with thyroid masses who attended to a Unit of the Department of ENT, Head and Neck Surgery of Govt. Medical College associated SMHS Hospital Srinagar in the first decade of this century are presented. Age of the patients ranged from 17 to 68 years peaking in the fourth decade of life (Figure 1 and Figure 2). Near 85% of the patients with thyroid masses were female and most of the cases (76%) euthyroid at the time of presentation. Depending upon the expertise of the pathologist, the FNA cytology has a good role in the preoperative diagnosis of thyroid masses especially the malignant types (Figure 3 and Figure 4). The specificity of FNA cytology in detecting malignant thyroid tumors in this study was 100% and the sensitivity was 73.08%. The overall diagnostic accuracy was 83.20%. 45.60% of the thyroid masses proved on excision biopsy to be malignant of which papillary carcinoma continued to be the most common malignant thyroid tumor followed by the medullary, the follicular and the undifferentiated types. Radionuclide scanning gave equivocal results in distinguishing between the benign and the malignant thyroid nodules in this study, but it was useful in evaluating indeterminate cases of FNA cytology. Magnetic resonance imaging of neck was used as an adjunctive imaging modality in assessing the extent of the primary malignant thyroid lesion, its direct extra-thyroidal spread and regional nodal metastases (Figure 5 and Figure 6). Different surgical techniques utilized in dealing with the thyroid masses included partial thyroidectomies and total thyroidectomy with or without modified neck dissection and the results are discussed.

Keywords

Thyroid Masses, Fine Needle Aspiration Cytology, Thyroid Scintiscan, Magnetic Resonance Imaging, Thyroidectomy, Excision Biopsy, Prognosticators

1. Introduction

The number of patients with thyroid masses attending the tertiary care hospitals in Kashmir for treatment is on rise. Differentiated thyroid cancer seems to afflict more and more of the young women every year [1] [2]. The epidemiology of the thyroid masses was studied in this series of patients and their thyroid status were determined. Technitium-99 pertechnetate scintiscanning patterns of thyroid masses were correlated with the histopathological findings; and also the accuracy of fine needle aspiration cytology in the diagnosis of thyroid masses evaluated. Surgical strategy in dealing with the thyroid masses especially the malignant ones was developed in the study and the prognosticators established.

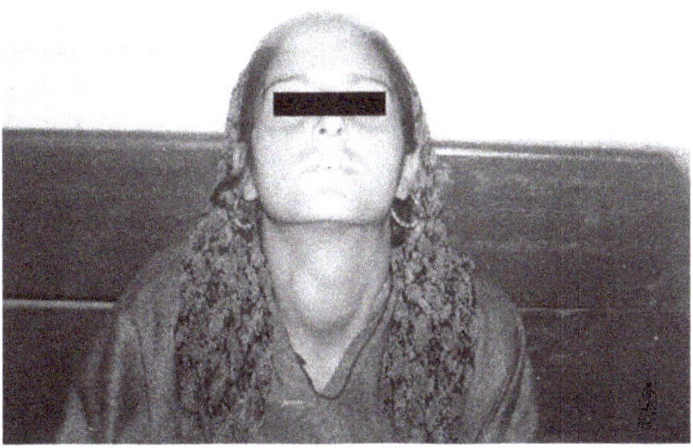

Figure 1. Papillary carcinoma of thyroid in a female of 37 years.

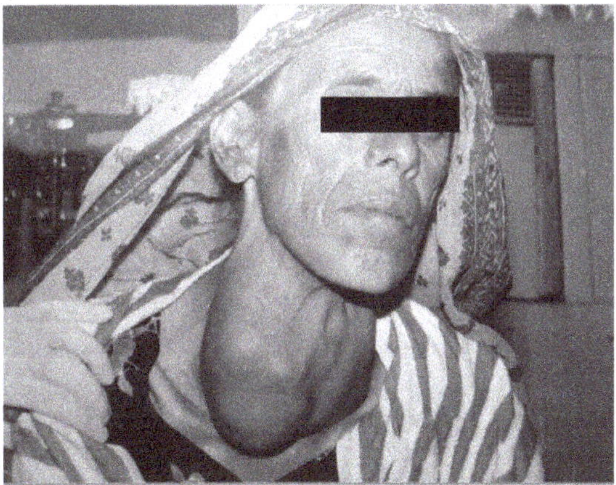

Figure 2. Multinodular goitre in an elderly female.

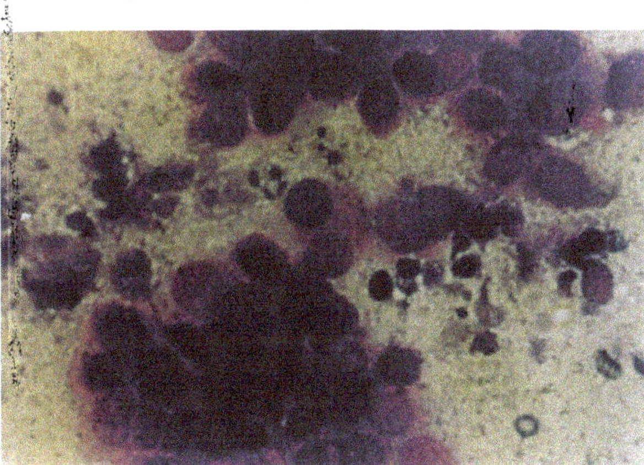

Figure 3. Photomicrograph of an FNA smear of papillary carcinoma of thyroid; Giemsa stain; ×400.

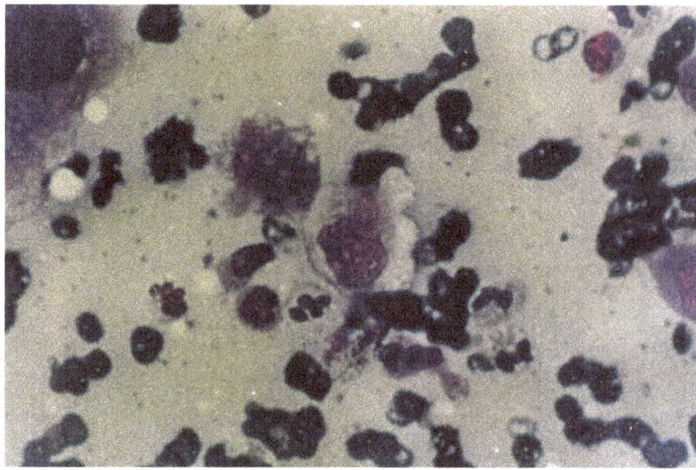

Figure 4. Photomicrograph of an FNA smear of anaplastic carcinoma of thyroid; Giemsa stain; ×400.

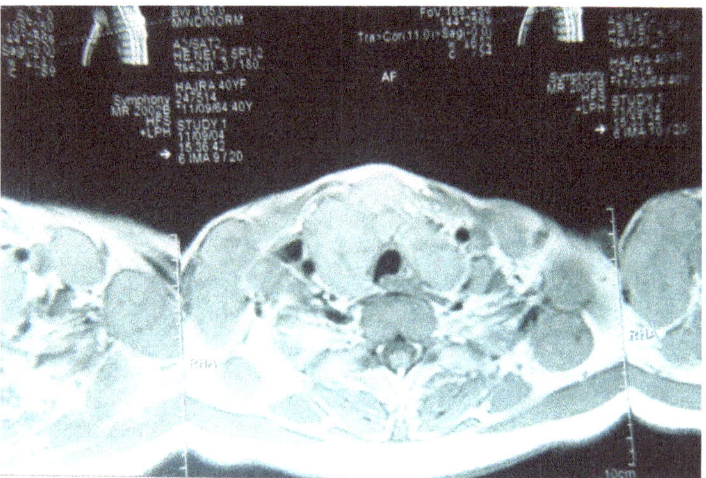

Figure 5. Axial MRI scan of neck showing capsular disruption of thyroid gland by papillary carcinoma, and multiple-level cervical nodal involvement.

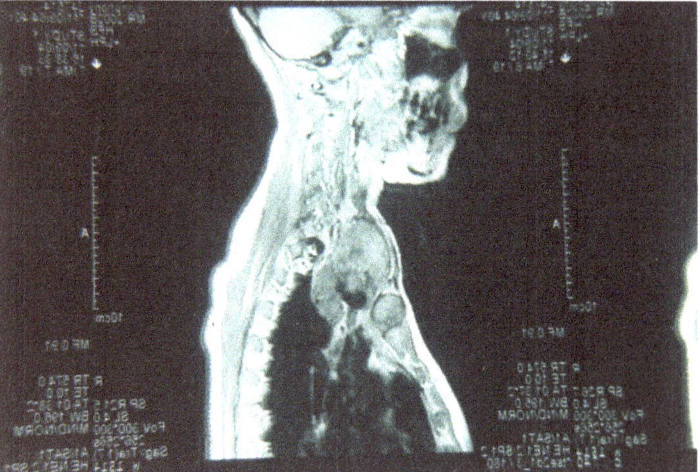

Figure 6. Sagittal MRI scan of neck showing superior mediastinal nodal involvement by papillary carcinoma of thyroid.

2. Material and Methods

The present prospective study is based on 125 patients with thyroid masses who were admitted in a Unit of the Department of ENT, Head & Neck Surgery in the Govt. Medical College associated SMHS Hospital Srinagar from the year 2000 to 2010 and were treated with different types of thyroid surgery. History of the disease was taken and the patients subjected to systemic examination and local examination of neck to know about the size and extent of the thyroid mass, and about the regional and distant metastasis in case of the suspected malignant masses. Fine needle aspiration cytology using Giemsa or haematoxylin stains was done in all of the patients. Bethesda system for reporting thyroid cytopathology was recommended late in the course of this study in the year 2007 [3]. Thyroid scintiscan using technetium-99 radionuclide was possible in only fifty unselected cases and the magnetic resonance imaging of the neck was done in all FNA positive carcinomas and all those false negatives who were subjected to completion thyroidectomy. FNA-documented benign masses of the thyroid in this study were generally managed by partial surgeries whereas the surgical strategy for the carcinomas was formulated on the basis of tumor cytology and the TNM extent (**Table 1**) on which the age and gender factors were imposed only in patients with differentiated thyroid cancer [4]. The revised ATA guidelines for the management of differentiated thyroid cancer were published in 2009 [5] and could not be applied. Solitary non-metastatic papillary carcinomas of thyroid in females under 45 years and with a maximum tumor diameter of less than 3 cm ($pT_1N_oM_o$ and small $pT_2N_oM_o$) were treated with lobectomy, serial measurements of thyroglobulin levels and six-monthly high resolution USG of neck and were followed for any distant metastases. Same treatment policy was applied to males with solitary non-metastatic papillary carcinomas of less than 1 cm ($pT_1N_oM_o$) in maximum diameter. Larger papillary carcinomas in either sex were subjected to total thyroidectomy with or without neck dissection as required to clear the disease. However, irrespective of the tumor size all patients of papillary carcinoma with multifocal disease, extra capsular spread, lymph node metastasis or distant metastasis were treated on similar lines. Near-total thyroidectomy though not recommended was exceptionally done in this study to save patients from severe hypoparathyroidism when it was otherwise a concern. Medullary carcinomas were treated with total thyroidectomy with neck dissection when indicated and serial serum calcitonin measurements, 6 monthly high resolution USG of neck and follow up for distant metastases. Two false negative cases of medullary carcinoma were initially treated with partial procedures. The only patient with undifferentiated carcinoma in this study was treated aggressively. All of the operative specimens were subjected to histopathological examination to confirm the diagnosis; establish the accuracy of fine needle aspiration cytology and thyroid scanning in diagnosing the thyroid disease, and correlating the findings so as to serve as a guide to more effective therapy for thyroid disease including completion thyroidectomy with or without neck dissection. The epidemiological data, findings of various investigations to facilitate diagnosis, and the results of surgery were noted in this study and are presented.

Table 1. TNM classification of thyroid carcinomas.

T:	**Primary Tumor**
T_0:	No evidence of primary tumor
T_1:	Tumor 1 cm or less in greatest dimension, limited to the thyroid
T_2:	Tumor more than 1 cm but not more than 4 cm in greatest dimension, limited to the thyroid.
T_3:	Tumor more than 4 cm in greatest dimension, limited to the thyroid.
T_4:	Tumor of any size extending beyond the thyroid capsule.
N:	**Regional Lymph Nodes**
N_0:	No regional lymph node metastasis
N_1:	Regional lymph node metastasis
N_{1a}:	Metastasis in ipsilateral cervical lymph node/nodes
N_{1b}:	Metastasis in bilateral, middle or contralateral cervical or mediastinal lymph node/nodes
M:	**Distant Metastasis**
M_0:	No distant metastasis
M_1:	Distant metastasis

3. Observations

Age and sex distribution: Age of the patients with thyroid masses ranged from 17 years to 68 years. The mean age of the affected patients was 35 years. The disease peaks in the fourth decade of life (40.80%). Thyroid masses were observed to be affecting females predominantly. Female to male ratio in this study was 5.94:1. **Table 2** depicts the age and sex distribution in 125 patients with thyroid masses.

Clinical Types: Solitary thyroid nodule with or without palpable cervical nodes was the commonest clinical type (92%) encountered followed by diffuse multinodular goitre, diffuse simple thyroid enlargement and palpable cervical lymph node mass with clinically normal thyroid gland in that order. **Table 3** shows clinical types of thyroid masses in 125 patients.

Fine needle aspiration cytology versus histopathological results: Fine needle aspiration cytology in this study showed 100% specificity in diagnosing malignant thyroid tumors (**Figure 7** and **Figure 8**) including 30 primary papillary carcinomas, 3 primary medullary carcinomas, one undifferentiated carcinoma, and one each of the regional secondary papillary and medullary carcinomas with non palpable primary. The diagnostic sensitivity of FNA cytology was 73.08%. Of 23 patients with "follicular neoplasm" reported on FNA there were 10 false negatives including 9 papillary carcinomas (with 4 follicular variants) and one medullary carcinoma; the remaining 13 were benign on HPE. One each of the three "follicular lesions" proved to be papillary carcinoma, follicular adenoma and a colloid goitre (**Figure 9**). Of 56 cases with colloid goitre reported on FNA cytology there were six false negatives of papillary carcinoma and one that of follicular carcinoma; the remaining 49 were true negatives. There were 3 reported cases of follicular adenoma on FNA which proved to be one each of papillary carcinoma, medullary carcinoma and a follicular adenoma. Of 2 patients with Hurthle cell neoplasm on FNA cytology one was papillary carcinoma and the other Hurthle cell adenoma. Histopathology confirmed 2 other FNA reports of Hurthle cell adenoma and Hashimoto's disease. The overall diagnostic accuracy of FNA cytology in this study was 83.20%.

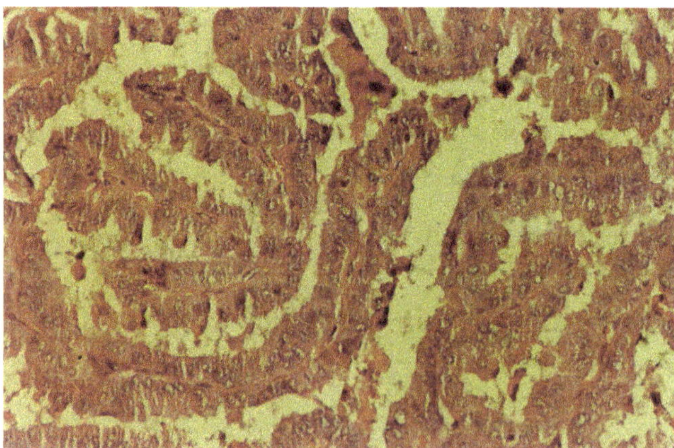

Figure 7. Photomicrograph of papillary carcinoma of thyroid showing papillary fronds and occasional "Orphan Annie eye" nuclei; Haemtoxylin-Eosin stain; ×400.

Table 2. Age and sex distribution in 125 patients with thyroid masses.

Age Group (Years)	No. of Patients	Male (%)	Female (%)
0 - 10	0 (0.00%)	0 (0.00%)	0 (0.00%)
11 - 20	8 (6.40%)	0 (0.00%)	8 (6.40%)
21 - 30	37 (29.60%)	6 (4.80%)	31 (24.80%)
31 - 40	51 (40.80%)	8 (6.40%)	43 (34.40%)
41 - 50	20 (16.00%)	1 (0.80%)	19 (15.20%)
51 - 60	7 (5.60%)	2 (1.60%)	5 (4.00%)
61 - 70	2 (1.60%)	1 (0.80%)	1 (0.80%)
Total	**125 (100%)**	**18 (14.40%)**	**107 (85.60%)**

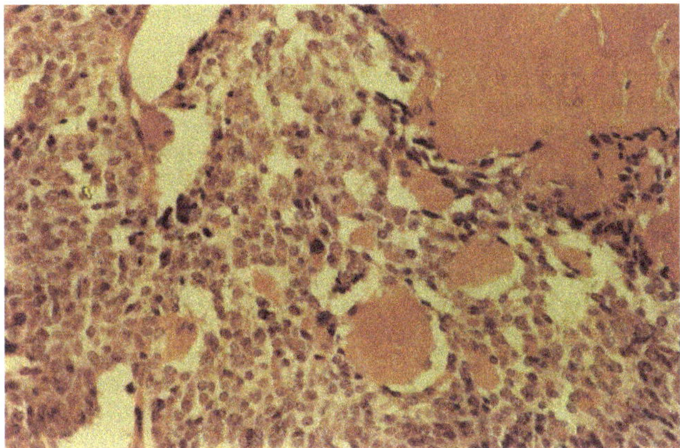

Figure 8. Photomicrograph of medullary carcinoma of thyroid showing solid pattern of growth, spindle cells and abundant deposits of amyloid; Haemtoxylin-Eosin stain; ×400.

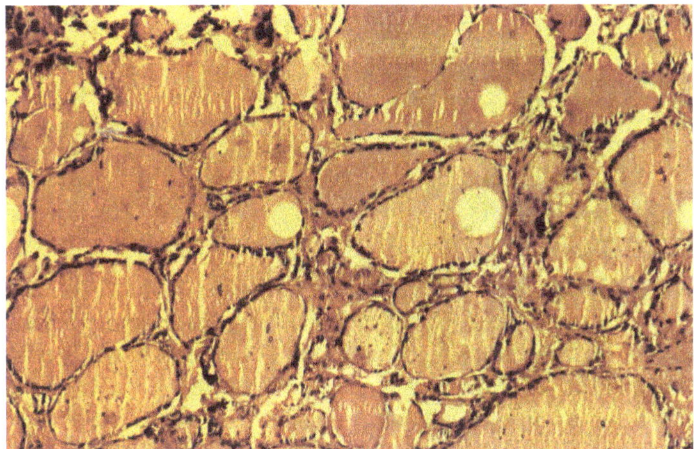

Figure 9. Photomicrograph of colloid goiter showing colloid follicles with flattened epithelium; Haemtoxylin-Eosin stain; ×400.

Table 3. Clinical types of the thyroid masses in 125 patients.

Clinical Type	No. of Patients	Percentage (%)
Solitary nodule with or without palpable neck nodes	115	92.00
Diffuse multinodular goitre	7	5.60
Diffuse simple thyroid enlargement	2	1.60
Palpable nodal mass with clinically normal thyroid	1	0.80
Total	**125**	**100.00%**

Radionuclide Scanning: A comparison between the results of technetium-99 pertechnetate scanning of 50 unselected cases of thyroid masses and their histopathological results was made to determine the role of thyroid scan in distinguishing between the benign and malignant thyroid nodules. **Table 4** summarizes these results.

Thyroid Hormone Status: Of 125 patients with thyroid masses 95 (76%) were euthyroid (normal T_3, T_4, TSH levels), 12 (9.60%) showed T_3 thyrotoxicosis (raised T_3 but normal T_4), 6 (4.80%) showed primary hypothyroidism (lowered T_3, T_4 but raised TSH), 6 (4.80%) showed reduced peripheral response (normal levels of thyroid hormones with clinical hypothyriodism) and 6 (4.80%) had biochemical thyrotoxicosis (high T_3, T_4 in absence of clinical thyrotoxicosis).

Table 4. Comparison of results of pre-operative technetium-99 pertechnetate thyroid scan with HPE in 50 patients with thyroid masses.

Technitium-99 Scan (Pre-op)	Histopathological diagnosis
Solitary cold nodule 33	Papillary carcinoma 10 (30.30%) Colloid goitre 9 (27.27%) Follicular adenoma 7 (1.22%) Medullary carcinoma 3 (9.09%) Hurthle cell adenoma 2 (6.06%) Adenomatous colloid goitre 2 (6.06%)
Enlarged lobe/gland with patches of decreased tracer uptake 7	Papillary carcinoma 3 (42.86%) Colloid goitre 2 (28.56%) Multinodulular goitre 1 (14.29%) Adenomatous colloid goitre 1 (14.29%)
Normal tracer uptake 3	Papillary carcinoma 2 (66.67%) Follicular adenoma 1 (33.33%)
Thyromegaly with a cold nodule 2	Papillary carcinoma 1 (50%) Multinodular goitre 1 (50%)
Increased tracer uptake in neck node with both lobes of thyroid appearing normal in size & shape 2	Papillary carcinoma thyroid metastasis level III node of R1 (50%) Papillary carcinoma thyroid with metastasis in level III node on L1 (50%)
Grossly enlarged left lobe with nodular calcification of both lobes of the thyroid gland 1	Papillary carcinoma of left lobe of thyroid gland 1 (100%)
Autonomous nodule in right lobe with suppressed rest of the gland 1	Papillary carcinoma of the left lobe 1 (100%)
Poorly visualized both lobes of thyroid 1	Papillary carcinoma of thyroid 1 (100%)

Treatment of Thyroid Masses: All of the 125 patients with thyroid masses were subjected to thyroid surgery. Benign masses were mostly treated with partial thyroidectomy techniques whereas the malignant cases were treated in accordance with the stage grouping of the tumor (**Table 5**). Of 31 patients reported on FNA cytology as papillary carcinomas with or without regional nodal metastases 10 (32.26%) were treated with total thyroidectomy alone; 11 (35.48%) were treated with total thyroidectomy and selective neck dissection; 2 (6.45%) with near total thyroidectomy; and 8 (25.80%) with lobectomy. All of the 4 (100%) FNA reported medullary carcinomas and a single case of undifferentiated carcinoma were treated with total thyroidectomy. There were 18 false negative papillary carcinomas, 2 false negative medullary carcinomas and one false negative follicular carcinoma in this study. Of 18 false negative papillary carcinomas 13 were treated with lobectomy as the initial treatment, 3 with enucleation and 2 with subtotal thyroidectomy. Of 2 false negative medullary carcinomas lobectomy was done in both as the initial treatment, and the only case of false negative follicular carcinoma in this study was initially subjected to subtotal thyroidectomy. Completion thyroidectomy as second stage operative procedure was performed in both of the false negative medullary carcinomas and the follicular carcinoma. Completion total thyroidectomy with or without selective neck dissection was also done in eight cases of false negative papillary carcinomas where a highly limited initial operative procedure such as enucleation was contemplated or where there was evidence of operative specimens with positive margins, multifocal or invasive lesion, mixed papillary-follicular histology or lymph node metastases. **Table 6** shows the types of operation done in 57 patients of thyroid carcinomas in the present study.

Follow up and prognosticators: Follow up period of the 57 operated patients with malignant thyroid tumors in this study ranged from 5 to 15 years. Of 49 operated patients of papillary carcinoma 46 (93.88%) survived disease free at 5 years. The other three died because of local failure, regional nodal recurrence and pulmonary metastasis respectively. Serial post operative thyroglobulin levels were persistently above the cut off level (77 ng/ml) in all of the 3 patients who died of the recurrent disease. The only patient of follicular carcinoma was alive at 5 years after surgery. Of 6 patients operated for medullary carcinoma 4 (66.67%) survived 5 years disease free. Disease recurred in neck nodes in the other 2 who were false negatives of FNA cytology at the time of presentation and were subjected initially to partial thyroidectomy followed by completion thyroidectomy and subsequently to modified neck dissection. Serial serum calcitonin levels were high above 10 pg/ml in the latter 2 patients who succumbed to the disease in the 5th post operative year.

Table 5. Staging of the thyroid carcinomas in 36 patients (modified TNM classification).

Type of Thyroid Carcinoma	Stage I		Stage II		Stage III		Stage IV	
	No. of Patients	Percentage %	No. of Patients	Percentage %	No. of Patients	Percentage %	No. of Patients	Percentage %
Papillary	20	64.52	7	22.58	4	12.90	-	-
Medullary	-	-	3	75.00	1	25.00	-	-
Undifferentiated	-	-	-	-	-	-	1	100

Table 6. Operative Procedures performed on 57 patients of thyroid carcinomas.

Type of Carcinoma No. of Patients)	Primary Operative procedure (No. of Patients)	Any Second Stage Operative Procedures (No. of Patients)
A. True Positive Carcinomas:		
a. Papillary carcinoma with or without regional nodal metastasis (31)	➢ Total thyroidectomy with selective neck dissection (11) ➢ Total thyroidectomy alone (10) ➢ Near total thyroidectomy (2) ➢ Lobectomy (8)	Revision surgery for regional nodal recurrence (2)
b. Medullary Carcinoma (4)	➢ Total thyroidectomy (4)	-
c. Undifferentiated carcinoma (1)	➢ Total thyroidectomy (1)	-
B. False Negative Carcinomas:		
a. Papillary carcinoma (18)	➢ Lobectomy (13) ➢ Enucleation (3) ➢ Subtotal thyroidectomy (2)	Completion total thyroidectomy alone or with selective neck dissection (8)
b. Medullary carcinoma (2)	➢ Lobectomy (2)	Completion thyroidectomy with type I modified radical neck dissection for nodal recurrence (2)
c. Follicular Carcinoma (1)	➢ Subtotal thyroidectomy (1)	Completion total thyroidectomy (1)

Complications associated with thyroid surgery: As expected hypothyroidism invariably occurs after total thyroidectomy and may occur after partial thyroidectomy procedures (19.77%) unless supplemented with levothyroxine. The hypothyroid state may proceed to myxoedema. Primary haemorrhage from left inferior thyroid artery was encountered in one patient (0.8%), transient hypocalcaemia occurred in 10.25% of the total thyroidectomy procedures and hypoparathyroidism was encountered in the same percentage of these patients. Of 125 operated patients right recurrent nerve paralysis complicated in one patient (0.8%), right external laryngeal nerve paralysis in one patient (0.8%), stitch abscesses in 5 (4%) and hypertrophic scar in 5 (4%).

4. Discussion

Thyroid masses commonly affect younger females. The mean age of the patients with thyroid masses in this study was 35 years, and near 86% of these patients were female. Female to male ratio was 5.94:1. Mazzafferi [6] in his series on the management of solitary thyroid nodules had female to male ratio of 4:1. The average age of 172 patients with thyroid masses reported by Shapiro *et al.* [7] was 36 years. 92% of the thyroid masses presented clinically as solitary nodules affecting predominantly the right lobe of the gland. Messaris [8] reported in his series of 568 patients of thyroid masses the right lobe involvement in near 57% of cases. Fine needle aspiration (FNA) cytology showed 100% specificity in diagnosing malignant thyroid tumours. The diagnostic sensitivity of FNA cytology in the present series of patients was 73.08% and the diagnostic accuracy was 83.20%. Being complementary to the false negative rate the low sensitivity was worrisome because in other words 21 malignant lesions in the series of 125 patients were simply missed—most of them (57%) from the FNA reported "follicular neoplasm" or "atypia of undetermined significance (follicular lesion)". In diagnosing thyroid masses with FNA cytology Afroze *et al.* [9] reported sensitivity of 61.9%, specificity of 99.3% and diagnostic accuracy of 94.5%; Kessler *et al.* [10] reported 79% sensitivity, 98.5% specificity and 87% diagnostic accuracy; and

Gupta *et al.* [11] reported 80% sensitivity, 86.6% specificity and 84% accuracy. Cibas and Ali report about the Bethesda system for thyroid cytopathology. This system recommends six diagnostic categories for thyroid masses which include the unsatisfactory, benign, "follicular lesion" or atypia of undetermined significance (AUS), "follicular neoplasm", suspicious for malignancy and malignant. According to these authors 35% of the "follicular neoplasms" prove not to be neoplasms but hyperplastic proliferation of follicular cells, and 15% to 30% prove to be malignant. The majority of "follicular neoplasm" cases turn out to be follicular adenomas or adenomatous nodules, both of which are more common than follicular carcinomas. Some of the "follicular neoplasms" are follicular variants of papillary carcinoma. For a definitive diagnostic procedure most of the patients with "follicular neoplasm" are managed by lobectomy. The "follicular lesion" or atypia of undetermined significance (AUS) result is obtained in 3% to 6% of thyroid FN aspirations. The recommended management is clinical correlation and repeated FNA at an appropriate interval. In most cases, a repeated FNA results in a more definitive interpretation. Only about 20% nodules are reported again as AUS. In some cases, however, the surgeon chooses not to repeat FNA but observe the nodule clinically or, alternatively to operate the patient because of concerning clinical and/or sonographic features. In the suspicious for malignancy category follicular variant of the papillary carcinoma of thyroid (PTC) can be difficult to distinguish from benign follicular nodule. Nodules reported to be "suspicious for malignancy" are resected by lobectomy or total thyroidectomy. 60% to 75% of these prove to be papillary carcinoma and the rest are follicular adenomas. Immunohistochemical analysis and flow cytometry in borderline cases is usually more helpful with medullary carcinoma and lymphoma than with PTC. The false negatives of the "benign" reports in the present series were 14.29%. The false negative rate of the benign FNA reports in the review studies quoted by Cibas and Ali was low (0% - 3%), but patients were nevertheless followed up with repeated assessments by palpation or ultra sound at 6 months to 18 months interval. If the nodule showed significant growth or suspicious sonographic changes, a repeated FNA was considered. Gharib *et al.* [12] comments that while FNA cytology is highly accurate in the diagnosis of nodular thyroid disease there can be difficulty in distinguishing some benign cellular adenomas from their malignant counter parts. Amrikachi *et al.* [13] reviewed 6226 fine needle aspiration biopsies from 1982 to 1998 and concludes that the major diagnostic problems are caused by diagnosis of malignancy based on one or two atypical cytological features or overlapping cytological features of follicular neoplasm with those of follicular variant of papillary carcinoma. Mehenna R. *et al.* [14] report about the impact of large nodule size and follicular varient of papillary carcinoma on false negatives in thyroid cytology.

A comparison between the radionuclide scanning of thyroid masses and the histopathological results of their operative specimens showed that thyroid scan is not quite specific in distinguishing between the benign and malignant masses in all of the scintiscan patterns including especially the solitary cold nodules which form the majority (92%) of these patterns. The diagnostic yield of malignant lesions in cold nodules in the present study was still better (39%) than reported by Ashcraft *et al.* [15] who in their review of 22 series of patients found 84% of the nodules were cold, 10% were warm and 5.5% were hot; and malignant disease was found in only 16% of the cold nodules. According to Mazzaferri radionuclide scanning of thyroid is not quite specific in diagnosing malignant tumors of thyroid but is useful for evaluating the undeterminate lesions of the FNA cytology which if 'cold' should be subjected to surgery or otherwise followed up.

Most of the patients (76%) with thyroid masses were euthyroid and only 4.80% showed primary hypothyroidism with raised TSH. Raised TSH as a factor for initiation or anaplastic transformation of relatively innocuous papillary carcinomas could neither by substantiated nor forfeited through this study. Brooks [16] comments that under the influence of pituitary thyroid stimulating hormone, a less malignant form of thyroid carcinoma (papillary) can become anaplastic over a long period. Ibanez *et al.* [17] gives similar suggestions. In the 54 patient series of Silverberg *et al.* [18] 6 originally papillary or follicular carcinomas later demonstrated anaplastic features, and 5 of these had earlier been treated with some form of radiation (external beam or ^{131}I) to the thyroid.

A modified TNM classification on which the age and the gender factors were imposed was utilized in staging the differentiated thyroid cancer. TNM classification irrespective of the age and gender of the patient was utilized for staging the medullary carcinoma; and the undifferentiated carcinoma of any size was treated as stage IV disease. Of 31 patients with papillary carcinoma 64.52% were in stage I disease, 22.58% were in stage II disease, 12.90% in stage III disease and none in stage IV disease. Of 4 patients with medullary carcinoma on FNA 75% were in stage II disease and 25% in stage III disease. The only patient with undifferentiated carcinoma was managed as stage IV disease. Risk factors such as age, distant metastasis, extent of the primary and its size (AMES) in the management of differentiated thyroid carcinoma were reported in detail by Cady and Rossi [19].

Benign thyroid masses in the present study were generally managed by conservative thyroidectomy procedures and the complications encountered were minimal. Greene [20] comments that all cold nodules should be removed because 20% of these will be found to be unequivocally malignant. The debate for selecting conservative thyroidectomy procedures or radical thyroidectomy operations in the treatment of differentiated carcinoma continues. Cady & Rossi observed that 90% of the patients with differentiated thyroid cancer are low risk and there was no statistically significant difference between the death rate of those treated with unilateral operations (1.6%) and those treated with bilateral operations (1.8%). However, in high risk patients of the differentiated thyroid carcinomas Hay quoted by above authors noted improved survival with bilateral operations in contrast to the unilateral operations. Besides, according to these authors serious morbidity including hypoparathyroidism in 32% of the operated patients' results from total thyroidectomy. Hundahl *et al.* [21] reviewed of 53,856 cases of thyroid carcinoma from 1985 to 1995 in which total thyroidectomy with or without lymph node dissection represented the dominant method of surgical treatment to patients with papillary and follicular carcinoma. At 5 years, variation in surgical treatment (*i.e.* lobectomy v.s more extensive surgery) failed to translate into compelling differences in survival for any subgroup of the differentiated carcinoma but longer follow up was required to evaluate this. Recent long term survival rate from high volume centres support a less aggressive management for papillary thyroid microcarcinoma (PTMC) than those advocated by existing guidelines [21] [23]. In a questionnaire distributed to Canadian otolaryngologists-head and neck surgeons and endocrinologists to determine the current management of papillary thyroid microcarcinoma [24] 47% of the respondents recommended hemi-thyroidectomy and 43% recommended total thyroidectomy for a newly diagnosed PTMC in low risk patients; observation was the preferred method for managing PTMC detected incidentally after hemi-thyroidectomy (76%). Respondents chose more aggressive treatment for male patients compared to female patients. WU *et al.* [25] found that after hemi-thyroidectomy for PTMC, if there were no complicating factors, 70% of the respondent OHN surgeons and endocrinologists recommended no further surgery, while 30% believed that completion thyroidectomy was necessary. The prognosis for PTMC remains excellent with disease specific mortality well under 1% [26]. Younger age appealed to influence prognosis favourably for all thyroid carcinomas. Contrary to the above studies Russel *et al.* [27] after examining eighty thyroid glands containing primary carcinomas observed that the thyroid carcinoma spreads from primary site to all parts of the gland through the intragrandular lymphatics. The lymph vessels in the capsule than collect and carry malignant cells to the pericapsular lymph nodes from which they pass into the cervical lymph nodes. As proved by the whole organ sub-serial sections, 87.5% of the 80 tumors extended into the isthmus, the opposite lobe, the pericapsular lymph nodes of the opposite lobe or 2 or all 3 of these structures. They suggest that for complete eradication of carcinoma of the thyroid gland, total thyroidectomy, including the excision of pericapsular lymph nodes is the treatment of choice. For removal of the proved metastasis in the regional lymph nodes radical neck dissection is indicated. Clark [28] in his study on the treatment of differentiated thyroid cancer suggests that total thyoidectomy is the treatment of choice because residual cancer would persist in the remaining thyroid tissue is at least 61% of patients if only lobectomy had been performed. Blood supply to the parathyroid glands can be preserved by ligating the branches of the inferior thyroid artery on the thyroid capsule rather than by ligating the main vessel proximally. By dissecting the vessels and parathyroid glands from the thyroid gland, the blood supply to the parathyroid glands is preserved. Stael *et al.* [29] recommended total thyroidectomy with therapeutic selective neck dissection when indicated to be safe and well tolerated approach in children with thyroid carcinomas. Medullary and the undifferentiated carcinomas in the present study were treated with total thyroidectomy and neck dissection for nodal disease. Flemming *et al.* [30] while summarizing the results of their study on the surgical strategy for the treatment of medullary carcinoma in Houston, Texas comments that the majority of patients with invasive medullary carcinoma of thyroid have metastasis to regional lymph nodes at the time of diagnosis as evidenced by the frequent finding of persistently elevated calcitonin levels after thyroidectomy and high rates of recurrence in the cervical lymph nodes. Their data provide the rationale for surgeons to perform more extensive nodal clearance at the time of initial thyroidectomy and to consider re-operative cervical lympadenectomy in patients with persistently elevated calcitonin levels after thyroidectomy. Bouvet *et al.* [31] also report about the surgical strategy for the treatment of medullary thyroid carcinoma. Completion thyroidectomy as a second stage operative procedure in the present study was done in most of the false negative carcinomas.

Serial postoperative thyroglobulin levels were above the cut off level (77 ng/ml) in all the 3 patients of papillary carcinoma who died of recurrent disease. Serial serum calcitonin levels were high above 10 pg/ml in 2 patients of medullary carcinoma who succumbed to disease in the fifth post operative year. Tubiana *et al.* [31] studied the long term results and prognostic factors in patients with differentiated thyroid carcinoma. A multivariate analysis of the prognostic factors was carried out on a series of 546 differentiated thyroid cancers followed for 8 to 40 years. For survival, the highest risk factor was associated with age; tumors diagnosed in patients younger than 45 years had the highest relapse free survival and total survival rates and slower growth rate. The second independent prognostic factor was histology. There was no difference between papillary and follicular well-differentiated tumours, but follicular moderately-differentiated had lower total survival and relapse free survival. The third factor was sex. Tumors tended to disseminate more in male than in female patients. The presence of palpable lymph nodes also had a significant independent impact on both total survival and relapse-free survival. Elevated levels of circulating thyroglobulin were observed in 12% of the patients who had been in complete remission for longer than 20 years. Lima N *et al.* [32] and Polachek *et al.* [33] laid emphasis on the prognostic value of serial thyroglobulin determinations after total thyroidectomy for differentiated thyroid cancer. Complications encountered after thyroid surgery in the present study were minimal. In the series of Mazzeferri *et al.* [34] the main complications of thyroid surgery were permanent hypoparathyroidism in 5% of the patients and permanent recurrent laryngeal nerve paralysis in 2%, almost always following total thyroidectomy for large and invasive tumours. Of 49 operated patients of papillary carcinoma in our study 93.88% survived disease-free at 5 years. Of 6 patients operated for medullary carcinoma 66.67% survived disease-free for 5 years. Bouvet *et al.* [35] describe in detail the surgical strategy, results of treatment and the prognosticators in medullary carcinoma of thyroid. The single case of undifferentiated carcinoma in this study died 2½ years after surgery because of local recurrence and airway obstruction. Results of the role of prognosticators in thyroid carcinoma in the present study are similar to those reported by Geissinger [36] and Gilliland *et al.* [37].

5. Conclusions

In this prospective study on 125 patients with thyroid masses treated surgically and followed up from 5 years to 15 years, following conclusions are drawn:

- Thyroid masses are more common in younger females. Peak age group affected by the thyroid masses in this study was the fourth decade of life (40.80%) and the mean age of the patients was 35 years. Female to male ratio was 5.94:1.
- 92% of the patients presented with a solitary nodule affecting the right lobe more often than the left.
- FNA cytology is highly specific in diagnosing thyroid malignancies (100%). The sensitivity of the FNA cytology in this study is 73.08% which is indicative of a significant false negativity. The overall diagnostic accuracy was 83.20%.
- Technetium-99 pertechnetate scintiscanning has adjunctive role in the diagnosis of thyroid masses but is not quite specific in diagnosing malignant tumors of thyroid. The chances of a cold nodule to be a papillarycarcinoma, colloid goitre or follicular adenoma are nearly equal. Thyroid scan may even be normal in patients having thyroid carcinoma. It is useful, however, in evaluating indeterminate cases of FNA cytology. MRI of the neck is rewarding in detecting the nodal involvement in thyroid B malignancy as well as assessing the extent of the primary and its direct extrathyroidal spread. Most of the patients (76%) with thyroid masses are euthyoird at the time of presentation.
- In the present study, 45.60% of the thyroid masses proved on excision biopsy to be malignant of which papillary carcinoma was the commonest followed by the medullary, the follicular and the undifferentiated carcinomas in that order.
- The risk factor considered in classifying the differentiated carcinomas in this study were the age, gender, tumor histology, tumor size, direct extrathyroidal spread, nodal involvement and distant metastasis. Most of the papillary carcinomas presented in stage I disease (64.52%) and stage II disease (22.58%). Only 12.90% of these presented in stage III disease. The only patient of undifferentiated carcinoma in this study was treated as stage IV disease.
- The surgical strategy in dealing with the differentiated thyroid cancer continues to be debatable between utilizing partial procedures on the one hand and radical thyroid techniques on the other. An exhaustive review of literature revealed evidence weighing more in favor of total thyroidectomy than partial thyroidectomy procedures for differentiated thyroid cancer.
- Benign thyroid masses were generally death with effectively by partial thyroidectomy procedures and the complications encountered were minimal. Completion thyroidectomy with or without neck dissection was opted for most of the patients which were reported initially benign on FNA but proved invasive malignant

tumors later after histopathological examination of the operative specimens.

- Medullary carcinomas were treated with total thyroidectomy, and neck dissection when indicated; and the only patient of undifferentiated carcinoma in this study was also treated with total thyroidectomy.
- Hypothyroidism is an expected consequence of the total thyroidectomy procedure. The other complications encountered after thyroid surgery in the present study included primary hemorrhage from the left inferior thyroid artery in one patient, unilateral external and recurrent nerve paralysis in one patient each, transient respiratory obstruction in the immediate post operative period in one, stitch abscess in 5 patients and scar hypertrophy in 5 patients.
- 5 years survival rate though admittedly insufficient to assess the results of treatment in differentiated thyroid cancer, however, most of the recurrences (69%) are reported to occur in first 5 years only. 95.79% of the patients with differentiated thyroid carcinomas followed up for 5 years in this study survived disease-free for that long period. 5 years survival rate for the medullary carcinoma cases was 66.67% and the only patient with undifferentiated carcinoma in this study survived barely 2½ years post treatment.
- Serial post operative thyroglobulin levels in the differentiated thyroid carcinomas and serial calcitonin levels in the operated medullary carcinomas are reliable prognosticators.

References

[1] Schottenfeld, D. and Gershman, S.T. (1978) Epidemiology of Thyroid Cancer. *CA: A Cancer Journal for Clinicians*, **28**, 66-86. http://dx.doi.org/10.3322/canjclin.28.2.66

[2] Davies, L. and Welch, H.G. (2006) Increasing Incidence of Thyroid Cancer in the United States, 1973-2002. *JAMA*, **295**, 2164-2167. http://dx.doi.org/10.1001/jama.295.18.2164

[3] Cibas, E.S. and Ali, S.Z. (2009) Bethesda System for Reporting Thyroid Cytopathology. *American Journal of Clinical Pathology*, **132**, 658-665. http://dx.doi.org/10.1309/AJCPPHLWMI3JV4LA

[4] Stell, P.M. and Maran, A.G.D. (2000) Surgical Treatment of the Differentiated Thyroid Cancer. Text Book of Head & Neck Surgery, 4th Edition, CRC Press, Florida, 470.

[5] Cooper, D.S., Doherty, G.M., Haugen, B.R., *et al.* (2009) Revised American Thyroid Association (ATA) Management Guidelines for Patients with Thyroid Nodules and Differentiated Thyroid Cancer. *Thyroid*, **11**, 1-16.

[6] Mazzaferri, E.L. (1993) Management of a Solitary Thyroid Nodule. *The New England Journal of Medicine*, **328**, 553-558. http://dx.doi.org/10.1056/NEJM199302253280807

[7] Shapiro, J.S., Nathan, B., Friedman, S.L., *et al.* (1970) Incidence of Thyroid Carcinoma in Grave's Disease. *Cancer*, **26**, 1261-1271. http://dx.doi.org/10.1002/1097-0142(197012)26:6<1261::AID-CNCR2820260613>3.0.CO;2-P

[8] Messaris, G., Kyriakou, K., Vasilopoulus, P., *et al.* (1974) The Single Thyroid Nodule and Carcinoma. *British Journal of Surgery*, **61**, 943-944. http://dx.doi.org/10.1002/bjs.1800611204

[9] Afroze, N., Kayani, N. and Hassan, S.H. (2002) Role of Fine Needle Aspiration Cytology in the Diagnosis of Palpable Thyroid Lesions. *Indian Journal of Pathology and Microbiology*, **45**, 241-246.

[10] Kessler, A., Gavriel, H., Zahav, S., *et al.* (2005) Accuracy and Consistency of Fine Needle Aspiration Biopsy in the Diagnosis and Management of Solitary Thyroid Nodules. *Israel Medical Association Journal*, **7**, 371-373.

[11] Gupta, M., Gupta, S. and Gupta, V.B. (2010) Correlation of Fine Needle Aspiration Cytology with Histopathology in the Diagnosis of Solitary Thyroid Nodule. *Journal of Thyroid Research*, **2010**, Article ID: 379051. http://dx.doi.org/10.4061/2010/379051

[12] Gharib, H. and Goellner, J.R. (1993) Fine-Needle Aspiration Biopsy of the Thyroid: An Appraisal. *Annals of Internal Medicine*, **118**, 282-289. http://dx.doi.org/10.7326/0003-4819-118-4-199302150-00007

[13] Amrikachi, M., Ramzy, I., Rubenfeld, S., *et al.* (2001) Accuracy of Fine Needle Aspiration of Thyroid. *Archives of Pathology & Laboratory Medicine*, **125**, 484-488.

[14] Mehanna, R., Murphy, M., Mccarthy, J., O'Leary, G., Tuthill, A., Murphy, M.S. and Sheahan, P. (2013) False Negatives in Thyroid Cytology: Impact of Large Nodule Size and Follicular Variant of Papillary Carcinoma. *Laryngoscope*, **123**, 1305-1309.

[15] Ashcraft, M.W. and Van Herle, A.J. (1981) Management of Thyroid Nodules II. Scanning Techniques, Thyroid Suppressive Therapy, and Fine Needle Aspiration. *Head and Neck Surgery*, **3**, 297-322. http://dx.doi.org/10.1002/hed.2890030406

[16] Brooks, J.R. (1973) The Solitary Thyroid Nodule. *The American Journal of Surgery*, **125**, 477-481. http://dx.doi.org/10.1016/0002-9610(73)90086-X

[17] Ibanez, M.D., Russell, W.O., Aboves-Scavedva, J., *et al.* (1966) Thyroid Carcinoma: Biologic Behavior and Mortality.

Cancer, **19**, 1039-1052.

[18] Silverberg, S.G., Hutter, R.V.P. and Foote, F.W. (1970) Fatal Carcinoma of the Thyroid: Histology, Metastases and Causes of Death. *Cancer*, **25**, 792-801. http://dx.doi.org/10.1002/1097-0142(197004)25:4<792::AID-CNCR2820250408>3.0.CO;2-P

[19] Cady, B. and Rossi, R. (1988) An Expanded View of Risk Group Definition in Differentiated Thyroid Carcinoma. *Surgery*, **104**, 947-953.

[20] Greene, R. (1956) Discerete Nodules of the Thyroid Gland with Special Reference to Carcinoma. Huntarian Lecture Delivered on 29th November, 1956.

[21] Hundahl, S.A., Flemming, I.D., Fremgen, A.M., *et al.* (1998) A National Cancer Data Base Report on 53, 856 Cases of Thyroid Carcinoma Treated in the US, 1985-1995. *Cancer*, **83**, 2638-2648. http://dx.doi.org/10.1002/(SICI)1097-0142(19981215)83:12<2638::AID-CNCR31>3.0.CO;2-1

[22] Hay, I.D., Hutchinson, M.E., Gonalez-Losada, T., *et al.* (2008) Papillary Thyroid Microcarcinoma: A Study of 900 Cases Observed in a 60 Year Period. *Surgery*, **144**, 980-988. http://dx.doi.org/10.1016/j.surg.2008.08.035

[23] Nixon, I.J., Ganlly, I., Patel, S.G., *et al.* (2012) Thyroid Lobectomy for Treatment of Well Differentiated Intrathyroid Malignancy. *Surgery*, **151**, 571-579. http://dx.doi.org/10.1016/j.surg.2011.08.016

[24] Merdad, M., Eskander, A., De Almeida, J., *et al.* (2014) Current Management of Papillary Thyroid Microcarcinoma in Canada. *Journal of Otolaryngology—Head and Neck Surgery*, **43**, 32. http://dx.doi.org/10.1186/s40463-014-0032-8

[25] Wu, A.W., Wang, M.B. and Nguyen, C.T. (2010) Surgical Practice Patterns in the Treatment of Papillary Thyroid Microcarcinoma. *Archives of Otolaryngology—Head and Neck Surgery*, **136**, 1182-1190. http://dx.doi.org/10.1001/archoto.2010.193

[26] Lee, J., Park, J.H., Lee, C.R., *et al.* (2013) Long Term Outcomes of Total Thyroidectomy versus Thyroid Lobectomy for Papillary Thyroid Microcarcinoma: Comparative Analysis after Propensity Score Matching. *Thyroid*, **23**, 1408-1415. http://dx.doi.org/10.1089/thy.2012.0463

[27] Russell, W.O., Ibane, M.L., Clark, L.C. and White, E.C. (1963) Classification, Intraglandular Dissemination, and Clinicopathological Study Based upon Whole Organ Sections of 80 (Thyroid) Glands. *Cancer*, **16**, 1425-1458. http://dx.doi.org/10.1002/1097-0142(196311)16:11<1425::AID-CNCR2820161106>3.0.CO;2-E

[28] Clark, O.H. (1982) The Treatment of Choice for Patients with Differentiated Thyroid Cancer. *Annals of Surgery*, **196**, 361-370. http://dx.doi.org/10.1097/00000658-198209000-00016

[29] Stael, A.P.M., Plukker, J.M., Rouwe, C.W., *et al.* (1995) Total Thyroidectomy in the Treatment of Thyroid Carcinoma in Childhood. *British Journal of Surgery*, **82**, 1083-1085. http://dx.doi.org/10.1002/bjs.1800820825

[30] Flemming, J.B., Lee, J.E., Bouvet, M., *et al.* (1999) Surgical Strategy for the Treatment of Medullary Thyroid Carcinoma. *Annals of Surgery*, **230**, 697-707.

[31] Tubiana, M., Schlumberger, M., Rougier, P., *et al.* (1985) Long Term Results and Prognostic Factors in Patients with Differentiated Thyroid Carcinoma. *Cancer*, **55**, 794-804. http://dx.doi.org/10.1002/1097-0142(19850215)55:4<794::AID-CNCR2820550418>3.0.CO;2-Z

[32] Bouvet, M., Schultz, P.N., Sharman, S.I., *et al.* (1970) Surgical Strategy for the Treatment of Medullary Thryroid Carcinoma. *Annals of Surgery*, **230**, 697-707.

[33] Lima, N., Cavaliere, H., Tomimori, E., *et al.* (2002) Prognostic Value of Serial Thyroglobulin Determinations after Total Thyroidectomy for Differentiated Thyroid Cancer. *Journal of Endocrinological Investigation*, **25**, 110-115. http://dx.doi.org/10.1007/BF03343973

[34] Polachek, A., Hirch, D. and Tzvetov, G. (2011) Prognestic Values of Post Thyroidectomy Thyroglubulin Levels in Patients with Differentiated Thyroid Cancer. *Journal of Endocrinological Investigation*, **34**, 855-860.

[35] Mazzaferri, E.L. and Jhiang, S.M. (1994) Long Term Impact of Initial Surgical and Medical Therapy on Papillary and Follicular Thyroid Cancer. *The American Journal of Medicine*, **97**, 418-428. http://dx.doi.org/10.1016/0002-9343(94)90321-2

[36] Geissinger, W.T., Horsley, J.S., Parker, F.P., *et al.* (1974) Carcinoma of the Thyroid. *Annals of Surgery*, **179**, 734-739. http://dx.doi.org/10.1097/00000658-197405000-00028

[37] Gilliland, F.D., Hunt, W.C., Morris, D.M., *et al.* (1997) Prognostic Factors for Thyroid Carcinoma. *Cancer*, **79**, 564-573. http://dx.doi.org/10.1002/(SICI)1097-0142(19970201)79:3<564::AID-CNCR20>3.0.CO;2-0

40

Assessment of Hearing Status by Pure Tone Audiogram—An Institutional Study

Ganesh Kumar Balasubramanian, Ramanathan Thirunavukkarasu, Ramesh Babu Kalyanasundaram, Gitanjali Narendran

Thanjavur Medical College, Thanjavur, India
Email: drganeshkumarb@gmail.com

Abstract

Aim: To assess the hearing status of the study subjects in terms of degree and type of hearing loss, and establish the burden of this disability in the society. Materials and methods: This is a prospective study conducted in patients who attend our OPD. After an otorhinolaryngeal examination, all the patients were subjected to pure tone audiometry using MAICA-MA52 audiometer. Results: Our study comprises 1012 males (64%) and 563 females (36%). Out of this, about 15% have conductive deafness and 42% have sensorineural hearing loss. About 29% suffer from mild hearing loss, 26% moderate and 11% severe hearing loss. The alarming information is that about 5% have total hearing loss of Sudden Sensorineural type (SSNHL). Conclusion: Pure tone audiometry is cost effective and easy to perform. Early diagnosis and timely intervention will reduce the morbidity of deafness in our country. Hence it is necessary to identify and treat sudden sensorineural hearing loss and noise induced hearing loss at an early stage.

Keywords

Pure Tone Audiogram, Conductive Deafness, Sudden Sensorineural Hearing Loss, Ototoxicity, Presbyacusis, Noise Induced Hearing Loss

1. Introduction

Hearing is an important and essential sense for verbal communication, language skills and personality development. Hearing loss is the second most common disability in India after the loco motor disability. More than 40 dB hearing impairment in patients above 15 years and more than 30 dB hearing impairment in patients below 14 years in the better ear are considered as hearing disability.

Hearing loss is classified as:

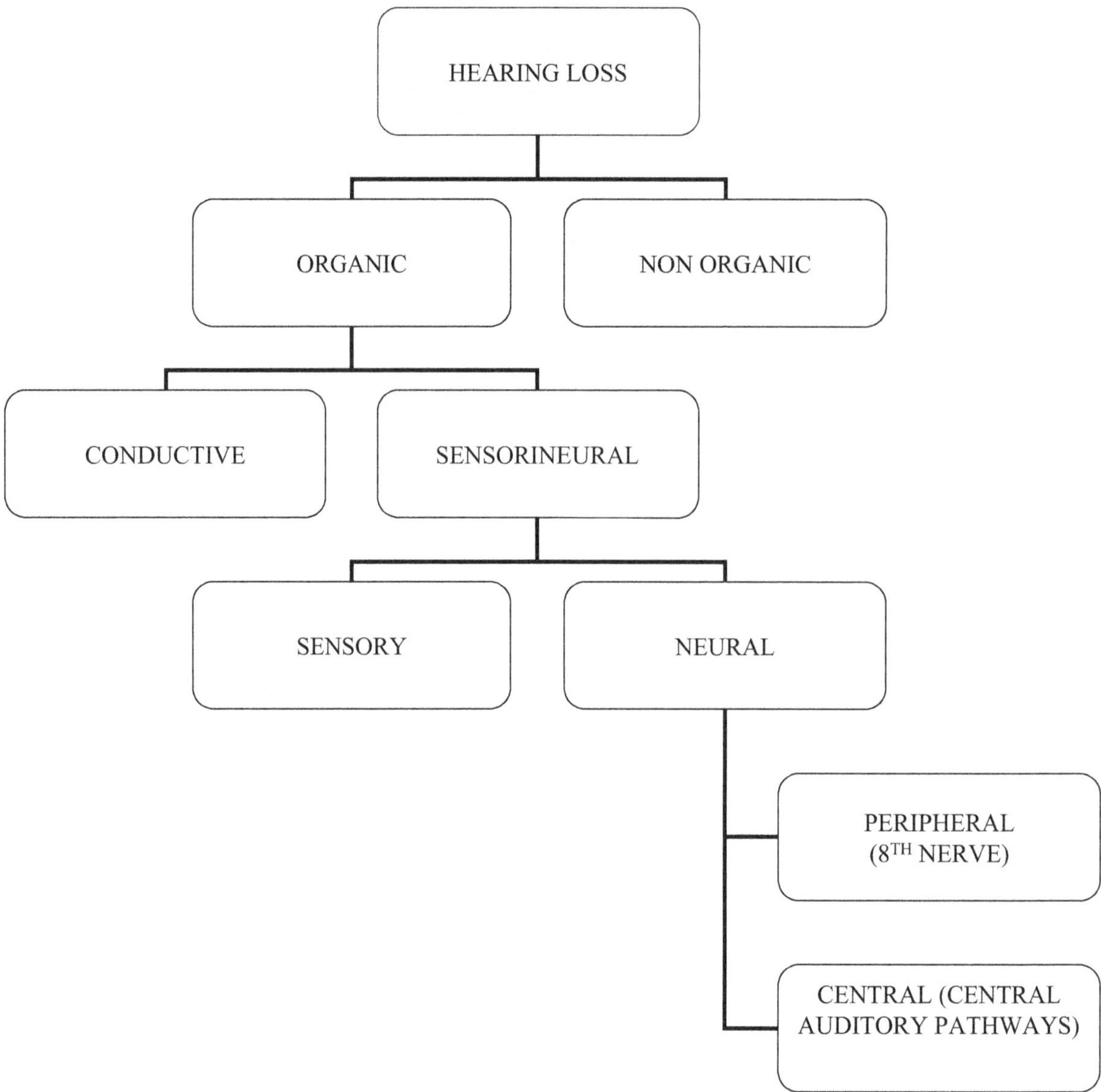

Conductive Hearing Loss: Any disease process which interferes with the conduction of sound to reach cochlea causes conductive hearing loss. The lesion may lie in the external ear, tympanic membrane, middle ear or ossicles up to stapedio-vestibular joint.

Sensorineural Hearing Loss: Results from lesions of the cochlea, 8th nerve or central auditory pathways. It may be present at birth (congenital) or start later in life (acquired).

According to WHO census, around 360 million have hearing disability and the majorities are adults (91%) and children are only 9%. Prevalence of hearing loss is more in the age group above 65 years [1]. Our study shows that age group of 50 years and above are involved more in number than other age groups.

National Institute on Deafness and other Communication Disorders (NIDCD) states that 15% of the population is having hearing loss due to loud noise in the working place or due to prolonged use of mobile phones [2]. Prolonged use of mobile phones for more than 30 minutes can cause 10 dB transient hearing loss [3]. As per the available information, about 6.3% of the Indian population is suffering from hearing impairment. Among these, the rural populations are more commonly affected than the urban population [4]. Hearing loss in children may affect their education due to the defective development of perceptual and linguistic abilities, because of reduced aural input [5]. Most common cause for hearing loss in children is serous otitis media or glue ear.

Sudden Sensorineural Hearing Loss (SSNHL) is defined as greater than 30 dB hearing impairment, over at least three contiguous frequencies, occurring over a period of 72 hours or less. Males are more commonly involved than females and the vulnerable age group is around 45 - 49 years. Presbyacusis or age related hearing loss is a slowly progressing one and involves both ears equally. Initially it affects the higher frequencies and later affects the lower frequencies also. The first sign is inability to understand the speech in noisy surrounding.

In pure tone audiogram, the tested frequency ranges from 250 Hz to 8000 Hz, and hearing level from −10 dB to 120 dB. This test is both qualitative and quantitative (Type and Severity of hearing loss). The degree of deafness is classified based on WHO (1980) classification with reference to ISO: R.389-1970 (International Calibration of Audiometers) as follows:

Normal Hearing	0 - 25 dB
Mild Hearing Impairment	26 - 40 dB
Moderate Hearing Impairment	41 - 55 dB
Moderately Severe Hearing Impairment	56 - 70 dB
Severe Hearing Impairment	71 - 90 dB
Profound Hearing Impairment	>90 dB

Aims and Objectives

The aims and objectives are to assess the hearing level, the degree and type of deafness in patients attending the outpatient department.

2. Materials and Methods

This is a prospective study conducted in our institution. Patients who attended the Department of Otorhinolaryngology and Head and Neck Surgery OPD from Jan-Dec 2014 (about 1575 patients) were taken for study. The age of patients varied from 10 to 70 years. All patients were subjected to pure tone audiometry (MAICA-MA52) after an otorhinolaryngeal examination. Both air conduction and bone conduction were measured with Hughson Westlake technique modified by Carhart & Jerger and plotted in graph. Most paediatric patients were subjected to tympanogram also. Male: Female ratio, age distribution, degree of deafness and type of deafness were evaluated.

3. Results and Analysis

Our study shows that 64% of males and 34% of females are involved. Among males, the 40 - 59 years age group is more commonly affected, this correlates with WHO data. Among females, the 20 - 39 years age group is more commonly affected (**Table 1**). Our study shows that 40 - 59 years age group is more commonly involved (38%), 20 - 39 years age group constitutes 30%, above 60 years constitutes 20% and the rest 12% is 10 - 19 years group.

This study reveals that 42% are suffering from sensorineural hearing impairment, 15% from conductive type, 14% shows mixed type and the rest 28% have normal hearing (**Table 2**).

In this study, about 29% have mild degree of deafness, 26% have moderate degree, 11% have severe degree, 6% suffer from profound to total deafness and the remaining 28% have normal hearing. Moderate degree of deafness is common above 40 years. In our study, profound and total deafness is evenly distributed in all age groups (**Table 3**).

4. Discussion

In our study the majority of patients belong to the male sex (64%). Among the males, 4th and 5th decades are more vulnerable age groups. Around 28% of the cases are unilateral. Pure tone thresholds in females are lower at higher frequencies compared to males, suggesting that aging process begins earlier in men. Conductive hearing loss is more common in younger individuals and as the age advances sensorineural hearing loss predominates. The majority of subjects with hearing loss belong to working age group. This is probably due to occupational noise exposure, stress and trauma. Subjects working in industries are more vulnerable for noise induced hearing loss.

Tucker has argued that hearing is an ability that may be apprehended, thus screening for hearing at school entry level, especially for suspected unilateral mild to moderate hearing loss should be considered [5]. Robinovich

Table 1. Sex distribution in different age groups.

Age Groups	Male	Female	Total	Percent
10 - 19 years	117	81	198	12%
20 - 39 years	236	232	468	30%
40 - 59 years	415	179	594	38%
60 years &above	244	71	315	20%

Table 2. Age wise distribution of type of hearing loss.

Age groups	Normal	Cond. HL	SN.HL	Mixed HL	Total
10 - 19 years	81	63	34	20	198
20 - 39 years	177	121	108	62	468
40 - 59 years	180	54	282	78	594
60 years & above	8	0	242	65	315

Table 3. Age wise distribution of degree of hearing loss.

Age groups	Normal	Mild HL	Moderate HL	Severe HL	Profound HL	Total
10 - 19 yrs	81	41	40	15	21	198
20 - 39 yrs	177	116	98	51	26	468
40 - 59 yrs	180	208	119	65	22	594
60 & above	8	92	153	40	22	315

has stated that early identification of hearing loss and adequate corrective measures help in better speech, language, social, psychological and educational development and a more satisfactory outcome [6].

More recently Dr. Frank Lin and his colleagues at Johns Hopkins University found a strong relationship between degree of hearing loss and risk of developing Dementia. Patients with mild degree have 2 times, moderate degree 3 times and severe degree has 5 times the risk than normal hearing individuals [7]. Hearing loss is an invisible handicap. Although it occurs in an increasing prevalence with age, hearing loss is often ignored during the diagnosis and treatment of cognitive and memory disorders in elderly patients.

Sudden sensorineural hearing loss is nowadays increasing in incidence. The causes may be infection, circulatory problems, meniere's disease, neoplasms, trauma, metabolic disorders, immunologic disorders or idiopathic. So in all cases of this type of hearing loss proper investigation regarding the etiology is very important. We did all relevant investigations and in many cases we found that viral infection is the culprit and some cases are idiopathic. The treatment includes systemic or oral steroids, hyperbaric oxygen therapy, antiviral drugs, vasodilators and chemorheologic agents. Most of the sudden sensorineural hearing loss patients presented with symptoms similar to eustachian tube catarrh. Because of this most patients presented with total hearing loss at the time of consultation. So in all cases of hard of hearing, audiological evaluation is mandatory and we have to do that at the first visit itself. Among all, pure tone audiometry is the most reliable, easy and cost effective method when compared to others.

Morbidity due to hearing loss in paediatric age group is inversely proportional to the literacy of parents. Most common causes for deafness in paediatric age group are Otitis Media with Effusion (OME), eustachian tube dysfunction, chronic suppurative otitis media and acute otitis media. For all these cases infection plays a major role, and it is more prevalent in low socioeconomic status and families with illiteracy. Infection is the most common cause for hearing loss in developing countries according to WHO data [8].

Tharwat and his colleagues, 1998, and Arts and others, 2002, stated that cochlear implants are needed for those patients with bilateral profound to total hearing loss who could not be benefitted with formal hearing aids and it is recommended especially in the younger age group [9].

In our study, most of the paediatric age group patients suffered from conductive type of deafness. Most common etiology for this is Otitis Media with Effusion. Pneumatic otoscopy is the diagnostic tool for this OME, but Tympanometry is the gold standard. Hence all those patients were subjected to impedence audiometry. Most of them were found to have Glue ear and received treatment and recovered completely. Treatment includes both medical and surgical management in the form of myringotomy and grommet insertion. Conductive type of hearing loss in adults are due to chronic suppurative otitis media and these are managed by mastoidectomy, if there is no improvement after the clearance of septic foci and medical management.

Auditory Neuropathy Spectrum Disorder (ANSD) is a type of hearing disorder in which the pure tone audiogram shows near normal hearing to profound hearing loss. But these groups can be confirmed by other tests, such as Oto Acoustic Emission (OAE) and Cochlear Microphonics (CM) which shows normal response and the Auditory Brain-Stem Response (ABSR) which shows abnormal or absent response. The site of lesion for this type of disorder is probably the inner hair cells of cochlea, spiral ganglia and the auditory nerve. Hyperbilirubinemia, anoxia/hypoxia, prenatal/neonatal infections, immune disorders are possible risk factors for this disorder [10]. So a detailed evaluation of antenatal, natal and postnatal history is important to identify this spectrum of disorders.

Noise induced hearing loss caused by exposure to recreational and occupational noise results in devastating disability that is virtually 100 percent preventable. This is the second most common form of sensorineural hearing deficit, after presbyacusis. Here the excessive sounds damage the stereocilia of the outer hair cells, therefore it is due to excessive wear and tear of delicate inner ear structures. Concurrent exposure to ototoxic drugs plays an additive effect. In olden days it was called as Boilermaker's disease. This type of hearing problems can be prevented by using earplugs or earmuffs. Noise induced hearing loss begins at higher frequencies (3000 - 6000 Hz) and produce bilateral symmetrical loss [11].

5. Conclusions

Pure tone audiometry is a simple and accurate method for the diagnosis of hearing impairment. Deafness prevention can be done only by mutual cooperation of both medical and non medical personnel. Majority of patients belong to the working age group. Hence early identification with timely intervention can reduce the morbidity of deafness in this age group which in turn helps to improve the productivity of the nation.

Hearing impairment leads to social isolation in elderly persons. An early and adequate diagnosis has an important role in adapting sound amplification devices and rehabilitation procedures for auditory function in elderly. In paediatric age groups, cochlear implant is possible if deafness is identified in the early stage. This in turn helps to improve their language and social and personality skills.

References

[1] Taneja, M.K. (2014) Deafness a Social Stigma: Physician Perspective. *Indian Journal of Otolaryngology and Head & Neck Surgery*, **66**, 353-358.

[2] Health Info Statistics and Epidemiology. Quick Statistics, National Institute on Deafness and other Communication Disorders (NIDCD). http://www.nidcd.nih.gov/health/statistics/pages/quick.aspx

[3] Ramya, C.S., Karthiyanee, K. and Vinutha, S. (2011) Effect of Mobile Phone Usage on Hearing Threshold: A Pilot Study. *Indian Journal of Otology*, **17**, 159-161. http://dx.doi.org/10.4103/0971-7749.94494

[4] National Programme for Prevention and Control of Deafness (NPPCD) Operational Guideline. http://mohfw.nic.in

[5] Tucker, S.M. (1995) Triagem e tratamento da surdez na pratica clinica. *Anais Nestle*, **50**, 18-24.

[6] Nogueria, J.C.R. and da Conceicao Mendonca, M. (2011) Assessment of Hearing in a Municipal Public School Student Population. *Brazilian Journal of Otorhinolaryngology*, **77** (6).

[7] Lin, F.R., Metter, E.J., O'Brien, J.R., Resnick, S.M., Zonderman, A.B. and Ferrucci, L. (2011) Hearing Loss and Incidence of Dementia. *Archives of Neurology*, **68**, 214-220. http://dx.doi.org/10.1001/archneurol.2010.362

[8] (2003) Prevention and Control of Deafness and Hearing Impairment Report on Intercountry Consultation, Colombo, Sri Lanka. World Health Organisation, Regional Office of South East Asia Report.

[9] Arts, H., Garber, A. and Zwolen, A. (2002) Cochlear Implants in Young Children. *Otolaryngologic Clinics of North America*, **35**, 925-942. http://dx.doi.org/10.1016/S0030-6665(02)00059-2

[10] Vignesh, S.S., Jaya, V. and Muraleedharan, A. (2014) Prevalence and Audiological Characteristics of Auditory Neu-

ropathy Spectrum Disorder in Paediatric Population: A Retrospective Study. *Indian Journal of Otolaryngology and Head and Neck Surgery*, **66** (3).

[11] Rabinowitz, P.M. (2000) Noise-Induced Hearing Loss Yale University School of Medicine, New Haven, Connecticut. *American Family Physician*, **61**, 2749-2756.

41

A Pierre Robin Syndrome with Absent Anterior 2/3 Tongue—A Case Report

K. Surender[1], K. Vasudev[1], B. Balaram[1], C. H. Vijay Raj[1], Lingaiah Jadi[2]

[1]Department of Pediatrics, Kakatiya Medical College, MGM Hospital, Warangal, India
[2]Department of ENT & HNS, Chalmeda Anand Rao Institute of Medical Sciences, Karimnagar, India
Email: surenderkagitapu@gmail.com

Abstract

The triad of micrognathia, glossoptosis and airway obstruction originally described in 1923 by Pierre Robin, is known as Robin sequence (or Pierre robin sequence "PRS"). PRS is characterized by micrognathia (small and symmetrical receded mandible), glossoptosis (tongue of variable size falls backwards into the post pharyngeal wall), and cleft palate (U or V shaped). We report a case of 2 hours old newborn presented with micrognathia, retrognathia, and glossoptosis and absent anterior two thirds of tongue.

Keywords

Micrognathia, Glossoptosis, Pierre Robin Sequence

1. Introduction

Robin sequence is an etiologically and phenotypically heterogeneous disorder [1]. PRS occurs as an isolated defect, as a part of recognized syndrome, or as a part of complex of multiple congenital anomalies. Diagnosis of a possible syndrome is very often critically important for correct management of a newborn affected with PRS [2] [3]. Isolated PRS is often a deformation resulting from intrauterine forces acting on the mandible, which restrict its growth and impact of the tongue between the palatal shelves. Some deformational cases of PRS have been associated with oligohydramnios. Because micrognathia results from intrauterine molding, mandibular catchup growth is expected after birth once intrauterine forces are removed. The most severe cases of micrognathia are unlikely to be isolated PRS caused by deformation. Therefore, catchup growth is unlikely.

2. Mini Review of Literature

In patients with PRS, 13% - 27.7% of other family members are affected with cleft lip with or without cleft palate [4] [5]. Jacobsen *et al.* screened 10 unrelated patients affected with PRS for *SOX9* and *KCNJ2* mutations and suggested that nonsyndromic PRS may be caused by both *SOX9* and *KCNJ2* dysregulation. Several lines of evidence for the existence of a 17q24 locus underlying PRS, including linkage analysis results, a clustering of translocation breakpoints 1.06 - 1.23 Mb upstream of *SOX9*, and microdeletions both approximately 1.5 Mb centromeric and approximately 1.5 Mb telomeric of *SOX9*, have been reported by Benko *et al.* [6] [7].

The proportion of cases that are isolated PRS varies in different studies. Hanson and Smith found that 25% of PRS cases had specific syndromes, another 35% had multiple anomalies without a specific recognized syndrome, and only 40% had isolated PRS [8]. Another study found that 74% of cases were isolated PRS [9].

While there is a great variation in severity, PRS is characterized by the following phenotypic features: micrognathia (small and symmetrical receded mandible), glossoptosis (tongue of variable size falls backwards into the post pharyngeal wall), cleft palate (U or V shaped) [10] [11]. Infants with PRS sequence often have airway obstruction, feeding difficulties, and challenges in gaining weight, and they may have associated anomalies, including hypotonia and limb reduction defects [12]. Congenital heart defects are present in up to 25% of the babies with PRS who die in early infancy. Patent ductus arteriosus (PDA) is the most common, followed by atrial septal defects, ventricular septal defects and coarctation of aorta. It has been reported that more than 20% of individuals will have developmental delay or cognitive impairment, and overall morbidity and mortality are higher in syndromic PRS or PRS with associated anomalies compared with isolated PRS [9].

3. Case Report

19 years old primi with no history of pregnancy induced hypertension, diabetes mellitus, premature rupture of membranes, oligohydromnios and polyhydromnios delivered a female baby by LSCS with birth weight of 2.5 kgs with history of birth asphyxia. On examination at 2 hours of age in hospital child is having micrognathia, retrognathia (**Figure 1**) and difficulty in breathing. On oral examination child is having "U" shaped cleft palate (**Figure 2**). Child has inspiratory stridor. Child had difficulty in maintaining saturation. We started on nasal prongs but child did not improved. Then we kept the baby in prone position with hood, then saturation maintained but there were repeated attacks of apnoea, so we thought to intubate the baby. But it was very difficult to intubate for us. We called for anesthetists to do the intubation, even for them it was difficult. With the help of otorhinolaryngologist (ENT Surgeon) we did VLS (Video-Laryngoscopy) to see the vocal cords (**Figure 3** and **Figure 4**). On close examination we concluded that infant is having not only posteriorly placed tongue but anterior two thirds of the tongue is not formed (**Figure 5**). We kept the child on supplemental oxygenation with hood in thermo neutral environment. As the child is not taking full feeds orally, we kept the child on parentral I.V. fluids and orogastric feeds. Child gradually maintained oxygen saturation at room air in prone position.

Child was started orogastric expressed breast milk feeds and gradually started taking palady feeds. The whole process took 3 weeks for the baby to stabilize and for discharge. Follow up after 1 week child is taking palady feeding, sleeping comfortably in prone position. Child started gaining weight. These children have feeding difficulties, they should be taken special interest in feeding with palady with calorie enrichment of milk.

PRS with absent anterior 2/3 of the tongue has not been reported till now. Hence we are reporting this case as a rare entity, after obtaining the informed consent from the patient's family.

4. Discussion

In infants with PRS, the tongue is displaced toward the posterior pharyngeal wall, resulting in obstruction at the level of the epiglottis. The tongue can act as a ball valve, leading to inspiratory obstruction. In addition to micrognathia, other mechanisms may contribute to airway obstruction in individuals with PRS, such as pharyngeal hypotonia and airway inflammation from associated gastro-oesophageal reflux. Patients with PRS may present in the immediate neonatal period with increased inspiratory work of breathing, cyanosis, and apnoea. Obstruction is more common in the supine position [13]-[15]. Chronic obstruction can lead to failure to thrive, carbon dioxide retention, pulmonary hypertension, and eventually right sided heart failure (corpulmonale). Air way obstruction is the main cause of feeding and growth issues in infants with PRS. Feeding problems can also be related to inadequate tongue control or pharyngeal hypotonia and complicated by presence of a cleft palate. Increased energy expenditure due to increased work of breathing may lead to failure to thrive if infant is not receiving adequate calorie intake [16].

The single initiating defect of this disorder may be hypoplasia of the mandibular area before 9 weeks in utero,

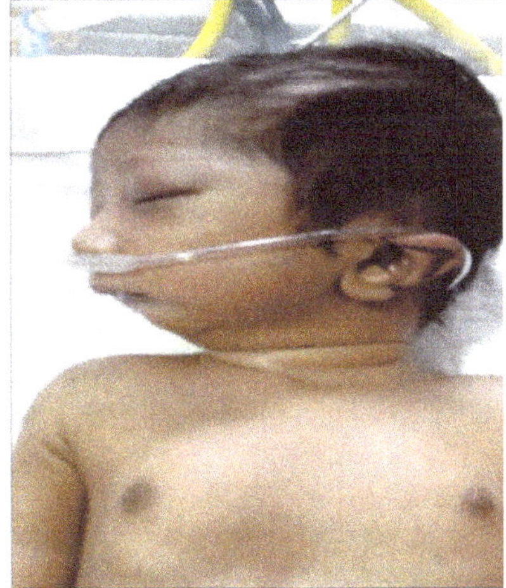

Figure 1. Showing micrognathia, retrognathia.

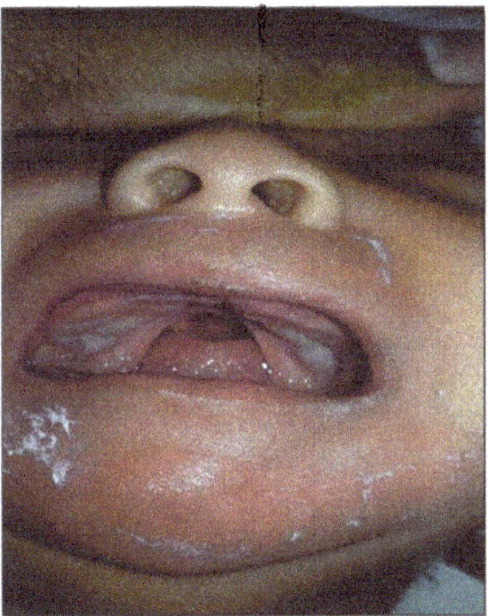

Figure 2. Showing "U" shaped cleft palate.

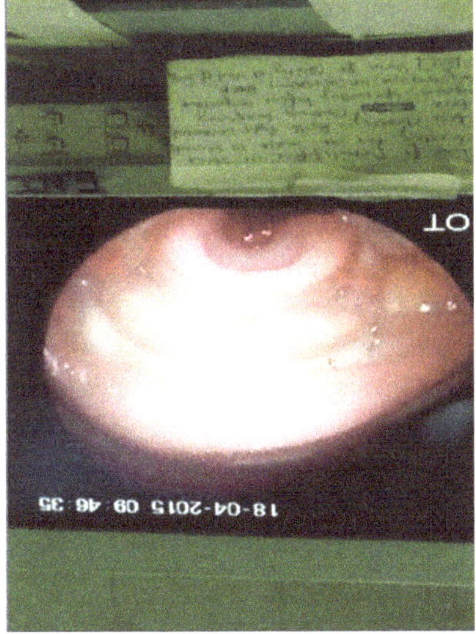

Figure 3. Difficult airway seen with VLS.

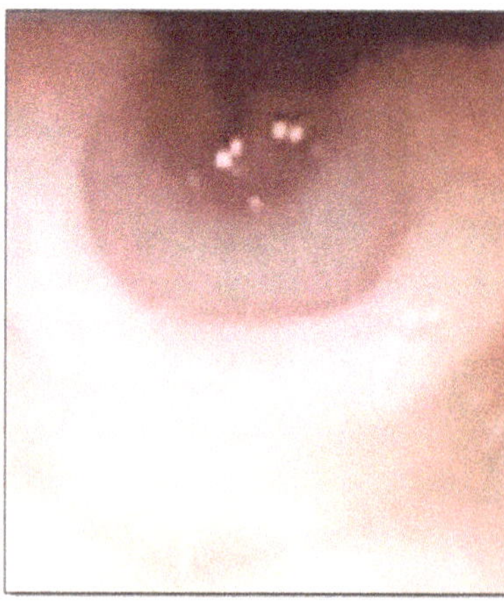

Figure 4. Close view of vocal cords with VLS.

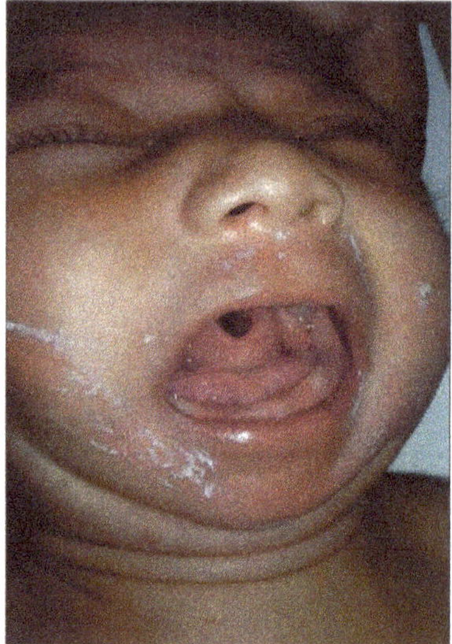

Figure 5. Showing absent anterior 2/3 tongue.

allowing the tongue to be posteriorly located and impairing the closer of the tongue to meet the midline [17] [18] (**Figure 6**) (Smiths text book of recognizable patterns of human malformations, 6th ed., page no. 262).

Anterior two-third of the tongue is formed by fusion of the tuberculum impar and the two lingual swellings. The anterior two-third of tongue is thus derived from the mandibular arch (**Figure 7**) (Inderbeer Singh text book of human embryology, 7th ed., page no. 162). From mandibular arch medial and lateral pterygoids, masseter, temporalis, mylohyoid, anterior belly of diagastric, tensor tympani, tensor palati are derived [17] [18].

In this case except anterior two-third of tongue all other derivatives of mandibular arch are developed. So when we see an infant is having PRS sequence then we have to check whether the baby is having isolated PRS sequence or syndromic baby having PRS sequence. We must be prepared for the expected complications like difficult airway and tongue abnormalities causing difficult breathing [18] [19].

The tongue in PRS is usually normal in size with foreshortened floor of the mouth and inspiratory obstruction. The infant should be in prone position to relive inspiratory obstruction. Some patients may need tracheostomy. Mandibular distraction procedures can improve mandibular size. Feeding requires great care, patience and palady feeding.

5. Conclusions

The new born baby presented with micrognathia, retrognathia and "U" shaped cleft palate with breathing difficulty, apnoea and inspiratory stridor. Respiration maintenance was difficult in supine position. Child maintained

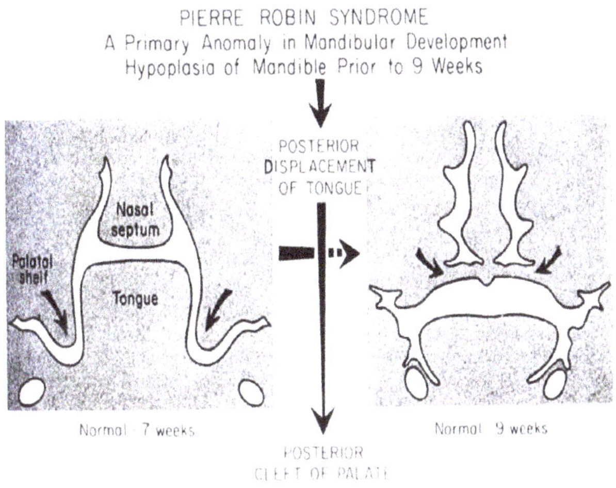

PIERRE ROBIN SYNDROME
A Primary Anomaly in Mandibular Development
Hypoplasia of Mandible Prior to 9 Weeks
POSTERIOR DISPLACEMENT OF TONGUE
Nasal septum
Palatal shelf
Tongue
Normal 7 weeks
Normal 9 weeks
POSTERIOR CLEFT OF PALATE

Figure 6. Diagrammatic depiction of development of mandible.

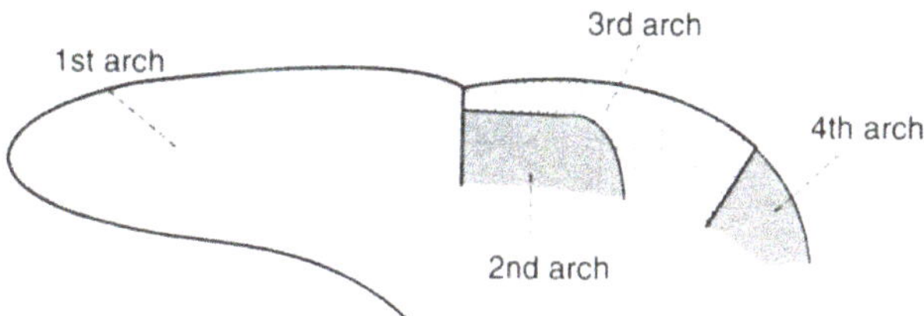

Figure 7. Diagrammatic depiction of development of Tongue.

saturation in prone position. With palady feeding child was improved. Absent anterior two-third of the tongue is the only additional finding, usually not a component of PRS.

For us to observe the morbid conditions like cognitive impairment, developmental delay, growth retardation, we need to follow up the child further.

References

[1] Pruzansky, S. (1969) Not All Dwarfed Mandibles Are Alike. *Birth Defects*, **5**, 120-129.

[2] Olasoji, H.O., Ambe, P.J. and Adesina, O.A. (2007) Pierre Robin Syndrome: An Update. *Nigerian Postgraduate Medical Journal*, **14**, 140-145.

[3] Shprintzen, R.J. (1992) The Implications of the Diagnosis of Robin Sequence. *Cleft Palate-Craniofacial Journal*, **29**, 205-209. http://dx.doi.org/10.1597/1545-1569(1992)029<0205:TIOTDO>2.3.CO;2

[4] Marques, I.L., Barbieri, M.A. and Bettiol, H. (1998) Etiopathogenesis of Isolated Robin Sequence. *Cleft Palate-Craniofacial Journal*, **35**, 517-525. http://dx.doi.org/10.1597/1545-1569(1998)035<0517:EOIRS>2.3.CO;2

[5] Holder-Espinasse, M., Abadie, V., Cormier-Daire, V., *et al.* (2001) Pierre Robin Sequence: A Series of 117 Consecutive Cases. *Journal of Pediatrics*, **139**, 588-590. http://dx.doi.org/10.1067/mpd.2001.117784

[6] Jakobsen, L.P., Ullmann, R., Christensen, S.B., *et al.* (2007) Pierre Robin Sequence May Be Caused by Dysregulation of SOX9 and KCNJ2. *Journal of Medical Genetics*, **44**, 381-386. http://dx.doi.org/10.1136/jmg.2006.046177

[7] Benko, S., Fantes, J.A., Amiel, J., Kleinjan, D.J., Thomas, S., Ramsay, J., *et al.* (2009) Highly Conserved Non-Coding Elements on Either Side of SOX9 Associated with Pierre Robin Sequence. *Nature Genetics*, **41**, 359-364. http://dx.doi.org/10.1038/ng.329

[8] Hanson, J.W. and Smith, D.W. (1975) U-Shaped Palatal Defect in the Robin Anomalad: Developmental and Clinical Relevance. *Journal of Pediatrics*, **87**, 30-33. http://dx.doi.org/10.1016/S0022-3476(75)80063-1

[9] Williams, A.J., Williams, M.A., Walker, C.A. and Bush, P.G. (1981) The Robin Anomalad (Pierre Robin Syndrome)—A Follow-Up Study. *Archives of Disease in Childhood*, **45**, 663-668. http://dx.doi.org/10.1136/adc.56.9.663

[10] Caouette-Laberge, L., Bayet, B. and Larocque, Y. (1994) The Pierre Robin Sequence: Review of 125 Cases and Evolution of Treatment Modalities. *Plastic and Reconstructive Surgery*, **93**, 934-942. http://dx.doi.org/10.1097/00006534-199404001-00006

[11] Marques, I.L., de Sousa, T.V., Carneiro, A.F., Peres, S.P., Barbieri, M.A. and Bettiol, H. (2005) Robin Sequence: A Single Treatment Protocol. *Jornal de Pediatria*, **81**, 14-22. [In Portuguese] http://dx.doi.org/10.2223/JPED.1277

[12] Evans, K., Hing, A.V. and Cunningham, M. (1331) Craniofacial Malformations, Micrognathia/Robin Sequence: Avery's Diseases of New Born. 9th Edition, 95.

[13] Singer, L. and Sidoti, E.J. (1992) Pediatric Management of Robin Sequence. *Cleft Palate-Craniofacial Journal*, **29**, 220-223. http://dx.doi.org/10.1597/1545-1569(1992)029<0220:PMORS>2.3.CO;2

[14] Myer, C.M., Reed, J.M., Cotton, RT, Willging, J.P. and Shott, S.R. (1998) Airway Management in Pierre Robin Sequence. *Otolaryngology—Head and Neck Surgery*, **118**, 630-635. http://dx.doi.org/10.1177/019459989811800511

[15] Benjamin, B. and Walker, P. (1991) Management of Airway Obstruction in Pierre Robin Sequence. *International Journal of Pediatric Otorhinolaryngology*, **22**, 23-27. http://dx.doi.org/10.1016/0165-5876(91)90094-R

[16] (2005) Robin Sequence: Smiths Recognizable Patterns of Human Malformation. 6th Edition, 262.

[17] Singh, I. and Pal, G.P. (2001) Human Embryology. 7th Edition, 161-162.

[18] Sadler, T. (2004) Head and Neck. Sun B. Langman's Medical Embryology. 9th Edition, Lippincott Williams & Wilkins, Philadelphia, 382-390.

[19] Gray, H. (1918) Anatomy of the Human Body. Lea & Febiger, Philadelphia. http://dx.doi.org/10.5962/bhl.title.20311

42

Treatment Outcomes in Head and Neck Cancer Patients 80 Years Old and over

Tomonori Terada, Nobuhiro Uwa, Kosuke Sagawa, Takeshi Mohri, Nobuo Saeki, Kota Kida, Kenzo Tsuzuki, Masafumi Sakagami

Department of Otolaryngology—Head and Neck Surgery, Hyogo College of Medicine, Nishinomiya City, Japan
Email: t-terada@hyo-med.ac.jp

Abstract

Background: With the recent aging of society, the need for medical treatment of elderly patients with head and neck cancer seems to have been increasing. Method: The present study analyzed all 103 patients with head and neck cancer ≥80 years, and we compared results with those of the previous generation (Group P; range: 75 - 79 years) comprising 104 patients treated in the same period. Results: We provided treatment just as wanted and could not choose it often. The reasons were oncological factors such as unresectable tumor or distant metastasis, refusal of treatment, and physical factors such as poor PS or number of comorbidities. Conclusion: Treatment choices should be based on the wishes and motivations of the patient and the medical assessment of physical function. When a patient ≥80 years old is treated, the high incidence of complications and severity of the disease should be considered.

Keywords

80 Years Old and over, Elderly Patients, Head and Neck Cancer, Treatment

1. Introduction

With the recent aging of society, the need for medical treatment of elderly patients with head and neck cancer seems to have been increasing. According to global health statistics announced on May 15, 2014 by the World Health Organization (WHO), the Japanese average lifespan was first among the participating 194 countries, at 84 years [1]. By sex, women were also first, at 87 years, and men were fifth at 80 years [1]. The Japanese average lifespan is expected to keep increasing, and Japanese society will thus continue to age, bringing increased opportunities to treat elderly patients with head and neck cancer. Because elderly individuals often have comorbidities and problems with social support in comparison with younger individuals, treatment according to policy may not take place [2] [3]. The present study was therefore performed to evaluate the situation for patients ≥80 years old with head and neck cancer.

2. Patients and Methods

From January 2000 to December 2011, a total of 918 patients with head and neck cancer visited the Department of Otolaryngology—Head and Neck Surgery at Hyogo College of Medicine. Of these, the present study analyzed all 103 patients ≥80 years old (11.2%). These patients comprised 81 men and 22 women, and mean age was 83.8 years (range, 80 - 93 years). Primary tumor sites were the larynx (40%), mesopharynx (17%), hypopharynx (13%), oral cavity (13%), nasopharynx (6%), salivary glands (6%), nasal cavity/paranasal sinuses (5%), and auditory organs (2%). The present study analyzed TNM stage, performance status (PS), multiple primary cancers, comorbidities, treatment, complications after treatment, and prognosis. In addition, we compared results with those of the previous generation (Group P) comprising 104 patients (95 men, 9 women)with a mean age of 76.7 years (range, 75 - 79 years)treated in the same period of January 2000 to December 2011, to investigate the influences of chronological age.

The Kaplan-Meier method was used to determine survival rates. Statistical analyses were performed using the chi-square test or non-parametric Mann-Whitney's U test. In all cases, values of $p < 0.05$ were regarded as statistically significant.

3. Results

3.1. TNM Stage

Cancer was often advanced, with Stage III in 18 cases (17.5%) and Stage IV in 40 cases (41.2%). The rate of advanced cancer for primary tumor sites was 34.1% for the larynx, 0% for the nasopharynx, 82.4% for the mesopharynx, 92.3% for the hypopharynx, 53.8% for the oral cavity, 100% for the salivary glands, 80% for the nasal cavity/paranasal sinuses, and 50% for the auditory organs. On the other hand, in Group P, Stage III was seen in 14 cases (13.5%), and Stage IV in 47 cases (45.2%). No significant difference was seen between groups (**Table 1**).

3.2. Performance Status (PS)

We assessed the daily living abilities of patients according to Eastern Cooperative Oncology Group (ECOG) PS at pretreatment [4] (**Table 2**). PS was 0 in 45 patients (43.7%), 1 in 34 patients (33.0%), 2 in 16 patients (15.5%), 3 in 5 patients (4.9%), and 4 in 3 patients (2.9%), and mean PS was 0.9 (**Table 1**). In Group P, mean PS was 0.63, and no significant differences were seen between groups.

3.3. Multiple Primary Cancers

Multiple primary cancers were present in 41 patients (39.8%) (**Table 1**), at a total of 55 sites overlap, and the most common sites were the head and neck, esophagus, lungs, and stomach, with 9 cases each. No significant difference in number of patients with multiple primary cancers was seen between groups.

3.4. Comorbidity

We applied the Chalson comorbidity index [5] and Cumulative Illness Rating Scale for Geriatrics (CIRS-G) [6] and chose the comorbidity that might have influenced the original selection of treatment from among nine items: 1) hypertension; 2) ischemic heart disease; 3) cerebrovascular disease; 4) diabetes; 5) respiratory disease (chronic obstructive pulmonary disease, asthma attack, interstitial pneumonia); 6) kidney failure requiring dialysis; 7) liver disease (liver cirrhosis); 8) mental disease (dementia, depression); or 9) hematological disease (myelodysplastic syndrome, idiopathic thrombocytopenic pupura).

Pretreatment comorbidity was found in 88 patients (85.4%). Hypertension was the most common (59.2%), followed by ischemic heart disease (33.0%), cerebrovascular disease (23.3%), diabetes (16.5%), respiratory disease (13.6%), and mental disease (11.7%). Fifteen patients showed no pretreatment comorbidity (14.6%), while one comorbidity was present in 32 patients (31.1%), two in 26 patients (25.2%), and three or more in 30 patients (29.1%). A significant difference in the number of comorbidities was evident between the subject group and Group P ($p < 0.01$) (**Table 1**).

Table 1. Patient characteristics in different age groups.

Characteristic	Subject group	Group P	Statistically significant
Patients (n = 207)	103	104	
Period	2000-2011	2000-2011	
Sex			
Male	81 (78.6%)	95 (91.3%)	p < 0.01
Female	22 (21.4%)	9 (8.7%)	
Age range (mean)	80 - 93 (83.8)	75 - 79 (76.7)	
Primary tumor sites			
Larynx	41	37	
Nasopharynx	6	4	
Mesopharynx	17	17	
Hypopharynx	13	18	NS
Oral cavity	13	13	
Salivary glands	6	4	
Nasal cavity/paranasal sinus	5	6	
Auditory organ	2	5	
TNM stage			
Stage I	20	24	
Stage II	25	19	NS
Stage III	18	1	
Stage IV	40	47	
Performance status (PS)			
PS 0	45	60	
PS 1	34	30	NS
PS 2	16	8	
PS 3	5	5	
PS 4	3	1	
Average PS	0.9	0.63	NS
Multile primary cancer			
None	62	61	
One	29	33	NS
Two	10	5	
Three or more	2	5	
Comorbidity			
None	15	25	
One	32	37	
Two	26	27	p < 0.01
Three or more	30	15	
Average	1.85	1.38	

NS: not significance.

Table 2. Eastern cooperative oncology group (ECOG) performance status.

Grade	
0	Fully active, able to carry on all pre-disease performance without restriction
1	Restricted in physically strenuous activity but ambulatory and able to carry out work of a light or sedentary nature, e.g., light house work, office work
2	Ambulatory and capable of all selfcare but unable to carry out any work activities. Up and about more than 50% of waking hours
3	Capable of only limited selfcare, confined to bed or chair more than 50% of waking hours
4	Completely disabled. Cannot carry on any selfcare. Totally confined to bed or chair
5	Dead

3.5. Initial Treatment

We performed radical standard treatment for 83 patients, palliative treatment for 8 patients, and no treatment at the request of the patient and their family for 12 patients. In Group P, we performed radical standard treatment for 93 patients, palliative treatment for 5 patients, and no treatment for 6 patients. No significant difference was evident between groups (**Table 3**).

Radical standard treatment was not able to be chosen due to oncological factors such as unresectable tumor or distant metastasis in 9 cases, declining treatment (opting to receive no treatment) in 8 cases, and physical factors such as poor PS or numerous comorbidities in 3 cases.

In the 83 cases for which radical treatment was performed, treatment could not be performed according to the policies of our institution in 19 cases (22.9%), including abbreviation of prophylactic neck dissection, abbreviation of postoperative radiation therapy and abbreviation of combination chemotherapy in radiation therapy. On the other hand, in Group P, patients unable to receive treatment according to our policy comprised only eight of the 93 cases (8.6%), showing a significant difference between groups ($p < 0.01$).

3.6. Achievement of Planned Initial Treatment

In the 91 cases in which radical standard or palliative treatment was performed, the planned initial treatment was unable to be achieved in 14 cases (15.4%), while 77 cases (84.6%) were able to complete the planned treatment (**Table 3**). Treatment difficulty was attributed to complications of treatment in eight cases, requests from patients for treatment cancellation in four cases, and physical reasons other than treatment complications in two cases. In Group P, among the 98 cases that received radical standard or palliative treatment, the planned initial treatment was not able to be completed in only 5 cases (5.1%), while 93 cases (94.9%) were able to complete the planned treatment, representing a significant difference between groups ($p < 0.05$).

Table 3. Treatment and prognosis in different age groups.

Characteristic	Subject group	Group P	Statistically significant
Patients (n = 207)	103	104	
Age range (mean)	80 - 93 (83.8)	75 - 79 (76.7)	
Initial treatment			
Radical standard	83 (80.6%)	93 (89.4%)	
RT alone	27	16	
RT + chemotherapy	26	26	
Operation	23	35	NS
Operation + RT	7	16	
Palliative	8 (7.8%)	5 (4.8%)	
Untreated	12 (11.7%)	6 (5.8%)	
Initial treatment (radical standard)			
According our policy	64	85	p < 0.01
Compromised and modified treatment	19	8	
Achievement of the planned initial treatment			
Achievement	77 (84.6%)	93 (94.9%)	p < 0.05
Omission	14	5	
Complication after treatment			
Appearance (treatment-related death)	24 (4)	19 (0)	NS
None	67	78	
Prognosis			
Disease specific 5 year survival rate	35.8%	53.9%	p < 0.01
Limited in case of the patients treated according to our policy	62.7%	63.2%	NS

RT: radiotherapy; NS: not significance.

3.7. Complications after Treatment

In the 91 cases that receive radical standard or palliative treatment, complications after treatment were identified in 24 cases (26.4%). The most common was pneumonia (aspiration, postoperative, or interstitial), occurring in 13 cases (54.1%). Others included sepsis, kidney failure, progression of dementia, cerebral infarction, fulminant hepatitis, disseminated intravascular coagulation, and chronic subdural hematoma, showing many serious complications. Four treatment-related deaths were recognized among these cases. On the other hand, in Group P, among the 98 cases that received radical standard or palliative treatment, complications after treatment were identified in 19 cases (19.4%). As in the subject group, serious complications had occurred, but no treatment-related deaths were encountered. No significant difference in the rate of complications after treatment was evident between groups (**Table 3**).

3.8. Prognosis

Disease-specific 5-year survival rates were 35.8% in the subject group and 53.9% in Group P (**Figure 1**), showing a significant difference between groups ($p < 0.01$). However, when we limited analysis to radical standard treatment completed according to the policy of our institution, disease-specific 5-year survival rates were 62.7% in the subject group and 63.2% in Group P, showing no significant difference between groups (**Figure 2**).

4. Discussion

Report of elderly individuals with head and neck cancer often consider patients around a cut-off of 70 or 75 years old and older [7]-[10]. Japanese people have among the longest life expectancies in the world, with an average lifespan of 84 years (men, 80 years; women, 87 years). Around the world, the number of countries with an average lifespan over 80 years old has expanded to 29 countries now. The average life expectancy for a 70-year-old Japanese is very long, at 19.5 years for women and 15.1 years for men, and that for an 80-year-old is 11.4 years for women and 8.5 years for men. On the basis of such information, when we examine elderly individuals with head and neck cancer, we think it appropriate to consider someone ≥80 years old as elderly. In Japan, treatment and associated problems for head and neck cancer patients ≥80 years old have been investigated in numerous studies [2] [3] [11]. The reason we chose a 75- to 79-year-old age group for comparison with the subject group was to clarify factors strongly influenced specifically by chronological age, as 75- to 79-year-old Japanese show no inferiority with younger patients for treatment choice, because Derks *et al.* [12] reported that they were able to provide standard treatment in 45- to 60-year-old head and neck cancer patients in 132 of 148 cases (89%), the rate was equal to Group P (75- to 79-year-old) in 93 of 104 cases (89.4%).

Comparing head and neck cancer patients ≥80 years old with 75- to 79-year-olds showed no significant differences in background factors such as disease classification, comorbidities, multiple primary cancers, or PS between groups (**Table 1**). These factors were thus thought to be little influenced by chronological age. The ratio of males to females and the number of comorbidities are affected by chronological age. In Japan, the ratio of woman was 8.7% for 75 - 79 years old and 21.4% for ≥80 years old. Because women have a longer average lifespan (87 years) than men (80 years old), the population differences between men and women ≥80 years old are large (approximately 6.1 million women compared to approximately 3.2 million men [13]). Sarini *et al.* [10] pointed out that the proportion of women is increased among elderly patients with head and neck cancer, that the ratios of woman. The number of comorbidities is also increased among patients ≥80 years old, with many cases showing more than three comorbidities, and conversely few cases showing none.

As for the disease-specific 5-year survival rate, a significant difference was seen between Group P (53.9%) and the subject group (35.8%). The proportion of patients receiving radical standard treatment did not differ significantly between groups. However, even if patients ≥80 years old were classified as suitable to receive radical standard treatment, many cases were unable to complete treatment according to the policies of our institution. When disease-specific 5-year survival rates were determined for those patients able to be treated according to institutional policies, results were comparable (subject group, 62.7%; Group P, 63.2%). In addition, for patients who achieved the planned initial treatment, subject group was significantly low in comparison with 94.9% of p group in 84.6% in subject group. Because treatment according to our policy appears difficult to initiate for patients ≥80 years old, and many of those patients who do start cannot complete treatment, the survival rates are poor.

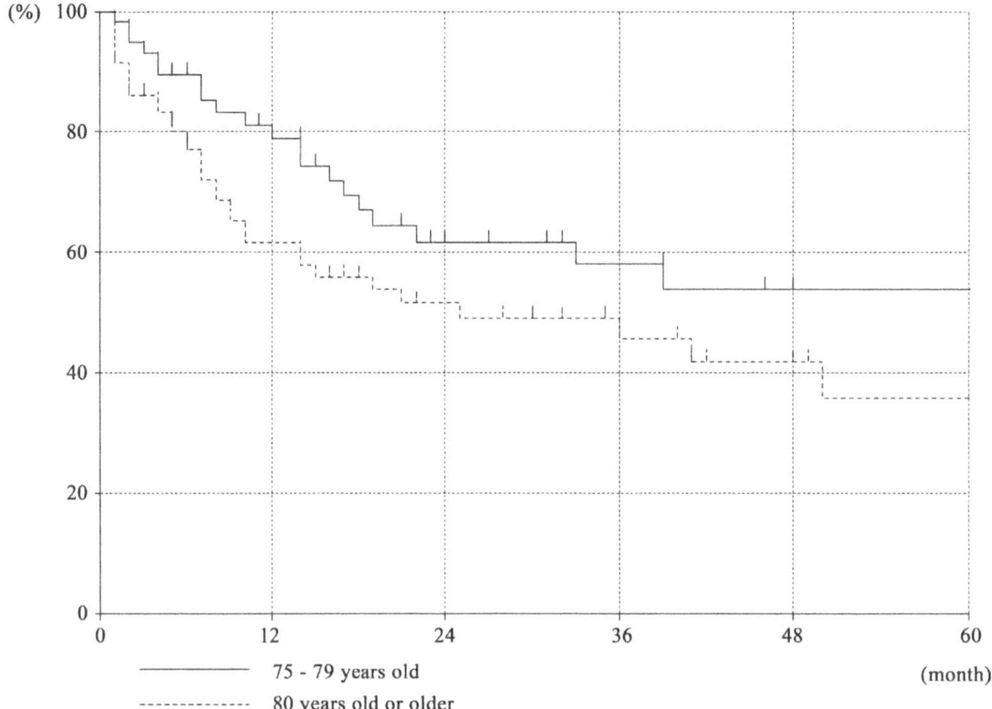

Figure 1. Disease specific survival rate in all cases.

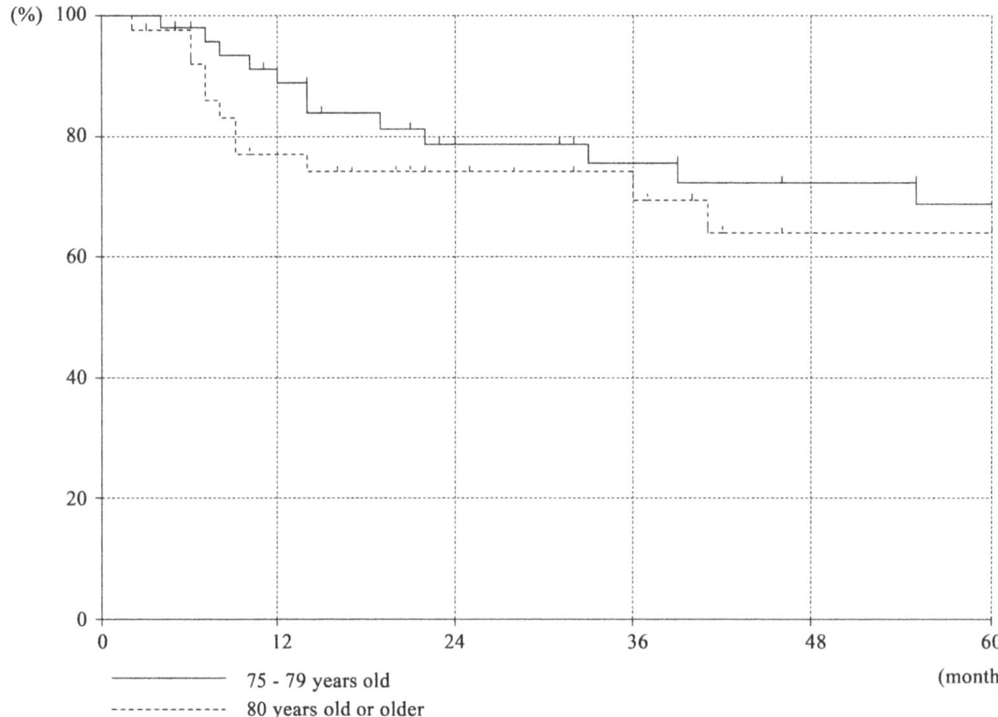

Figure 2. Disease specific survival rate in the limited cases treated according to the policy of our institution.

If an elderly patient ≥80 years old can complete radical standard treatment, the prognosis seems comparable to that of a younger patient. Therefore, as noted in past reports [3] [11] [13], choice of treatment should not be based on chronological age, but instead simply according to standard policy where possible. Under the present conditions, we provided treatment just as wanted and could not choose it often. The reasons were oncological factors such as unresectable tumor or distant metastasis, refusal of treatment, and physical factors such as poor PS or number of comorbidities. Chaibi *et al.* [14] reported that cases in which the CIRS-G score is high typically cannot receive intensive treatment. Furthermore, Derks *et al.* [13] reported that they were able to provide standard treatment in 70- to 79-year-old head and neck cancer patients in 59 of 79 cases (75%), compared to only 14 of 39 cases (36%) among patients ≥80 years old.

When a patient exceeds 80 years old, surpassing the average lifespan for a man, a feeling of satisfaction that the patient and family were able to accomplish some degree of longevity may arise. The desire for life may subsequently fade, and the patient may not accept the risk of complications that accompanies aggressive treatment to achieve radical cure and may instead decline treatment. When the patient and family do not expect to undergo aggressive treatment based on their outlook on life and death, sufficient information must be provided about symptoms and functional disorders that may arise in the future, and decisions on treatment policy need to be made. With regard to the drop in the acceptance of treatment among the elderly, Monden *et al.* [3] made similar points. Among patients ≥80 years old who did not receive radical curative treatment, cases in which the patient or family declined aggressive treatment comprised 50%. The will of the patient and family to undergo treatment may thus greatly influence decisions on treatment among elderly head and neck cancer patients ≥80 years old. We need to make an effort to give elderly patients an incentive to undergo aggressive treatment.

It is necessary to pay full attention when we choose treatment for head and neck cancer patients ≥80 years old, because complications after treatment can be serious and treatment-related death was recognized in four patients. Precise judgment of whether the patient can endure the treatment by examining physical function and comorbidities is crucial to limit the high incidence and severity of complications after treatment.

5. Conclusions

From January 2000 to December 2011, we evaluated 103 cases of head and neck cancer patients ≥80 years old who visited our institution. We analyzed TNM stage, PS, multiple primary cancers, comorbidities, treatment, complications after treatment, and prognosis.

We think that the desire for treatment of the patient and family greatly influences decisions on treatment policy in head and neck cancer patients ≥80 years old. We need to make an effort to give elderly patients an incentive to undergo aggressive treatment.

Treatment choices should be based on the wishes and motivations of the patient and the medical assessment of physical function. When a patient ≥80 years old is treated, the high incidence of complications and severity of the disease should be considered.

References

[1] World Health Organization (WHO) in Internet, World Health Statistics 2014, Mortality and Burden of Disease, by Life Expectancy. http://apps.who.int/ghodata/

[2] Suzuki, M., Matayoshi, N., Hasegawa, M., *et al.* (2008) Treatment Outcomes in Head and Neck Cancer Patients Aged 80 or over. *Japanese Journal of Head and Neck Cancer*, **34**, 594-599. http://dx.doi.org/10.5981/jjhnc.34.594

[3] Monden, S., Nishikawa, K., Morishita, T., *et al.* (2003) Head and Neck Cancer Treatment in the Elderly—Evaluation and Management of Complications. *Nippon Jibiinkoka Gakkai Kaiho*, **106**, 7-16. http://dx.doi.org/10.3950/jibiinkoka.106.7

[4] Oken, M.M., Creech, R.H., Tormey, D.C., *et al.* (1982) Toxicity and Response Criteria of the Eastern Cooperative Oncology Group. *American Journal of Clinical Oncology*, **5**, 649-655. http://dx.doi.org/10.1097/00000421-198212000-00014

[5] Charlson, M.E., Pompei, P., Ales, K.L., *et al.* (1987) A New Method of Classifying Prognostic Comorbidity in Longitudinal Studies: Development and Validation. *Journal of Chronic Diseases*, **40**, 373-383. http://dx.doi.org/10.1016/0021-9681(87)90171-8

[6] Miller, M.D., Paradis, C.F., Houck, P.R., *et al.* (1992) Rating Chronic Medical Illness Burden in Geropsychiatric Practice and Research: Application of the Cumulative Illness Rating Scale. *Psychiatry Research*, **41**, 237-248. http://dx.doi.org/10.1016/0165-1781(92)90005-N

[7] Milisavljević, D., Stanković, M., Zivić, M., *et al.* (2012) Head and Neck Cancer Surgery in Elderly: Complications and Survival Rate. *Collegium Antropologicum*, **36**, 13-17.

[8] Van der Schroeff, M.P., Derks, W., Hordijk, G.J., *et al.* (2007) The Effect of Age on Survival and Quality of Life in

Elderly Head and Neck Cancer Patients: A Long-Term Prospective Study. *European Archives of Oto-Rhino-Laryngology*, **264**, 415-422. http://dx.doi.org/10.1007/s00405-006-0203-y

[9] Bernardi, D., Barzan, L., Franchin, G., *et al.* (2005) Treatment of Head and Neck Cancer in Elderly Patients: State of the Art and Guidelines. *Critical Reviews in Oncology/Hematology*, **53**, 71-80. http://dx.doi.org/10.1016/j.critrevonc.2004.08.001

[10] Sarini, J., Fournier, C., Lefebvre, J.L., *et al.* (2001) Head and Neck Squamous Cell Carcinoma in Elderly Patients: A Long Term Retrospective Review of 273 Cases. *Archives of Otolaryngology—Head & Neck Surgery*, **127**, 1089-1092. http://dx.doi.org/10.1001/archotol.127.9.1089

[11] Saikawa, M., Ebihara, T. and Yoshidumi, T. (2000) Treatment for Head and Neck Cancer in Patients at the Age of 80 or Older. *Journal of the Japan Broncho-Esophagological Society*, **51**, 93-97.

[12] Derks, W., Leeuw, R.D., Hordijk, G.J., *et al.* (2005) Reasons for Non-Standard Treatment in Elderly Patients with Advanced Head and Neck Cancer. *European Archives of Oto-Rhino-Laryngology*, **262**, 21-26. http://dx.doi.org/10.1007/s00405-004-0744-x

[13] Statistics Japan in Internet, Ministry of Public Management, Estimate of the Population, by the Population for a Specific Age Group. http://www.stat.go.jp/index.htm

[14] Chaïbi, P., Magné, N., Breton, S., *et al.* (2011) Influence of Geriatric Consultation with Comprehensive Geriatric Assessment on Final Therapeutic Decision in Elderly Cancer Patients. *Critical Reviews in Oncology/Hematology*, **79**, 302-307. http://dx.doi.org/10.1016/j.critrevonc.2010.08.004

Permissions

All chapters in this book were first published in IJOHNS, by Scientific Research Publishing; hereby published with permission under the Creative Commons Attribution License or equivalent. Every chapter published in this book has been scrutinized by our experts. Their significance has been extensively debated. The topics covered herein carry significant findings which will fuel the growth of the discipline. They may even be implemented as practical applications or may be referred to as a beginning point for another development.

The contributors of this book come from diverse backgrounds, making this book a truly international effort. This book will bring forth new frontiers with its revolutionizing research information and detailed analysis of the nascent developments around the world.

We would like to thank all the contributing authors for lending their expertise to make the book truly unique. They have played a crucial role in the development of this book. Without their invaluable contributions this book wouldn't have been possible. They have made vital efforts to compile up to date information on the varied aspects of this subject to make this book a valuable addition to the collection of many professionals and students.

This book was conceptualized with the vision of imparting up-to-date information and advanced data in this field. To ensure the same, a matchless editorial board was set up. Every individual on the board went through rigorous rounds of assessment to prove their worth. After which they invested a large part of their time researching and compiling the most relevant data for our readers.

The editorial board has been involved in producing this book since its inception. They have spent rigorous hours researching and exploring the diverse topics which have resulted in the successful publishing of this book. They have passed on their knowledge of decades through this book. To expedite this challenging task, the publisher supported the team at every step. A small team of assistant editors was also appointed to further simplify the editing procedure and attain best results for the readers.

Apart from the editorial board, the designing team has also invested a significant amount of their time in understanding the subject and creating the most relevant covers. They scrutinized every image to scout for the most suitable representation of the subject and create an appropriate cover for the book.

The publishing team has been an ardent support to the editorial, designing and production team. Their endless efforts to recruit the best for this project, has resulted in the accomplishment of this book. They are a veteran in the field of academics and their pool of knowledge is as vast as their experience in printing. Their expertise and guidance has proved useful at every step. Their uncompromising quality standards have made this book an exceptional effort. Their encouragement from time to time has been an inspiration for everyone.

The publisher and the editorial board hope that this book will prove to be a valuable piece of knowledge for researchers, students, practitioners and scholars across the globe.

List of Contributors

Saloni Shah
Civil Hospital, B.J. Medical College, Ahmedabad, India

Rajesh Vishwakarma
ENT Department, Civil Hospital, B.J. Medical College, Ahmedabad, India

Spero H. Raoul Hounkpatin, Fabien A. C. Gounongbe, Marius C. Flatin, Karl A. F. B. Dossou-Kpanou and Elvire Dossoumou
1Faculté de Médecine, Université de Parakou, Parakou, Benin

François Avakoudjo, Sonia Lawson Afouda and Wassi Adjibabi
Faculte des Sciences de la Santé de Cotonou, Université d'Abomey-Calavi, Cotonou, Bénin

Dayse Távora-Vieira
Otolaryngology, Head & Neck Surgery, School of Surgery, University of Western Australia, Perth, Australia
Fremantle Hospital, Fremantle, Australia

Gunesh P. Rajan
Otolaryngology, Head & Neck Surgery, School of Surgery, University of Western Australia, Perth, Australia
Fremantle Hospital, Fremantle, Australia

Suman Arasikere Panchappa, Dhinakaran Natarajan, Thangaraj Karuppasamy, Alaguvadivel Jeyabalan, Radhakrishnan Kailasam Ramamoorthy, Sivasubramanian Thirani and Rajaganesh Kutuva Swamirao
Department of ENT, Madurai Medical College, Madurai, India

Hakim Chabbak, Amine Rafik and Abdessamad Chlihi
National Center for Burns and Plastic Surgery, Casablanca, MoroccoNational Center for Burns and Plastic Surgery, Casablanca, Morocco

Subrat Kumar Behera and Sharath Govindappa
Department of ENT, S.C.B. Medical College, Cuttack, India

Niranjan Mishra
Department of OMFS, S.C.B. Medical College, Cuttack, India

Anoop Attakkil, Vandana Thorawade, Mohan Jagade, Rajesh Kar, Kartik Parelkar, Dnyaneswar Rohe, Poonam Khairnar and Reshma Hanowate
Department of ENT, Grant Medical College & Sir J.J. Hospital, Mumbai, India

Carolina Durao and Sofia Decq Motta
Otolaryngology Department, Hospital Prof. Doutor Fernando Fonseca, Amadora, Portugal

Ana Hebe, Ricardo Pacheco, Pedro Montalvão and Miguel Magalhães
Otolaryngology Department, Portuguese Oncology Institute of Lisbon, Francisco Gentil, Portugal

Vaishali Shah and H. Ganapathy
ENT Department, Apollo Main Hospital, Chennai, India

Ram Gopalakrishnan
Infectious Diseases Department, Apollo Main Hospital, Chennai, India

N. Geetha
Pathology Department, Apollo Main Hospital, Chennai, India

Devkumar Rangaraja
Department of ENT, Grant Medical College & Sir J.J. Hospital, Mumbai, India

Bhaskar Mitra, Subhalakshmi Sengupta, Anshita Rai, Jay Mehta, Aruna Rai Quader, Subhendu Roy and Anita Borges
Drs. Tribedi & Roy Diagnostic Laboratory, Kolkata, India

Rajanala Venkata Nataraj, Mohan Jagade, Kartik Parelkar, Reshma Hanawte, Arpita Singhal, Dev Rengaraja, Kiran Kulsange, Kartik Rao and Pallavi Gupta
Department of Ear, Nose & Throat and Head & Neck Surgery, Grant Government Medical College, Mumbai, India

Loay Al-Ekri and Abdulkarim Alsaei
Department of ENT, Head & Neck Surgery, Salmaniya Medical Complex, Manama, Kingdom of Bahrain

Yana Yuriyvna Gomza
1Otorhinolaryngology Department, National O.O. Bogomolets Medical University, Kiev, Ukraine

Ralph Mösges
Institute of Medical Statistics, Informatics and Epidemiology, University Hospital of Cologne, Cologne, Germany

Noemí Aguirre
Pediatrics Resident, Pontifical Catholic University of Chile, Santiago, Chile

Francisca Córdova
School of Medicine, Pontifical Catholic University of Chile, Santiago, Chile

Francisca Jaime
Pediatrician, Resident of Pediatric Gastroenterology and Nutrition, Pontifical Catholic University of Chile, Santiago, Chile

Ximena Fonseca
Otorhinolaryngologist, Assistant Professor, Pediatrics Division, Medical School, Pontifical Catholic University of Chile, Santiago, Chile

Pamela Zúñiga
Hematologist-Oncologist, Assistant Professor, Pediatrics Division, Medical School, Pontifical Catholic University of Chile, Santiago, Chile

Paula Prieto-Oliveira
Inter-Institutional Grad Program on Bioinformatics, University of São Paulo, São Paulo, Brazil

Sérgio Vitorino Cardoso
Department of Oral Pathology, School of Dentistry, Federal University of Uberlândia, Uberlândia, Brazil

Florence Zumbaio Mistro and Sérgio Kignel
Department of Semiology, School of Dentistry, Fundação Hermínio Ometto, Araras, Brazil

Suzana Cantanhede Orsini Machado de Sousa
Department of Oral Pathology, School of Dentistry, University of São Paulo, São Paulo, Brazil

Marco Túllio Brazão-Silva
Department of Oral Diagnosis, School of Dentistry, School of Health Sciences, University of the State of Amazonas, Manaus, Brazil

Olajide Toye Gabriel
Department of Ear, Nose and Throat Surgery, Federal Teaching Hospital, Ido Ekiti, Nigeria

Usman Aminu Mohammed and Eletta Adebisi Paul
Department of Ear, Nose and Throat Surgery, Federal Medical Centre, Bida, Nigeria

Saroj Mali, Divij Sonkhya, Mohnish Grover and Nishi Sonkhya
Department of ENT, SMS Medical College and Hospital, Jaipur, India

Aisha Larem, Sally Sheta, Abdulsalam Al-Qahtani and Hassan Haidar
Department of Otolaryngology, Hamad Medical Corporation, Doha, Qatar

Ajinkya Kelkar
Department of Otolaryngology and Head and Neck Surgery, Yashwantrao Chavan Hospital, Pune, Maharashtra, India

Kalpesh Patil
Department of Paediatric Surgery, Yashwantrao Chavan Hospital, Pune, Maharashtra, India

Essam A. Abo el-Magd
Departments of Otorhinolaryngology, Faculty of Medicine, Aswan University, Aswan, Egypt

Yousseria Elsayed Yousef
Pediatric Nursing, Faculty of Nursing, Sohag University, Sohag, Egypt

Osama M. El-Asheerr
Pediatrics, Faculty of Medicine, Assiut University, Assiut, Egypt

Karema M. Sobhy
Public Health, Faculty of Medicine, Aswan University, Aswan, Egypt

Ramesh Babu Kalyanasundaram, Ganesh Kumar Balasubramanian, Ramanathan Thirunavukkarasu and Prabhakharan Saroja Durairaju
Department of ENT and Head & Neck surgery, Thanjavur Medical College, Thanjavur, India

Hassanin Abdulkarim, Hassan Haidar, Maryam Abdulraheem, Ahmad Abualsoud and A. Salam Alqahtani
Department of Otorhinolaryngology, Head & Neck Surgery, Hamad Medical Corporation, Doha, Qatar

Ahmed Elsotouhy
Department of Radiology, Hamad Medical Corporation, Doha, Qatar

Isabel López-Sánchez, José-Ramón Alba-García and Cristina Vázquez-Romero
ENT Department, General and University Hospital, Valencia, Spain

Miguel Armengot-Carceller
Rhinology Unit, ENT Department, General and University Hospital.Valencia University, Valencia, Spain

Weizhong Ernest Fu, Ming Yann Lim and Li-Chung Mark Khoo
Department of Otolaryngology, Tan Tock Seng Hospital, Singapore City, Singapore

Khoon Leong Chuah
Department of Pathology, Tan Tock Seng Hospital, Singapore City, Singapore

Chaganti Padmavathi Devi, Karri Maruthi Devi and Madabhushi Venugopal
Guntur Medical College, Guntur, India

Mulukutla Partha Akarsh
Siddhartha Medical College, Vijayawada, India

Kartik Parelkar, Smita Nagle, Mohan Jagade, Poonam Khairnar, Madhavi Pandare, Rajanala Nataraj, Reshma Hanwate, Bandu Nagrale and Devkumar Rangaraja
Department of ENT, Grant Govt Medical College & Sir J J Group of Hospitals, Mumbai, India

Waheed Rahman, Rashid Sheikh*, Hassen Mohammed and Zeynel Abidin Dogan
Department of Otorhinolaryngology and Head & Neck Surgery, Hamad Medical Corporation, Doha, Qatar

Jun Myung Lee, Nam Gyu Ryu and Ick Soo Choi
Department of Otorhinolaryngology-Head and Neck Surgery, Inje University College of Medicine, Ilsanpaik Hospital, Goyang, Korea

R. V. Nataraj, Jagade Mohan, Chavan Reshma, Parelkar Kartik, Hanawte Reshma, Singhal Arpita, Kulsange Kiran, Rengaraja Dev, Rao Kartik and Gupta Pallavi
Department of Ear, Nose & Throat and Head and Neck Surgery, Grant Government Medical College, Mumbai, India

Brian Schwab, Michele Gandolfi, Erica Lai, Erin Reilly, Lorie Singer and Ana H. Kim
Department of Otolaryngology, New York Eye and Ear Infirmary of Mount Sinai, New York, USA

Jeffrey Hsu and Melin Tan-Geller
Montefiore Medical Center, New York, USA

Vijayalakshmi Subramaniam
Department of Otorhinolaryngology, Yenepoya Medical College, Yenepoya University, Mangalore, India

Rashmi Jain
Department of Ophthalmology, Yenepoya Medical College, Yenepoya University, Mangalore, India

Sivan Yegnanarayana Iyer Saraswathy
Department of Community Medicine, PSG Institute of Medical Sciences & Research, Coimbatore, India

Varun Mishra
Information Technology Consultant, Bangalore, India

Vipa Boonkitticharoen
Department of Diagnostic and Therapeutic Radiology, Ramathibodi Hospital, Mahidol University, Bangkok, Thailand

Boonchu Kulapaditharom, Phurich Praneetvatakul and Thongchai Bhongmakapat
Department of Otolaryngology, Ramathibodi Hospital, Mahidol University, Bangkok, Thailand

Noppadol Larbcharoensub
Department of Pathology, Ramathibodi Hospital, Mahidol University, Bangkok, Thailand

Ganesh Kumar Balasubramanian, Ramanathan Thirunavukkarasu, Ramesh Babu Kalyanasundaram and Gitanjali Narendran
Thanjavur Medical College, Thanjavur, India

Itzhak Braverman and Galit Avior
Unit of Otolaryngology-Head & Neck Surgery, Hadera, Israel

Alex Nemirovsky and Adi Klein
Pediatric Department Hillel Yaffe Medical Center, Hadera and The Faculty of Medicine, The Technion, Haifa, Israel

Miriam Sarid
Western Galilee College, Acco, Israel

Zexing Cheng and Juebo Yu
Department of Otolaryngology, Yangzhou First People's Hospital, Yangzhou, China

Xiaoming Tang
Department of Computed Tomography and Interventional Radiology, Yangzhou First People's Hospital, Yangzhou, China

Jagdish Prasad Purohit, Chandra Bhan, Bhoopendra Singh, Ajay Pratap Singh, Siva Selvaraj, Manish Pandey and Vijay Krishna Sharma
Department of ENT, Head and Neck Surgery, MLB Medical College, Jhansi, India

M. S. Sheikh
Associate Professor of ENT, Government Medical College Srinagar, Kashmir, India

S. Bunafsha
Medical Interne, Women's Medical College Hospital, Uttara Model Town, Dhaka, Bangladesh

S. Gul Afshan
Externe, Women's Medical College, Dhaka, Bangladesh

Ganesh Kumar Balasubramanian, Ramanathan Thirunavukkarasu, Ramesh Babu Kalyanasundaram and Gitanjali Narendran
Thanjavur Medical College, Thanjavur, India

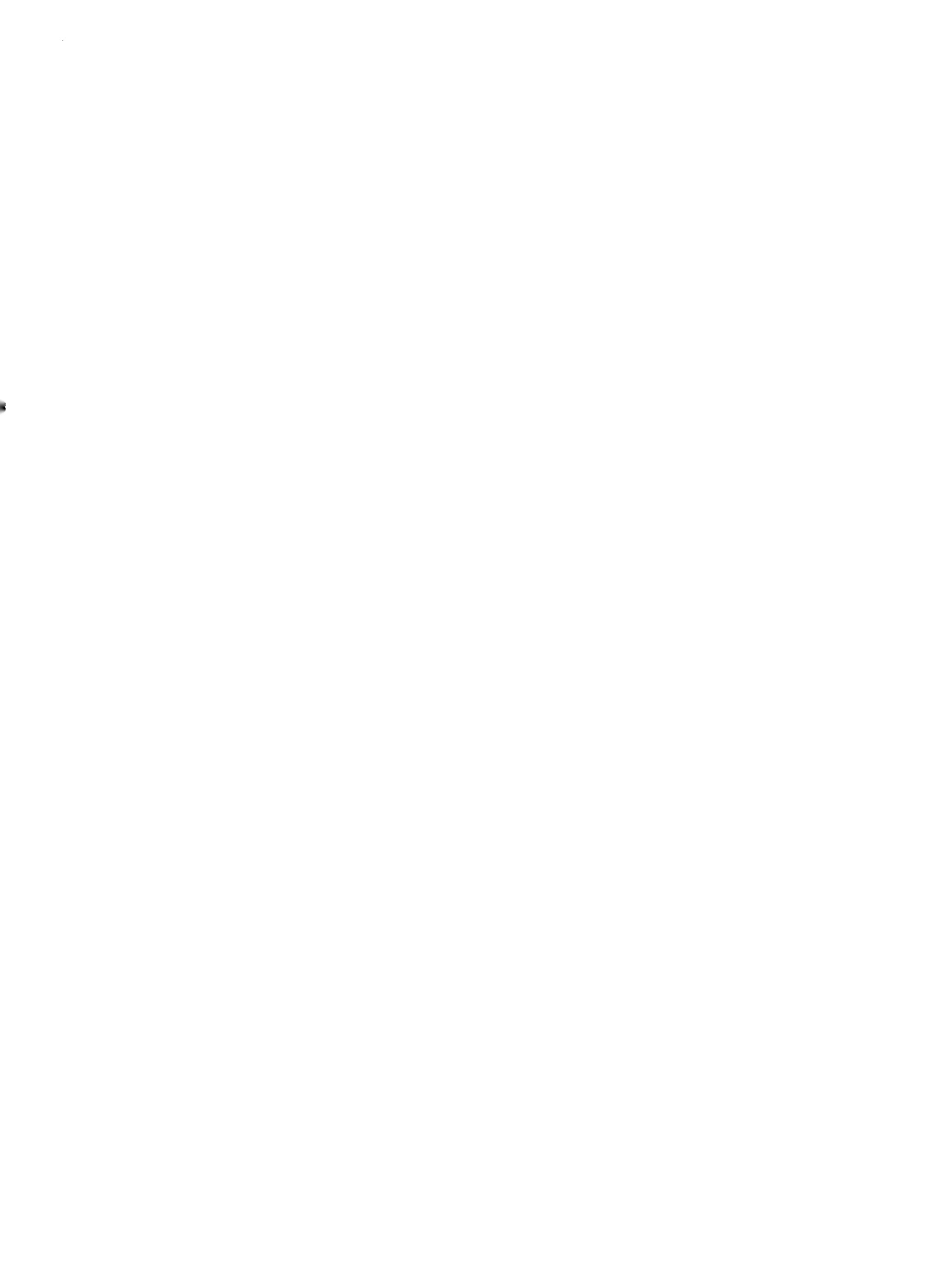

www.ingramcontent.com/pod-product-compliance
Lightning Source LLC
Chambersburg PA
CBHW080455200326
41458CB00012B/3979
9781632424419